National Health
and Nutrition
Examination Survey

PHYSICIAN
EXAMINATION
PROCEDURES
MANUAL

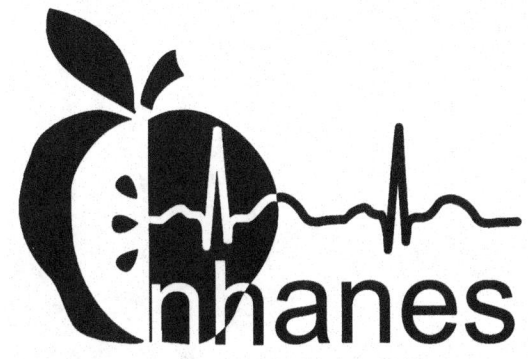

January 2003

TABLE OF CONTENTS

TABLE OF CONTENTS (continued)

TABLE OF CONTENTS (continued)

List of Appendixes

List of Tables

List of Tables (continued)

List of Exhibits

TABLE OF CONTENTS (continued)

List of Exhibits (continued)

List of Exhibits (continued)

TABLE OF CONTENTS (continued)

List of Exhibits (continued)

TABLE OF CONTENTS (continued)

List of Exhibits (continued)

TABLE OF CONTENTS (continued)

List of Exhibits (continued)

TABLE OF CONTENTS (continued)

List of Exhibits (continued)

TABLE OF CONTENTS (continued)

List of Exhibits (continued)

1. OVERVIEW OF THE NATIONAL HEALTH AND NUTRITION EXAMINATION SURVEY

This chapter provides a general description of the health examination surveys conducted by the National Center for Health Statistics (NCHS) and the current National Health and Nutrition Examination Survey (NHANES). It also provides an overview of the tasks that staff perform during the survey.

1.1   History of the National Health and Nutrition Examination Programs

This NHANES is the eighth in a series of national examination studies conducted in the United States since 1960.

The National Health Survey Act, passed in 1956, gave the legislative authorization for a continuing survey to provide current statistical data on the amount, distribution, and effects of illness and disability in the United States. In order to fulfill the purposes of this act, it was recognized that data collection would involve at least three sources: (1) the people themselves by direct interview; (2) clinical tests, measurements, and physical examinations on sample persons; and (3) places where persons received medical care such as hospitals, clinics, and doctors' offices.

To comply with the 1956 act, between 1960 and 1984, the National Center for Health Statistics (NCHS), a branch of the U.S. Public Health Service in the U.S. Department of Health and Human Services, has conducted seven separate examination surveys to collect interview and physical examination data.

The first three national health examination surveys were conducted in the 1960s:

1.   1960-62 – National Health Examination Survey I (NHES I)

2.   1963-65 – National Health Examination Survey II (NHES II)

3.   1966-70 – National Health Examination Survey III (NHES III)

(Revised October 2005)

NHES I focused on selected chronic disease of adults aged 18-79. NHES II and NHES III focused on the growth and development of children. The NHES II sample included children aged 6-11, while NHES III focused on youths aged 12-17. All three surveys had an approximate sample size of 7,500 individuals.

Beginning in 1970 a new emphasis was introduced. The study of nutrition and its relationship to health status had become increasingly important as researchers began to discover links between dietary habits and disease. In response to this concern, under a directive from the Secretary of the Department of Health, Education and Welfare, the National Nutrition Surveillance System was instituted by NCHS. The purpose of this system was to measure the nutritional status of the U.S. population and monitor nutritional changes over time. A special task force recommended that a continuing surveillance system include clinical observation and professional assessment as well as the recording of dietary intake patterns. Thus, the National Nutrition Surveillance System was combined with the National Health Examination Survey to form the National Health and Nutrition Examination Survey (NHANES). Four surveys of this type have been conducted since 1970:

1.   1971-75 – National Health and Nutrition Examination Survey I (NHANES I)

2.   1976-80 – National Health and Nutrition Examination Survey II (NHANES II)

3.   1982-84 – Hispanic Health and Nutrition Examination Survey (HHANES)

4.   1988-94 – National Health and Nutrition Examination Survey (NHANES III)

NHANES I, the first cycle of the NHANES studies, was conducted between 1971 and 1975. This survey was based on a national sample of about 28,000 persons between the ages of 1-74. Extensive data on health and nutrition were collected by interview, physical examination, and a battery of clinical measurements and tests from all members of the sample.

NHANES II began in 1976 with the goal of interviewing and examining 28,000 persons between the ages of 6 months to 74 years. This survey was completed in 1980. To establish a baseline for assessing changes over time, data collection for NHANES II was made comparable to NHANES I. This means that in both surveys many of the same measurements were taken in the same way, on the same age segment of the U.S. population.

While the NHANES I and NHANES II studies provided extensive information about the health and nutritional status of the general U.S. population, comparable data were not available for many of the ethnic groups within the United States. Hispanic HANES (HHANES), conducted from 1982 to 1984, produced estimates of health and nutritional status for the three largest Hispanic subgroups in the United States—Mexican Americans, Cuban Americans, and Puerto Ricans—that were comparable to the estimates available for the general population. HHANES was similar in design to the previous HANES studies, interviewing and examining about 16,000 people in various regions across the country with large Hispanic populations.

NHANES III, conducted between 1988 and 1994, included about 40,000 people selected from households in 81 counties across the United States. As previously mentioned, the health status of minority groups is often different than the health status and characteristics of nonminority groups, so black Americans and Mexican Americans were selected in large proportions for NHANES III. Each group comprised 30 percent of the sample. NHANES III was the first survey to include infants as young as 2 months of age and to include adults with no upper age limit. To obtain generalizeable estimates, infants and young children (1-5 years) and older persons (60+ years) were sampled at a higher rate than previously. NHANES III also placed an additional emphasis on the effects of the environment upon health. Data were gathered to measure levels of pesticide exposure, presence of certain trace elements in the blood, and amounts of carbon monoxide present in the blood. A home examination was incorporated for those persons who were unable or unwilling to come to the exam center but would agree to an abbreviated examination in their homes.

In addition to NHANES I, NHANES II, Hispanic HANES, and NHANES III, several other HANES projects have been underway since 1982. These projects have been a part of the HANES Epidemiologic Follow-up Survey, a multiphase survey conducting follow-up interviews with the NHANES I population in order to provide longitudinal data on the health of the U.S. population.

1.2   Overview of the Current NHANES

This NHANES follows in the tradition of past NHANES surveys, continuing to be a keystone in providing critical information on the health and nutritional status of the U.S. population.

The major difference between the current NHANES and previous surveys is that the current NHANES is conducted as a **continuous, annual survey**. Each single year and any combination of consecutive years of data collection comprises a nationally representative sample of the U.S. population. This new design allows annual statistical estimates for broad groups and specific race-ethnicity groups as well as flexibility in the content of the questionnaires and exam components. New technologic innovations in computer-assisted interviewing and data processing result in rapid and accurate data collection, data processing, and publication of results.

The number of people examined in a 12-month period will be about the same as in previous NHANES, about 5,000 a year from 15 different locations across the nation. The data from the NHANES are used by government agencies, state and community organizations, private researchers, consumer groups, companies, and health care providers.

1.2.1   Data Collection

Data collected on the current NHANES survey began early in 1999 and will continue for approximately 6 years at 88 locations (stands) across the United States. The survey was preceded by a pretest in the spring of 1998 and a dress rehearsal was conducted in early 1999.

Approximately 40,000 individuals of all ages in households across the U.S. will be randomly selected to participate in the survey. The study respondents include whites as well as an oversample of blacks and Mexican-Americans. The study design also includes a representative sample of these groups by age, sex, and income level. Adolescents, older people, and pregnant women are also oversampled in the current NHANES.

The overall goals of the NHANES are to:

- Estimate the number and percentage of persons in the U.S. population and designated subgroups with selected diseases and risk factor;

- Monitor trends in the prevalence, awareness, treatment, and control of selected diseases;

- Monitor trends in risk behaviors and environmental exposure;

- Analyze risk factors for selected diseases;

- Study the relationships between diet, nutrition, and health; and

- Explore emerging public health issues and new technologies.

Selected persons are invited to take part in the survey by first being interviewed in their homes. Household interview data are collected via computer-assisted personal interviewing (CAPI) and include demographic, socioeconomic, dietary, and health-related questions. Upon completion of the interview, respondents are asked to participate in a physical examination. The examination is conducted in a specially equipped and designed Mobile Examination Center (MEC), consisting of four trailers. The MEC houses the state-of-the-art exam equipment and is divided into rooms to assure the privacy of each study participant during the exams and interviews. The examination includes a physical and dental examination conducted by a physician and a dentist, laboratory tests, a variety of physical measurements, and other health interviews conducted by highly trained medical personnel.

The household interviews and MEC exam combined will collect data in the following important health-related areas:

- Cardiovascular and respiratory disease;

- Vision;

- Hearing;

- Mental illness;

- Growth;

- Infectious diseases and immunization status in children;

- Obesity;

- Dietary intake and behavior;

- Nutritional status;

- Disability;

- Skin diseases;

- Environmental exposures;

- Physical fitness; and

- Other health-related topics.

1.3   Sample Selection

A sample is defined as a representative part of a larger group. Since it is impossible to interview and examine everyone in the U.S. for NHANES, a representative sample is taken of the U.S. population. By studying a representative sample of the population, it is assumed that the findings would not have been too different had every person in the U.S. been studied. Because generalizations about the population will be made, it is extremely important that the sample be selected in a way that accurately represents the whole population. Statisticians calculate the size of the sample needed and take into consideration the geographic distribution and demographic characteristics of the population, such as age, gender, race, and income.

An introductory letter is sent to each household in the sample. A few weeks after the letter goes out, interviewers visit each listed household and use carefully designed screening procedures to determine whether any residents are eligible for the survey. If eligible residents are present, the interviewer then proceeds to introduce the study, presents the Sample Person (SP) a survey brochure, and obtains a signed consent for the household interview. The brochure contains detailed information on the survey, the household interview, and the MEC examination.

A signed consent form must be obtained from each eligible individual before the household interview can be conducted. A refusal to sign the consent form is considered a refusal to participate in the survey. After the interview is completed, the interviewer then explains the MEC exam, obtains another signed consent form for the MEC exam, and contacts the field office to schedule a MEC appointment for the SP. All SPs aged 12 years and older must sign the Examination Consent forms to participate in the MEC examination. Parental consent is also required for SPs under 18 years of age. SPs aged 7-11 years old are asked to sign the Examination Assent Form. An additional consent form is required for consent to future general research for both adults (ages 18+) and parents of children under 18 years. This consent form gives permission to store a small sample of blood and urine for future specimen testing. A refusal to sign the MEC consent or assent form is considered a refusal to participate in the examination phase of the survey. Examinations will not be performed on sample persons who do not sign a consent form.

1.4 Field Organization for NHANES

There are two levels of field organization for this study – the home office staff and the field staff.

- **Home Office Staff from Westat** – Project staff from Westat are responsible for overseeing the field teams and field work.

- **Field Office (FO) Staff** – For this survey, an office will be opened at every survey location (stand). Each field office will have a Study Manager (SM), Office Manager (OM), a Field Manager (FM), and one Assistant Office Manager (AOM).

  - The **Study Manager (SM)** is responsible for the overall management of operations at a stand.

  - The **Office Manager (OM)** is responsible for the stand office operations and is the main conduit for the flow of work and information between the MEC and the household interviewing staff. S/he will supervise one or more local office clerks hired to assist with office activities. The OM reports to the SM.

  - The **Field Manager (FM)** has primary responsibility for the supervision of the household interviewers. The FM also assists the SM and supervises the activities of the Assistant Office Managers. S/he will deal with administrative issues, ISIS problems, and preparations for the next stand.

  - The **Assistant Office Managers (AOMs)** are primarily responsible for data entry into the Integrated Survey Information System (ISIS), editing data collection materials, and verification of interviewer work. The AOMs report to the FM and also work closely with the OM.

- **Household Interviewers** – This staff is primarily responsible for identifying and enrolling the survey participants, conducting the household interviews, and appointing the study participants for the MEC exam. Specifically, household interviewers will locate occupied residential dwelling units, administer the Screener to select eligible sample persons, obtain signed consents to the household interview, conduct the interviews, set up examination appointments, obtain consents for the MEC exam, conduct field reminders for MEC appointments, and assist in rescheduling broken, cancelled, and no-show appointments.

  Several times a week, household interviewers visit the field office and report to the field manager. During the course of the study, interviewers also interact on a daily basis with other field office staff and home office staff.

- **MEC Staff** – This staff of health professionals conducts the health exams. The survey includes two exam teams.

There are 16 individuals on each traveling team: 1 MEC manager, 1 MEC coordinator, 1 licensed physician, 1 licensed dentist, 3 medical technologists, 4 health technologists, 2 MEC interviewers, 2 dietary interviewers, and 1 phlebotomist. In addition, local assistants are recruited, trained, and employed at each stand to assist the exam staff. A data manager also travels with each team.

The following section describes the steps that are always completed prior to the opening of a stand and an overview of the tasks that interviewers are expected to perform. Highlighted items are basic concepts critical to the conduct of the study.

Steps completed prior to interviewing include:

- Statisticians scientifically select certain segments in the sampling area. A segment is an area with definite boundaries, such as a city block or group of blocks containing a cluster of households.

- Twelve weeks before data collection begins, NHANES staff list the segments. Listing is the systematic recording on special forms of the address of every dwelling unit (DU) located within the segment. Commercial buildings and other structures not intended as living quarters are not listed.

- A sample of dwelling units is selected from the listing forms. This sample is the group of addresses that interviewers visit in order to conduct interviews.

- Immediately before data collection begins, an advance letter is sent to each dwelling unit with a mailing address. This letter briefly describes the study and inform the household that an interviewer will contact them in the near future.

The tasks interviewers perform when they arrive at a stand include:

1. After the successful completion of training, interviewers are given an assignment of sampled dwelling units to contact. Each assignment consists of prelabeled Household Folders, prelabeled Neighbor Information Forms, and the appropriate Segment Folder.

2. Using addresses on the Household Folders and listing/mapping materials in the Segment Folder, interviewers locate these dwelling units.

3. If a selected address is not a dwelling unit or is not occupied, interviewers complete the "Vacant/Not a DU Section" on the Screener Non-Interview Form.

4. In an occupied residential dwelling unit, interviewers contact an adult who lives in the selected household and administer the Screener using a laptop computer.

The Screener is an interview that lists all the individuals who live in the household, divides the household into families, and collects all the demographic characteristics necessary to immediately determine if there are persons in the household eligible for further interviewing.

All instructions necessary to determine eligibility and to select sample persons (SPs) are programmed in the CAPI Screener.

5. If all persons in a household are ineligible, no further work is done with the case. When eligible household members are identified, interviewers continue to conduct all the necessary tasks associated with the case.

6. In eligible households, the interviewer obtains a signed interview consent form prior to completing the medical history and/or the family questionnaire.

7. Next, the appropriate medical history CAPI interview is administered to eligible respondents. The questions asked depend on the age of the SP.

8. In each household containing children aged 1-5, floor and window sill dust samples are obtained. These samples provide information on lead levels in the household environment.

9. A Family questionnaire is also administered to one adult family member from each eligible family in the household.

10. Next, an appointment is scheduled for each SP, coordinating the MEC schedule and the SP schedule.

11. Interviewers then obtain signed consent form(s) for each SP for the examination, call the field office to confirm the examination appointment(s), and give each SP an appointment slip.

12. If there is more than one eligible family in a household, this process is repeated with each additional family.

13. Interviewers record the result of each contact or attempted contact with the household on the Call Record located in the Household Folder.

14. Interviewers also support the survey by conducting field reminders prior to MEC appointments and reschedule broken, cancelled, or no-show MEC appointments.

15. If an interviewer is unable to complete any of the questionnaires or procedures for any SP, an SP Card is completed. This card documents the problems encountered in completing one or more tasks.

16. Interviewers check for missed DUs and/or structures when instructed to do so. If any are found, the Missed DU or Missed Structure Procedures is implemented and appropriate forms will be completed.

17. When an interview has been completed, interviewers edit their work, carefully reviewing all forms for completeness and legibility.

18. Interviewers report in person to the FM at the stand office for regularly scheduled conferences, usually every other day. During these conferences, interviewers discuss completed cases, discuss problems with incomplete cases, receive new case assignments, and report time, expenses, and production.

19. To insure the accuracy and completeness of the survey, all interviewer work is edited by the field office staff, and then validated by recontacting respondents. After this review, supervisors provide interviewers with feedback concerning the quality of the work.

20. At the end of each stand field period, interviewers return all interviewing materials to the supervisor.

1.5   Exams and Interviews in the Mobile Examination Center (MEC)

Examinations and interviews are conducted in a mobile examination center (MEC), which is composed of four specially equipped trailers. Each trailer is approximately 48 feet long and 8 feet wide. The trailers are set up side-by-side and connected by enclosed passageways. During the main survey, detachable truck tractors drive the trailers from one geographic location to another.

Exhibit 1-1 shows a floor plan for the MEC. The interior of the MEC is designed specifically for this survey. For example, the trailers are divided into specialized rooms to assure the privacy of each study participant during exams and interviews. Many customized features have been incorporated including an audiometry room that uses a soundproof booth, a wheelchair lift, and a wheelchair-accessible bathroom available to assist participants with mobility problems. Exhibit 1-2 shows the locations of the various exams within the MEC.

1.5.1   Exam Sessions

The MEC operates 5 days a week and includes weekday, evening, and weekend sessions. Two 4-hour sessions are scheduled each day with approximately 10-12 SPs per session. During a stand, work weeks rotate to offer a variety of MEC appointments on weekday mornings, afternoons, and evenings, and every weekend.

Exhibit 1-1. Floor plan of the MEC

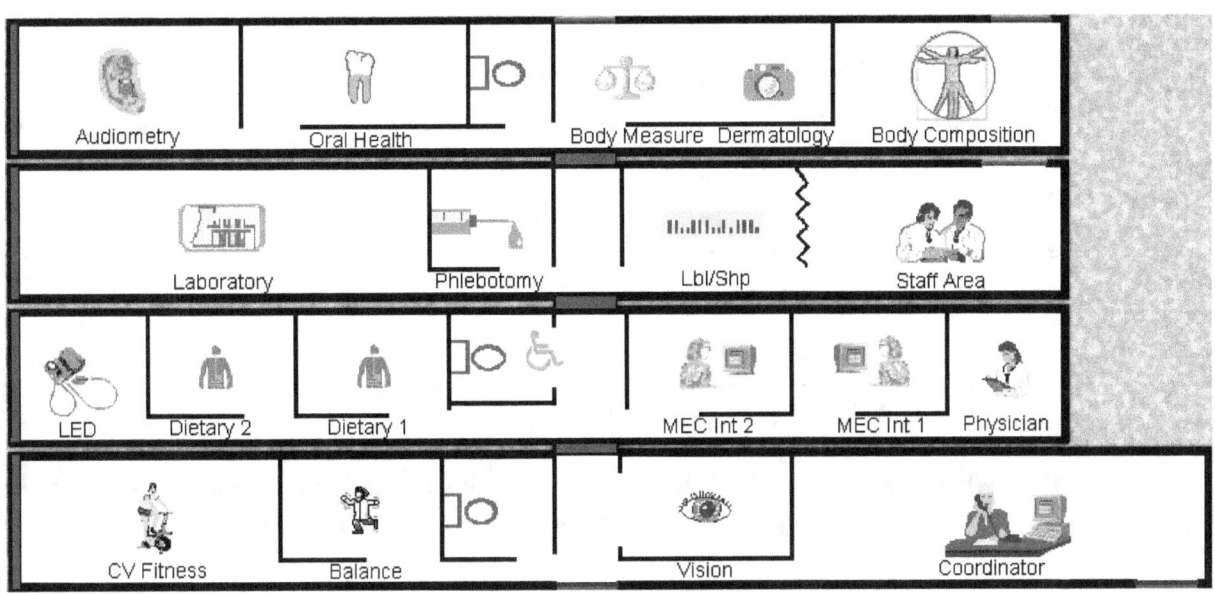

Exhibit 1-2. MEC exams and rooms

Trailer	Room	Room Use
Trailer 1	Reception area	Welcoming and waiting area for SPs
	Vision room	Vision tests
	Balance	Balance test
	Fitness	Cardiovascular fitness
Trailer 2	Physician	Physical examination
	MEC Interview	Health interview
	MEC Interview	Health interview
	Dietary Interview	Dietary interview
	Dietary Interview	Dietary interview
	Lower Extremity Disease	Testing for lower extremity pulses and sensitivity
Trailer 3	Venipuncture	Drawing of blood samples, MRSA collection and physical activity monitor
	Laboratory	Processing of urine and blood samples
	Label/shipping area	Lab area for labeling and shipping specimens
	Staff lounge	Staff area that houses main computer system
Trailer 4	Total Body Composition	Total body composition scans and bioimpedance
	Body Measures	Body measurements and dermatology
	Dental	Dental exam
	Audiometry/Tympanometry	Hearing tests

1.5.2   Exam Team Responsibilities

There are 16 individuals on each exam team. In addition, a local assistant will be hired to assist the staff in managing examinee flow. One data manager also travels with each team. The duties of the exam team members are summarized below:

- One MEC manager supervises the exam staff, manages the facility, and supports exam operations.

- One coordinator directs the flow of SPs through the MEC examination process. The coordinator manages all SP appointments, verifies that all components are completed for each SP, and exits SPs from the MEC.

- One physician conducts the medical examination and records results, reviews the results of the complete blood count and pregnancy test, and serves as the safety officer for the MEC.

- One dentist conducts the dental exam and calls the results to a health technologist who records the findings.

- Two health (MEC) interviewers administer questionnaires for physical and mental health information.

- Two dietary interviewers administer the dietary questionnaire. The interviewers record a 24-hour dietary recall of the types and amounts of foods consumed by the SP in the last 24 hours.

- Four health technologists with radiologic technology or other health training take and record body measurements, perform balance tests, vision tests, cardiovascular fitness tests, muscle strength assessments, lower extremity measures, total body composition (DEXA) scans, bioimpedance (BIA) tests, administer hearing tests, and collect skin images. In addition, the technologists record findings for the dental examiner.

- Three medical technologists conduct clinical laboratory tests on biological and environmental specimens, record the results of the tests, and prepare and ship specimens to various laboratories.

- One phlebotomist administers the phlebotomy questionnaire draws blood from SPs, and recruits SPs for special studies.

- The data manager (DM) assists in the setup and testing of computer systems and telecommunications hookups at the FO and MEC. S/he also coordinates the maintenance and repair of computer systems at the FO and MEC with the home office and external venders and acts as the FO and MEC systems "help desk" person. The data manager reports to the SM on administrative matters and the HO for ISIS-related matters.

Each staff member is part of a team of professional persons with specific assignments that must be completed in order to accomplish the overall objective of the survey. Each individual must be aware of and respect the job demands placed upon other staff members, maintain an attitude of tolerance and consideration for fellow members of the team, and willingly perform extra tasks that may be assigned to support other staff members in the performance of their duties. MEC staff members may be requested to perform tasks not directly related to their specific professional skills in order to implement the overall data collection plan.

1.5.3   Examination Components

The full examination for an adult takes approximately 3½ hours, but the actual length depends on the SP's age. Some exams are done only on certain age groups so the exam profiles vary, even among adult SPs. The exam components are described briefly below and summarized in Exhibit 1-3:

- **Anthropometry**

  The purpose of the anthropometry component is to provide: (1) nationally representative data on selected body measures, (2) estimates of the prevalence of overweight and obesity, (3) data to study the association between body measures and such health conditions and risk factors as cardiovascular disease, diabetes, hypertension, and activity and dietary patterns, and (4) data to monitor growth and development in children. A total of 11 body measurements are collected, but the number and type of measures varies with the age groups.

- **Balance**

  Balance disorders, disequilibrium, and dizziness from vestibular disorders constitute a major public health problem. Primary disorders may be hidden by their consequences, such as falls, while subtle dysfunction may underlie difficulties in learning, writing, reading, and in everyday activities. The main objectives of the balance test are to obtain prevalence data, examine the relationship between balance disorders and other factors, and to characterize normal and disordered balance and spatial orientation. The standard Romberg test is used to measure postural sway.

- **Bioelectrical Impedance Analysis (BIA)**

  The purpose of the BIA exam is to monitor secular trends in overweight prevalence, describe the prevalence of obesity, and examine the relationship between overweight and obesity and other examination measures. BIA measures the electrical impedance of body tissues and is used to assess fluid volumes, total body water, body cell mass, and fat-free body mass.

Exhibit 1-3. Examination components

Component	Ages
Anthropometry	All
Audiometry/Tympanometry	20-69 (half-sample)
Balance	40+
Bioimpedance (BIA)	8-49
Cardiovascular Fitness	12-49
Dermatology	20-59
Dietary Interview	All
Lower Extremity Disease	40+
MEC Interview	8+
Mental Health	8-19 years (also includes parents of 8-15-year-olds); 20-39 years (half-sample)
MRSA sample collection	1+
Oral Health	2+
Physical Activity Monitor	6+
Physician Exam	All
Total Body Composition	8+
Urine Collection	6+
Venipuncture	1+
Vision	12+
Volatile Organic Compounds (VOC)	20-59 (random subsample)

■ **Cardiovascular Fitness**

Evaluation of physical fitness provides nationally representative data on measures of physical fitness, and estimates of the prevalence of persons at risk due to sedentary habit and poor physical fitness. Cardiovascular fitness is assessed with a submaximal treadmill test on examinees aged 12 through 49 years.

■ **Dermatology (Skin Disorders)**

The specific aims of this component are: (1) to monitor the prevalence, secular trends and impact of selected skin conditions that were last assessed in NHANES I (1971-75); (2) to identify risk factors for selected skin conditions that can be used to increase understanding of disease etiology and prevention; and (3) to create a data resource that can be used to develop a CDC National Skin Cancer Prevention and Control Agenda. The MEC dermatology exam involves standardized photography of selected sites on the body. This component will focus on two specific skin diseases: psoriasis and hand dermatitis. The major goal is to determine the prevalence of these two conditions.

- **Dietary Interview**

  The goal of the dietary component is to estimate total intake of foods, food energy and nutrients, nonnutrient food components, and plain drinking water by the U.S. population; and assess dietary behaviors and the relationship of diet to health. Quantitative dietary intake data is obtained for all subjects by means of a 24-hour dietary recall interview using a computer-assisted dietary data entry system. A second 24-hour recall will be conducted on all SPs by telephone through a phone center operation at the home office. In 2003, a self-administered form, the Food Frequency Questionnaire, will be offered to SPs who complete the MEC dietary interview. It will be mailed from and returned to the home office.

- **Hearing**

  The goals of the hearing exam are to obtain normative data on the hearing status of the adult U.S. population, and to evaluate certain covariates that may be related to hearing loss, such as occupational exposure. The hearing component tests adults by performing pure tone audiometry and tympanometry. Because pure tone screening by itself may not be sensitive enough to detect middle ear disease, tympanometry is conducted to provide an estimate of tympanic membrane compliance.

- **Laboratory**

  The laboratory component includes the collection and processing of various biological and environmental specimens including blood for subjects 1 year and older, urine for subjects 6 years and older. On-site pregnancy testing excludes pregnant women from other examination components such as DEXA, BIA, and cardiovascular fitness testing. Complete Blood Counts (CBCs) are also performed in the MEC laboratory. All other specimen testing is performed by Federal, private, and university-based laboratories under contract to NCHS.

- **Lower Extremity Disease (LED)**

  The purpose of this component is to determine the prevalence of LED and its risk factors. Simple and reproducible measures of lower extremity arterial disease are obtained. Peripheral neuropathy is evaluated by measurement of cutaneous pressure sensation in the feet. Foot deformities permit the estimation of prevalence of those at high risk for the late-stage complications of LED.

- **MEC Interview**

  The MEC Interview consists of questionnaire sections designed to obtain information on health behaviors, specific conditions, medical history, and risk factors. The information collected in the interview is intended to assist researchers in analyzing the data collected in the other examination components. The interview is administered to all age-eligible subjects, or a suitable proxy, using computer-assisted interviewing software.

- **Mental Health**

  The mental health assessment is used to estimate the prevalence of selected disorders in the U.S. and to describe the degree of comorbidity between mental health disorders and other medical conditions and biological risk factors. Assessments are made during the MEC Interview using relevant portions of the Diagnostic Interview Schedule for Children (DISC) and the Composite International Diagnostic Interview (CIDI) for adults.

- **Methicillin-Resistant *S. Aureus* (MRSA) Sample Collection**

  A nasal swab specimen collection for Methicillin-Resistant Staphylococcus aureus (S. aureus) is obtained on SPs aged 1+ years for the purpose of estimating the prevalence of MRSA in the population. Antimicrobial resistance to S. aureus has increased so dramatically, particularly in the hospital setting, that currently only one treatment option exists for this organism. NHANES is the first population-based prevalence study of MRSA. No other population-based studies or national surveillance efforts are available to provide reliable national estimates for this problem.

- **Oral Health**

  This component monitors oral health status, risk factors for disease, and access to preventive and treatment services. The exam consists of a series of subcomponents which assess dentition and periodontal disease.

- **Physical Activity Monitor**

  The purpose of physical activity monitor component (PAM) is to assess the physical activity levels of NHANES examinees 6+ years of age. NHANES examinees wear a physical activity monitor (PAM) to examine physical activity patterns over a 7-day monitoring period and then mail it back to the home office. The monitors detect locomotion-type activities such as walking or jogging. The monitors provide a means of capturing non-structured activities that are often difficult for survey respondents (SPs) to self-report. Physical activity data are linked to other household interview and health component data and are used to track changes that occur in body weight, functional status, bone status, and health status over time.

- **Physician Exam**

  Blood pressure assessment and discussion of testing for sexually transmitted disease are the primary elements of the physician's exam. The purpose of assessment of blood pressure is to monitor prevalence and trends in major cardiovascular conditions and risk factors and to evaluate prevention and treatment programs targeting cardiovascular disease. The physician discusses the purpose of STD testing and arranges for SPs to select a unique password with which to phone NCHS and obtain test results.

- **Total Body Composition**

  This component is composed of the BIA and Dual Energy X-ray Absorptiometry (DEXA). The purpose of the DEXA scan is to gain insights into age, gender, and racial/ethnic differences in the skeleton relative to other measures of body composition such as total muscle and fat mass, as well as behavioral factors such as diet and activity. A total body scan using dual energy X-rays is performed to provide measures of bone mineral content, bone mineral density, muscle and fat mass.

- **Vision**

  The vision examination consists of a near vision acuity test, a distance vision acuity test, an eyeglass prescription determination (when appropriate), and an automated refraction measurement. Information from the component may be used to estimate the prevalence of visual acuity impairment and distribution of refractive error in the U.S. population. Data are also used to evaluate screening strategies for visual impairment and eye disease, and evaluate functional impairment related to vision.

- **Volatile Organic Compounds (VOC)**

  Information on levels of exposure to a selected group of volatile organic compounds is collected on a subsample of the survey population to assist in determining whether regulatory mechanisms are needed to reduce the levels of hazardous air pollutants to which the general population is exposed.

1.5.4   Sample Person Remuneration

All examinees receive remuneration for the MEC visit as well as payment for transportation expenses. The MEC visit remuneration is age-related and includes an extra incentive if the SP fasts prior to the exam. SPs who complete the physical activity monitoring component also receive an incentive. In addition, remunerations are offered to SPs who complete the dietary phone interview and the Food Frequency Questionnaire.

1.5.5   Report of Exam Findings

Examinees receive the results of many of the tests and exams conducted in the MEC, though some results are used only for research and are not reported.

One report, a Preliminary Report of Findings, is produced for the SP on the day of their examination and includes results that are immediately available and require no further evaluation or interpretation. Just prior to the examinee's departure from the MEC, the coordinator prints a report that includes height, weight, and body mass index, complete blood count, blood pressure, and results from the audiometry, cardiovascular fitness, lower extremity disease, vision, and dental exams. The MEC physician reviews the blood pressure and complete blood count test results for abnormalities and discusses any problems with the SP (or their parent). The dentist also discusses the dental recommendations with the SP. Approximately 12-16 weeks after the exam, NCHS mails the remainder of the examination results to the SP after appropriate clinical or quality reviews are completed. Seriously abnormal results are reported to the SP via telephone by NCHS before the remaining findings are mailed.

Certain tests, such as those for sexually transmitted diseases (chlamydia, gonorrhea, syphilis, Herpes simplex 1 and 2, bacterial vaginosis, and Trichomoniasis) and human immunodeficiency virus (HIV) are released only to the sample person using a specially devised procedure requiring a unique password.

To further assist sample persons, an in-house NCHS survey response team is available to answer calls from NHANES participants regarding the results from the Report of Finding System. The response team effort works both as a triage mechanism and a surveillance system. A receipt and control record is kept on all sample person inquiries. Also available at no cost to sample persons is an 800 toll-free telephone number which can be accessed during regular scheduled business hours. The response team members include a physician, a nurse with a doctorate degree, and other staff who are trained to answer specific questions.

Tests and procedures conducted in the MEC are not considered diagnostic exams and are not a substitute for an evaluation by a medical professional. No clinical treatments or health interventions of any type are performed in the MEC. If a health problem is discovered during the course of the MEC exam, the physician offers to contact the examinee's personal healthcare provider or recommend a local physician or clinic for follow-up care. If a sample person is found to have a serious condition requiring immediate attention, the local rescue squad may be summoned or the SP will be advised to seek immediate medical treatment.

1.5.6   Dry Run Day

At the beginning of the examination period, one-half day is devoted to calibrating instruments, practicing MEC procedures, and collecting biological specimens that serve as blind quality control samples. A dry run day is scheduled immediately prior to the first exam day of every stand to make sure that all equipment is operational, supplies are adequate, and the facility is working properly. Any problems are corrected quickly before the "real" examinations begin. All procedures in the dry run are completed as though the actual exam session was being conducted. The only difference is that the examinees are actual volunteers who are not part of the sample for the survey. Volunteers may include local residents, local officials, or field employees or guests of NCHS.

1.6   Integrated Survey Information System (ISIS)

The Integrated Survey Information System (ISIS) is a computer-based infrastructure designed to support all survey operations including sample management, data collection, data editing, quality control, analysis, and delivery of NHANES data. With a collection of customized subsystems, the ISIS links the Field Office, Mobile Examination Center, Westat home office, and NCHS during field operations. Each component in NHANES such as Dietary Interview has a computer application for direct data entry. Data collected in the Dietary Interview room of the mobile examination center is directly entered in the ISIS system computers. In addition, data from biomedical equipment such as the blood pressure monitor in the CV Fitness room is directly downloaded to the ISIS system where it is displayed on the computer screen and stored in the system database.

1.7   Confidentiality and Professional Ethics

All information regarding this study must be kept strictly confidential except as required by law. This includes location of survey sites. Since this study is being conducted under a contract with the National Center for Health Statistics, the privacy of all information collected is protected by two public laws: Section 308(d) of the Public Health Service Act (42 U.S.C.242m) and the Privacy Act of 1974 (5 U.S.C. 552a).

Each person working on the study must be continuously aware of the responsibility to safeguard the rights of all the individuals participating in the study. Each participant should be treated courteously, not as a sample number. Never divulge names or any other information about study participants except to the research team. Refrain from any discussions about study participants, in or out of the MEC, which might be overheard by people not on the survey staff. All of the members of the research team are under the same legal, moral, and ethical obligations to protect the privacy of the SPs participating in the survey. No participant names will be included in any reports prepared about the survey and neither NCHS nor the contractor is allowed to release information that would identify study participants without the consent of the participants.

Cooperation from the public is essential to the success of survey research. A great deal of effort is expended in obtaining cooperation from many national, regional, state, and local officials and the general public. It is the responsibility of every field employee to build on the integrity of the survey to encourage continued access to study participants during current and future surveys. Professional conduct, both on and off the job, is extremely important.

Each staff member has a responsibility for promoting good public relations. The Public Health Service and the contractor will be judged by the actions of the staff both on and off duty; consequently staff must be discreet in speech and action. Personal appearance and behavior must be governed by these same considerations. Please be aware of the audience at all times and avoid statements or actions that could shed an unfavorable light on the survey.

Staff will be asked to sign a pledge of confidentiality before the survey begins. This pledge states that they are prohibited by law from disclosing any information while working on the survey to anyone except authorized staff of NCHS and the contractor, and that they agree to abide by the contractor's Assurance of Confidentiality.

2. OVERVIEW OF PHYSICIAN'S EXAMINATION

Data obtained by physicians for the survey database include blood pressure (BP) measurements and heart rates (HR). These measurements are the data source for reporting the national standard for blood pressure and heart rate from the NHANES. Additional tasks carried out by the MEC physicians include asking specific safety and medical exclusion questions to determine sample persons' (SPs) eligibility for the cardiovascular (CVF) fitness treadmill testing. The physicians discuss the sexually transmitted disease (STD) testing done on the survey, as well as bacterial vaginosis (BV) with women 14-49 years old. The physicians instruct SPs about how to obtain their STD test results confidentially. When physicians determine that data obtained during the mobile examination center examination indicates a medical referral, they refer SPs to health care providers in the local community.

Specific physician training focuses on standardizing BP and HR measurements, and safety exclusion decisionmaking for cardiovascular fitness (CV) testing. Clear and complete instruction for the physician aids standardized, accurate data collection across both MEC teams, and emphasizes the importance of following the protocol for the purpose of systematic, prioritized survey data collection.

2.1　　　Medical Policy Regarding the Examination

The purpose of the NHANES study is to collect data on the health status of the United States population. Treatment is **not** within the role of the MEC physician, and any findings that are of concern to physicians are noted and included in referrals. In most instances, the examining physician will not be licensed within the state in which the examinations are being conducted. The liability insurance obtained for Westat physicians does not cover any type of treatment procedure except stabilization in an emergency.

NHANES survey staff have no control over, nor connection with local health care systems. Any involvement beyond routine referral is ineffective and interferes with the purpose of the study. Referral of examinees is included in the MEC procedures for ethical reasons although referral is **not** within the purpose of the study. Before SPs depart the MEC, they are provided with a report of the findings that become available while they are in the MEC. They are provided a final report of all findings approximately 3 months after their MEC examination. These are in the form of written reports and they are mailed to the SPs.

2.2 The Role of the Physician in NHANES

Physicians function as mobile examination center (MEC) team members with the primary function of collecting blood pressure, heart rate and pulse data, ascertaining information specified by the protocol to determine whether SP's should be included or excluded from CV testing, and counseling SPs regarding STD and HIV testing. They are the primary care providers during medical emergencies. If there is a life threatening or medical emergency the MEC physician provides immediate intervention and referral as needed. MEC physicians do not provide diagnosis or treatment of medical conditions, nor is the MEC a medical treatment facility.

2.2.1 Presence in MEC during MEC Examinations

Examinations do not occur on the MEC without the presence of a physician. Physicians report to the mobile examination center at least 5 minutes before examinations are scheduled to begin. They leave the MEC only when all examination and interview protocol procedures have been completed and all SPs have left the MEC.

2.2.2 Response to Medical Emergencies

If an examinee becomes ill or disabled during the examination session, the physician renders only the level of care necessary to keep the examinee out of immediate danger. Arrangements are made to transport SPs to an appropriate medical facility. An ambulance is called if a potentially life threatening condition develops, or if indicated for any SP. Further details about medical emergencies are included in Chapter 6.

2.2.3   Maintenance of Emergency Equipment and Supplies

Physicians maintain emergency equipment and supplies for use in the MEC. They inventory supplies, restock supplies as needed, and ensure that all emergency equipment, medications and supplies are current and in proper working order. Emergency procedures and supplies are described in detail in Chapter 6.

2.3   Physicians' Examination

The physicians' examination is described in detail in Chapter 4, Physician Protocol. The physicians' examination consists of measuring blood pressure and heart rate or pulse depending on the age of the SP. In addition, the physician asks specific questions to determine eligibility for CVF testing and discusses the implications of STD testing. In addition, SP's 14-49 are asked to self-collect vaginal swabs for Human Papillomavirus (HPV), Trichomonas, and Bacterial Vaginosis (BV). Women aged 50-59 are asked to self-collect vaginal swabs for HPV. The physician instructs the SP in these procedures. The physician exam also includes a set of exclusionary questions for those SPs who consent to have their blood tested for prostate specific antigen (PSA). The blood to test the antigen is drawn during the venipuncture, which could occur either before or after the SP sees the physician for the physician exam. In either case, the physician asks a set of questions that would exclude the SP from the PSA testing if the SP answers Yes to any one of the questions. If the SP does not agree to have his blood tested for PSA, then the physician codes the PSA section of the exam as a refusal, and the laboratory removes the PSA blood sample from the specimens.

2.3.1   Measurement of Blood Pressure and Pulse

Physicians count heart rates on all SPs through 4 years of age. Radial pulse is counted on SPs from 5 years of age through age 7 and blood pressure and pulse is measured on all SPs 8 years of age and above. The specific protocol used for blood pressure measurements is described in Chapter 4, Physician Protocol.

2.3.2   Review for Exclusion and Inclusion of Cardiovascular Fitness Treadmill Testing

SPs who are 12 years of age through 49 years of age are eligible for CV testing. CV testing uses stringent inclusion and exclusion criteria. The physicians use a standardized protocol to assure that SPs having even minimal risk are excluded from CV testing. Physicians use the protocol to ascertain that SPs meet all the required criteria before allowing SPs to do CV testing. The specific protocol used for exclusion and inclusion of SPs in CV testing is described in Chapter 4, Physician Protocol.

2.3.3   Counseling for STD and HIV

All SPs who are 14-17 years of age are tested for chlamydia, gonorrhea, and herpes type 2; SPs who are 18-39 are tested for chlamydia, gonorrhea, Herpes type 2, syphilis, and HIV; and SPs aged 40-49 are tested for Herpes Type 2, syphilis, and HIV. Female SPs who are 14-49 are also tested for Human Papilloma Virus (HPV), trichomonas, and Bacterial Vaginosis (BV). Female SPs 50- 59 are tested for HPV. Physicians counsel SPs about the survey specific STD and BV testing and tell them how to get their test results. The specific protocol used for STD/HIV and BV counseling is described in Chapter 4, Physician Protocol.

2.3.4   Referrals

Physicians are responsible for monitoring out of range data values as defined by the component protocols. If data values exceed predefined limits, the ISIS system flags these data for review. Physicians are responsible for discussing out of range values with SPs and making referrals to outside physicians if necessary. Physicians' procedures for managing referrals are described in Chapter 5.

2.4   Maintenance of Physician's Examination Room

Physicians are individually responsible for the maintenance of the physician's examination room and all equipment and supplies required for their examination. At the beginning of a stand physicians inventory supplies and equipment. They prepare the examination room by opening and setting up all supplies and equipment. They determine that adequate supply levels are available and that all equipment is in proper working order. At the end of each examination session physicians clean and properly store all equipment and restock supplies as needed. At the end of each stand physicians inventory equipment and supplies and pack up equipment and supplies. Details about equipment maintenance and supplies are included in Section 3, Equipment and Supplies.

3. EQUIPMENT AND SUPPLIES

3.1   Description of Equipment

Equipment is selected that meets the requirements for obtaining the required data and creates the best opportunity for minimal data collection error. All equipment is regularly subjected to quality control checks. Equipment required for blood pressure and heart rate measurement is a stethoscope, and an inflation system including an arm blood pressure cuff and a manometer. A stopwatch is used for standardizing time between individual BP measurements. Quality control procedures for physician equipment are described in detail in Chapter 8, Physician Equipment Quality Control.

3.2   Sphygmomanometer

The inflation system consists of a latex inflation bag, a Calibrated® V-Lok® cuff, a Latex Inflation Bulb, and an Air-Flo® Control Valve. The pressure gauge is a Baumanometer® calibrated mercury true gravity wall model.

3.2.1   The Baumanometer® Calibrated Manometer

Upon receipt from the factory, these manometers are precisely calibrated to true gravity, and are guaranteed by the manufacturer to remain scientifically accurate. Regular inspection is necessary to eliminate extraneous conditions that could cause the blood pressure measurement to be erroneously read. The mercury-gravity manometer consists of a calibrated cartridge glass tube that is optically clear, easy to clean, and abrasion resistant. The mercury reservoir at the bottom of the tube communicates with a compression cuff through a rubber tube. When air pressure is exerted on the mercury in the reservoir by pumping the pressure bulb, the mercury in the glass tube rises and indicates how much pressure the cuff applies against the artery. The measurement markings on the glass tubes are ceramic lines; they are fused to the surface of the glass, and cannot be removed with chemicals, solvents, or even by abrasion.

The manometer is connected to the wall for ease of accurate visualization while the physician is seated next to the SP. The physician inspects the manometer before each blood pressure measurement. The mercury meniscus shape is examined and if the shape of the mercury meniscus (top of the column of mercury) is not a smooth, well-defined curve, the equipment is replaced. If the mercury does not rise easily in the tube, or if the mercury column bounces noticeably as the valve is closed, the equipment is replaced as the atmospheric pressure within the tube is likely altered rendering the manometer inaccurate. The physicians never attempt to repair the equipment. The level of the mercury in the calibrated glass tube is expected to be at the zero line when the manometer is on a level surface with the inflation system disconnected. If the level of the mercury is above or below the zero line, there may be too much mercury in the reservoir, a mercury leak, or dirt in the mercury or in the calibrated glass tube. To correct this, the physician takes the manometer off the wall, tips the manometer gently to the right, and then to the erect position. If the meniscus of the mercury column does not return to zero, the equipment is replaced.

3.2.2   Calibrated® V-Lok® Cuff

The Calibrated® V-Lok® compression cuff is made of urethane-coated Dacron, an unyielding material that exerts an even pressure on the inflatable bladder inside the cuff. The compression cuffs have Velcro fasteners that adhere to them to keep the cuff in position when placed on the arm. The physicians measure the circumference of the arm and the correct cuff size is precisely determined according to the measured arm size. The size of the arm, not the SP's age, determines the cuff to be used. The size of the cuff and the bladder used influences the accuracy of the blood pressure readings. If the cuff is too narrow, the observed blood pressure is overestimated (higher than it really is), and if it is too wide, the reading may be underestimated (lower than it really is). The four cuff sizes used are child, adult, large arm, and thigh. The cuff sizes are discussed in detail in Chapter 4, Physician Protocol.

The function of the pressure bulb is to create pressure in the system to allow inflation of the bladder. The pressure control valve controls the rate at which the system is deflated. The cuffs, pressure bulb, control bulb, manometer, and manometer tubing are checked each day before use for cracks, tears, and air leaks.

3.2.3   Littman™ Classic II S.E. Stethoscope

The stethoscopes used for listening to Korotkoff sounds are Littman™ Classic II SE for adults and Littman™ Classic II pediatric for children. These stethoscopes are typically used in clinical settings for general physical examinations. They have a bell and diaphragm chestpiece, and an acoustical *rating by the manufacturer* of 7 on a scale of 1-10, with a rating of 10 having the best acoustical attributes. The construction uses a single-lumen rubber tubing connection between the eartubes and the chestpiece. The eartubes are permanently set at an anatomically correct angle, and the plastic ear covers come in different sizes allowing the user to match the best ear canal size to achieve an acoustically sealed ear fit. All parts of the stethoscope can be cleaned for use between SPs. The bell of the stethoscope is used to auscultate the Korotkoff sounds for blood pressure measurements. The techniques for obtaining blood pressure data are described in detail in Chapter 4.

3.3   Maintenance of Equipment

Physicians maintain all equipment used in their component. The following sections specifically state the requirements that physicians follow to check equipment and maintain equipment used for the physician examination.

3.3.1   Mercury Sphygmomanometer

The mercury manometer is calibrated when it is manufactured; recalibration is unnecessary. However, regular inspection is necessary to eliminate conditions that could cause the blood pressure measurement to be read as erroneously high or low. Physicians must adhere to the following instructions related to BP equipment maintenance.

Check the shape of the meniscus (top of the column of mercury) - it should be a smooth, well-defined curve. If the shape of the mercury meniscus is not a smooth, well-defined curve, replace the equipment. This is caused by dirt in the mercury or the glass tube. Check that the mercury rises easily in the tubing and that the mercury column does not bounce noticeably when the valve is closed. If the mercury does not rise easily in the tube, or if the mercury column bounces noticeably as the valve is closed, replace the equipment as this indicates alteration of the atmospheric pressure within the tube.

Disconnect the inflation system from the blood pressure (BP) cuff and check that the meniscus of the mercury in the glass manometer tube is zero. The level of the mercury in the calibrated glass tube should always be at the zero line when the manometer is on a level surface with the inflation system disconnected. If the level of the mercury is above or below the zero line, there may be too much mercury in the reservoir, a mercury leak, dirt in the mercury or in the calibrated glass tube. Move the manometer gently from side to side. If the top of the mercury column does not return to zero when returned to the upright position, replace the equipment.

Check for cracks in the glass tube. Check the cap at the top of the calibrated glass tube to make sure it is securely in place. Check the cuff, pressure bulb, and tubing for cracks or tears. Check the pressure control valve for sticks or leaks. Use the following procedure to check for air leaks:

- Connect the inflation system and wrap it around the calibration cylinder;

- Inflate to 250 mm Hg;

- Open valve and deflate to 200 mm Hg and close valve; and

- Wait for 10 seconds; if mercury column drops more than 10 mm Hg, there is an air leak in the system.

Never attempt to repair the equipment yourself. Contact the MEC manager to have equipment sent for repair or replacement. The manometer will be sent to Baum for repair or replacement. Chapter 8 provides specific daily, weekly, and stand equipment quality control procedures.

Contact for repair or replacement of manometer:

W. A. Baum Co. Inc.
Copiague, New York 11726
Phone: 516-226-3940
Fax: 516-226-3969

3.3.2 Littman Stethoscope

Check the stethoscope for cracks in the rubber and for tight earpiece attachment. Check that the head of the stethoscope is securely attached to the rubber tubing. Check that the head can be easily rotated so that either the bell or the diaphragm can be accessed. The bell head is always used to auscultate the Korotkoff sounds for BP measurement. Chapter 8 provides specific daily, weekly, and stand equipment quality control procedures.

3.3.3   Blood Pressure Cuffs

Check the inflation cuff for cleanliness, and wipe between each use with disinfectant wipes. Check the inflation cuff as an integral component of the inflation system. Chapter 8 provides specific daily, weekly, and stand equipment quality control procedures.

3.4   Mercury Spills or Leaks

A mercury manometer is used to measure blood pressures. The mercury is encased in a glass tube, and unless exposed to the atmosphere, is harmless. Mercury is a metallic substance that gives off a toxic vapor when exposed to the atmosphere. Temperature, ventilation, and sunlight affect the level of the vapor's concentration. Mercury vapors will permeate the skin surface and are poisonous when inhaled. Check the cap at the top of the calibrated glass tubing. If it is not securely closed, the mercury could leak out. Loss of air and mercury will occur if the glass tube is broken. Care should be taken in handling the manometer to prevent this. If the tube appears cracked, check for any spilled mercury and replace the equipment if necessary.

3.4.1   Required Procedure for Handling Spilled or Leaking Mercury

The following procedure is required for handling spilled or leaking mercury:

- Contact the MEC manager immediately to report the incident and receive instructions. The Mercury Spill Kit contains all the materials needed for clean up.

- The MEC manager will determine what action should be taken. If necessary, the local hazardous materials contact may be called to report such spills. The local hazardous materials agency may want to make a followup visit to the facility to check for levels of mercury in the exposed area.

- Do not touch the mercury with bare hands or attempt to vacuum or clean up the spill.

■ The procedures for cleaning up the mercury are different depending on the surface where the spill is detected.

■ If the spill is small the following procedure may be used:

- Leakage or spillage on a hard surface (e.g., hard floor, table, etc.,)

    1. Get the Mercury Spill Kit from the physician's exam room.

    2. Put on the green protective gloves.

    3. Use the mercury (HG Absorb) sponge.

    4. Remove the sponge from the plastic zip-closable bag.

    5. Dampen the sponge with water.

    6. Wipe the area contaminated with mercury. Do this slowly to allow for complete absorption of all free mercury. The chemical layer (Hg Absorb powder) on the sponge will absorb the mercury droplets.

    7. After finishing with the Hg Absorb sponge, place it back into its plastic zip-closable bag.

    8. Place the manometer case and mercury sponge into separate plastic bags and secure with tape. Return to the MEC manager.

    9. Complete a Mercury Spill Report Form.

    10. Obtain replacement equipment.

- Leakage and/or spillage on a soft or absorbent surface (e.g., rug, etc.):

    1. Get the Mercury Spill Kit from the physician's exam room.

    2. Put on the green protective gloves.

    3. Turn off heat or air conditioning to avoid spreading vapors to other rooms in the MEC.

    4. Open a window if possible to ensure adequate ventilation to the outside for the room where the spill occurred.

    5. Use the mercury (Hg Absorb) sponge, if possible. See directions above.

    6. Wet the MERCSORB☐ powder with water. Mercury will react with powder, forming a metal/mercury amalgam.

7. Wipe or sweep wetted powder over all cracks and hard to reach locations for maximum pickup.

8. Pick up amalgam by sponging or by using the small sweep and dustpan provided in the Mercury Spill Kit.

9. Complete a Mercury Spill Report Form.

10. Obtain replacement equipment.

4. PHYSICIAN PROTOCOL

4.1   General Overview

Physicians are the data collectors in the MEC for blood pressure, heart rate, and pulse measurements for the survey. The protocol for these measurements is described in detail in Section 4.2 of this chapter. Physicians are the MEC examiners who review specified health-related data and ask questions for cardiovascular fitness to determine whether SPs meet inclusion or exclusion criteria for cardiovascular fitness testing. The questions are listed in Appendix G and the procedures for this part of the protocol are described in Section 4.3 of this chapter. Physicians also may ask "Shared Exclusion" questions. These shared exclusion questions are asked by the first person to examine the SP. The purpose of having questions that are shared between examiners is to minimize examination time by excluding questions from any component that have already been asked in another examination component. This process saves time in each component and prevents replication of questions for SPs. These questions are asked to determine whether SPs should be included or excluded from body composition testing or muscle strength testing. Physicians are the designated MEC examiners to discuss sexually transmitted diseases, Bacterial Vaginosis, and Human Immunodeficiency Virus testing with SPs. The protocol for discussion differs by age groups and is described in detail in Section 4.4 of this chapter. MEC physicians are the designated examiners to discuss pregnancy results with SPs. Physicians also review several examination data results to determine the need for referrals. The referral procedure, including referral for pregnancy, is described in detail in Chapter 5, Referrals.

4.2   Blood Pressure, Heart Rate, and Pulse Measurements

Physicians count heart rates on all SPs through 4 years of age. Radial pulse is counted on SPs from 5 through 7 years of age and blood pressure and pulse is measured on all SPs 8 years of age and above. Physicians record the survey blood pressure measurements. The protocol for blood pressure measurement follows procedures developed by the American Heart Association. Physicians and backup physicians are certified in blood pressure measurement through a training program that includes didactic information, video practice listening to Korotkoff sounds, and practice in listening to blood pressures using volunteers with a certified instructor. Certification is achieved when physicians meet all requirements of the training program. Recertification is accomplished quarterly.

4.2.1   SPs Included for Blood Pressure, Heart Rate, and Pulse Measurements

Heart rates are measured on all children up to and including 4 years of age. Radial (brachial if necessary) pulses are measured on SPs 5 years old and above. Blood pressures are measured on all SPs 8 years old and above.

4.2.2   SPs Excluded from Blood Pressure, Heart Rate, and Pulse Measurements

SPs are excluded from blood pressure measurement if they have any condition that could potentially cause them harm or discomfort or would prevent accurate blood pressure measurement. Conditions that may affect BP are noted, but these conditions do not exclude SPs from BP measurement. SPs are asked if they have had any food, coffee, cigarettes, or alcohol in the past 30 minutes. Although intake of coffee and cigarettes could affect blood pressure, this information is not used to exclude SPs from blood pressure measurement. There are no protocol specific reasons for excluding SPs from heart rate or pulse measurement.

4.2.3   Procedures for Measuring Blood Pressures, Heart Rates, and Pulses

These sections are written as instructional procedures for physicians to follow when measuring BPs, heart rate, and pulse. Physicians are taught during an intense training to follow these procedures exactly when measuring blood pressures, listening to heart rates, and counting pulses.

4.2.3.1   Position SP for Blood Pressure Measurements

Ask the SP to sit in a chair and rest quietly for 5 minutes prior to blood pressure measurement. The arm and back should be supported and the legs should be uncrossed with both feet flat on the floor. The arm should be bared and unrestricted by clothing with the palm of the hand turned upward and the elbow slightly flexed. The arm should be positioned so that the midpoint of the upper arm is at the level of the heart. The location of the heart is taken as the junction of the fourth intercostal space and the lower left sternal border. The mercury manometer should be positioned at the eye level of the examiner so the mercury meniscus can be easily read without parallax. Small or short SP's may have to sit on a book or pillow to raise their body to the correct position. If necessary, place SP's feet on a box or other item to stabilize their feet in a flat position. Very tall SPs may need to place their arm on a book or pillow to bring their upper arm to the correct position.

4.2.3.2   Selecting the Arm for BP Measurement

For the purpose of standardization, both pulse and blood pressure are measured in the right arm unless specific conditions prohibit the use of the right arm, or, if SPs self-report any reason that the blood pressure procedure should not use the right arm. If the measurements cannot be taken in the right arm, they are taken in the left arm. Use of the right or left arm must be noted during ISIS data entry. BP measurements are not done on any arms that have rashes, small gauze/adhesive dressings, casts, are withered, puffy, have tubes, open sores, hematomas, wounds, arteriovenous (AV) shunt, or any other intravenous access device. Also, women who have had a unilateral radical mastectomy do not have their blood pressure measured in the arm on the same side as the mastectomy was performed. In all cases, if there is a problem with both arms, the blood pressure is not taken.

4.2.3.3   Locating the Pulse Points

Locating the Radial Pulse: Position SP with the right palm upward. Palpate the radial pulse on the flexor surface of the wrist laterally with the pads of your index and middle fingers.

Locating the Brachial Pulse: Position SP with the right palm turned upward and the arm slightly bent at the elbow. With the pads of your index and middle fingers, palpate the brachial pulse in the groove between the biceps and triceps muscles above the elbow. This is the point where the center of the cuff bladder is placed. The brachial pulse is then palpated in the medial aspect of the antecubital fossa. This is the point where the bell of the stethoscope is placed. If the brachial pulse cannot be felt in the arm, check the radial pulse. If no radial or brachial pulse is palpable on the right arm, use the left arm. If a radial pulse is apparent, whether or not the brachial pulse can be felt, the blood pressure measurement should be attempted.

4.2.3.4   Cuff Size and Application

It is important to select an appropriate size cuff that properly fits the SP's arm. The length and width of the bladder inside the cuff should encircle at least 80 percent and 40 percent of an adult's arm, respectively. The length and width of the cuff should encircle 100 percent of the arm in children less than 13 years old. *The index lines on the cuff are **not used in this study**.* The appropriate size cuff to be used is determined as outlined below:

- Using a centimeter tape, determine the <u>midpoint</u> of the upper arm by measuring the length of the arm between the acromium and olecranon process (between the shoulder and elbow).

- Mark the <u>midpoint</u> of this measurement with a cosmetic pencil.

- Measure the circumference of the bare upper arm at the <u>midpoint</u>.

- Find the arm circumference under column 4 in Table 4-1.

- Use the cuff size from column 1 associated with the arm circumference in column 4. (Example: If the arm circumference at <u>midpoint</u> is 36 cm, use the large adult cuff.)

- Position the rubber bladder over the brachial artery at least 1" above the crease of the elbow. For long thin arms, the cuff should be placed in the middle of the arm. Place the marker on the inner part of the cuff directly over the brachial artery.

- Cuff should be wrapped in a circular manner. Do not wrap the cuff in any spiral direction.

- Check the fit of the cuff to ensure that it is secure but not tight.

Table 4-1.   Arm circumference and acceptable cuff size

Cuff Size	Bladder width (cm)	Bladder length (cm)	Arm circumference[1]
Child	9	17	17-21.9
Adult	12	22	22-29.9
Large adult	15	32	30-37.9
Adult thigh	18	35	38-47.9

[1] Adapted from Human Blood Pressure Determination by Sphygmometry, American Heart Association.

4.2.3.5 Determine the Maximum Inflation Level (MIL)

- Determine the maximum inflation level (MIL) after the SP has been seated and resting quietly for approximately 3 minutes.

- The MIL or palpatory method provides an approximation of the systolic blood pressure to determine the highest level to which the cuff should be inflated when the actual measurement is made. The MIL is determined as follows:

  - Locate the radial pulse in the right arm (Section 4.2.3.3).

  - Inflate the cuff quickly to a pressure of 70 – 80 mm Hg. Then inflate the cuff in increments of 10 mm Hg until the radial pulse is no longer palpable (palpated systolic). Continue inflating the cuff in increments of 10 mm Hg to a final measure that is 30 mm Hg above the pressure where the pulse was last palpated. This number is the MIL. Note this measurement for recording.

  - Rapidly deflate the cuff, confirm the return of the pulse, and disconnect the tubing.

  - If you were unable to obtain the MIL, wait 1 minute and repeat the process.

  - Enter the MIL in the *MIL Field* in the ISIS system.

4.2.3.6 Heart Rate Measurements for SPs Through Age 4

For all SPs through the age of 4 years, only the heart rate is recorded. Count the heart rate by listening to the heart at approximately the 4th intercostal space, midclavicular line. Use the bell device of the pediatric stethoscope.

- Remove all clothing over the left chest wall.

- The heart rate should be recorded after the child rests for 4 minutes.

- If the SP is extremely active or crying, allow an additional maximum of 2 minutes for the child to become quiet before counting the heart rate.

- If the child can sit in a chair without an adult, have the child sit quietly in the chair until the heart rate is counted.

- If the child needs to be held, ask the adult who accompanies the child to hold the child in an upright position, without "squeezing" any portion of the body, especially the abdomen.

- Count the rate for 30 seconds and record the rate in the ISIS *Heart Rate Field*.

- Note regularity and record in the ISIS *Regular Field*.

4.2.3.7 Pulse Measurements for All SPs Ages 5 Through 7

For all SPs 5 through 7 years of age, only the radial pulse rate is recorded.

- The pulse may be taken after the SP has been seated and resting quietly for approximately 4 minutes.

- With the elbow and forearm resting comfortably on a table and the palm of the hand turned upward find the radial pulse and count for 30 seconds.

- The number of beats in 30 seconds is recorded.

- The *rhythm field* is defaulted to "Regular." If there is an irregular rhythm, click on the radio button indicating regular, and check the box to specify "Irregular."

  - If the SP is between the ages 12 through 49, the system will enable a space to enter the number of irregular beats that occurred in 60 seconds.

  - Count the pulse again for 60 seconds and record the number of missed beats during that period. Enter this number in the appropriate box. If there are 4 or more missed beats in 60 seconds, the system will block the SP from the Cardiovascular Fitness Component.

4.2.3.8 Seated Blood Pressure Readings

Both blood pressure and pulse are taken and recorded on SPs 8 years old and above. Three consecutive blood pressure readings are obtained, using the same arm. If a blood pressure measurement is interrupted or you are unable to get one or more of the readings, a fourth attempt may be made. Wait at least 30 seconds between readings. Open the thumb valve completely and disconnect the manometer tubing from the cuff between each reading to reduce the pressure in the cuff to zero.

4.2.3.9   Procedure

- The following procedures are used for seated blood pressure readings:

  - Place earpieces of the stethoscope into the ear canals, angled forward to fit snugly.

  - Confirm that the stethoscope head is in the low-frequency (bell) position. The bell is recommended because it may be better suited to hear the low frequency Korotkoff sounds. Position the bell of the stethoscope over the brachial artery and hold it firmly in place, making sure that the head makes contact with the skin around its entire circumference. If possible, avoid allowing the cuff, tubing or bell to come in contact with each other.

  - Position the bell of the stethoscope over the brachial artery pulsation just above and medial to the antecubital fossa.

  - Rapidly and steadily, inflate the cuff to the MIL.

  - When the MIL is reached, open the thumb valve and smoothly deflate the cuff at a constant rate near 2-mm Hg per second (one mark per second) while concurrently listening for Korotkoff sounds.

  - Keep the center of the manometer at eye level.

  - Watch the top of the mercury column (meniscus) as the pressure in the bladder falls and note the level of the manometer pressure when the first repetitive sounds are heard (Phase I) and when they disappear (Phase V).

  - Continue steady deflation at 2 mm Hg per second for at least another 10 mm Hg. past where the last sounds were heard.

  - Rapidly deflate the cuff and disconnect the manometer tubing between measurements to ensure the cuff deflates completely to zero.

  - Enter Phase I (the level of the pressure on the manometer at the first appearance of repetitive sounds) as the systolic blood pressure reading.

  - Enter Phase V (the point at which the last muffled sound is heard) as the diastolic blood pressure reading.

  - If phase I or phase V occurs between the millimeter marks on the glass column, round upward to the nearest digit.

  - Wait for at least 30 seconds between readings, with the SP resting quietly.

  - Take a second set of measurements and enter the systolic and diastolic pressures in the system.

- Disconnect the manometer tubing and wait 30 seconds between readings with the SP resting quietly.

- Take the third measurement and record the systolic and diastolic pressures in the system.

- The system will automatically calculate the average based on predetermined guidelines.

- If enhancement techniques were needed, enter this in the system for that reading.

- If you are unable to get a blood pressure reading for some reason, deflate the cuff and enter this in the system as "Could Not Obtain."

- Four measurements can be attempted if necessary. Wait 30 seconds and proceed with the fourth measurement.

4.2.3.10   Averaging Rules for Determining Mean Blood Pressure

■   ISIS calculates the blood pressure average using the following protocol:

- If only one blood pressure reading was obtained, that reading is the average.

- If there is more than one blood pressure reading, the first reading is always excluded from the average.

- If only two blood pressure readings were obtained, the second blood pressure reading is the average.

- If all diastolic readings were zero, then the average would be zero.

  ■   Exception: If there is one diastolic reading of zero and one (or more) with a number above zero, the diastolic reading with zero is not used to calculate the diastolic average.

- If two out of three are zero, the one diastolic reading that is not zero is used to calculate the diastolic average.

4.2.3.11   Procedures to Enhance the Brachial Pulse Sounds

■   If you are having difficulty hearing the blood pressure sounds, two methods can be used to increase the intensity and loudness of the sounds:

-    Elevate the SP's arm before and during inflation, and then lower the arm after the cuff has been inflated. Blood pressure is then determined in the usual manner.

-    Inflate the cuff, and then have the subject open and close his/her fist several times. Blood pressure is then determined in the usual manner.

■   When an enhancement method is used to measure BPs, check *"enhancement" field* on the data entry screen for that measurement.

4.2.3.12   Additional Blood Pressure Measurement Guidelines

■   If a BP measurement was interrupted, use the following guidelines:

-    The maximum number of cuff inflations for each SP is five, counting all MIL attempts and blood pressure attempts. The rationale for this is twofold: to minimize the discomfort to the SP of frequent cuff inflations and to accomplish data collection for this measurement within the time allowed.

-    If the blood pressure sounds are not heard during the first measurement, review your technique, check stethoscope position for loose connections or tubing kinks, and maintain a quiet environment. Relocate the brachial pulse and apply the bell headpiece directly over the pulse point. See the procedures in the above section for enhancing the Korotkoff sounds at the brachial pulse. Check enhancement techniques in the box on the blood pressure screen.

-    If the difference between the MIL and the 1st systolic measurement is less than 10 mm Hg or greater than 50 mm Hg, the system will prompt the examiner to obtain a new MIL. In this case, return to the first screen, do another estimate of the MIL, and record the new MIL in the system. The first and second BP measures are then obtained in the usual manner. Due to the limit of five inflations, the third BP measure (and the subsequent 4th measurement) should be marked as "Could not Obtain".

4.2.3.13   Hard Edit Limits for Blood Pressure

A hard edit is a limit imposed by the system that prevents data entry above or below the specified instrument or measurable limits. When entries are recorded that are outside these limits, the system displays a message that the value is out of range and sends a "popup message" asking that the value be re-entered. The system will not allow entries that are outside the specified hard edit limits. The hard edits imposed by the system are listed below:

- Systolic blood pressure and maximum inflation level cannot be greater than 300 mm Hg. This is the upper range of the measurement device. The mercury manometer has a minimum and maximum scale of 0 to 300, respectively. It is impossible to get a reading above or below this level.

- Systolic and diastolic blood pressure and maximum inflation level can be even numbers only. This is a function of the measurement device. The manometer displays the readings in increments of 2.

- Systolic blood pressure must be greater than diastolic blood pressure.

- If there is no systolic blood pressure, there can be no diastolic blood pressure. (There can be a systolic measurement without a diastolic measurement.)

- Systolic blood pressure cannot be zero (diastolic blood pressure can be zero).

4.2.3.14   Soft Edit Limits for Blood Pressure

A soft edit is a limit imposed by the system if a value is outside the predefined edit limits for the SP being measured. The predefined edits are based on NHANES III data. When measures outside these values are recorded, the system displays a "popup" message warning that the limit is out of range, and asks if the measurement is correct. The person entering the data has the option of editing or accepting that data value. Soft edits are placed on heart rate, pulse, and on systolic and diastolic blood pressures. The soft edits applied by the system are listed below.

- The difference between systolic BP and diastolic BP cannot be less than 20 mm Hg or greater than 100 mm Hg.

- Maximum inflation level should be greater than systolic blood pressure

- Systolic BP minimum and maximum ages 8-19   76 to 130 mm Hg

- Diastolic BP minimum and maximum ages 8-19   20 to 85 mm Hg

- Systolic BP minimum and maximum ages 20-49   86 to 160 mm Hg

- Diastolic BP minimum and maximum ages 20-49   50 to 100 mm Hg

- Systolic BP minimum and maximum ages 50+   90 to 200 mm Hg

- Diastolic BP minimum and maximum ages 50+   50 to 106 mm Hg

- Pulse minimum and maximum all ages, males and females   40 to 190 beats/minute

4.3   SP Exclusion from Cardiovascular Fitness Examination (CV Fitness)

The MEC facility and the MEC staff are not part of a medical facility, although there are provisions for life threatening emergency treatments if necessary. All examinations focus on obtaining the required survey data in the most accurate manner that best protects SPs from undue risk. Exclusions from any mobile examination center component are done systematically and by rigorous protocol rules. Physicians follow protocol rules for all exclusions and do not make out-of-protocol decisions about excluding SPs from any examination.

The primary criterion guiding exclusion of SPs from CV Fitness (submaximal treadmill testing) is SP safety. In addition, SPs may be excluded from the CV Fitness component due to physical limitations that would affect the accuracy of data obtained during treadmill testing. Physicians' questions focus on areas that identify conditions that could affect SP safety and data accuracy.

To accurately determine SPs who are at risk for negative cardiovascular events during treadmill testing, the protocol requires physicians to ask questions related to cardiovascular symptoms, other related and comorbid medical conditions, and medications typically prescribed for cardiovascular disease. When SPs respond positively to any one question or medication in these categories, they are, for reasons of their own safety, excluded from the cardiovascular fitness testing. Likewise, blood pressure is another indicant of a potential cardiovascular condition; therefore, both upper and lower limits of systolic and diastolic blood pressure measurements are set by protocol. When those blood pressures are recorded, the system automatically excludes SPs from treadmill testing. Disability and glaucoma exclusions are set by the protocol for safety reasons and for accurate treadmill performance testing results, respectively. All exclusions from the Cardiovascular Fitness component are based on medical conditions, medications, physical limitations, heart rate, blood pressure, and irregular heart beat. Appendix G lists the exclusion questions asked by the physician that result in exclusion of SPs from treadmill testing. Appendix D lists the medications that result in exclusion from the CV Fitness component. These medications are updated quarterly.

4.3.1   Conditions for Exclusion from Cardiovascular Fitness Testing

SPs are asked questions about past and current medical conditions by the household interviewer during the Household Questionnaire part of the Household interview. The conditions resulting in exclusion from the treadmill test include: pregnancy, BPs outside the specified minimum and maximum for the age category, history of previous myocardial infarction, coronary heart disease, stroke, emphysema, and certain physical function or development problems that would make it difficult or unsafe to complete treadmill testing without undue risk to SPs. The following sections describe how information is obtained for each of the exclusion categories.

4.3.1.1   Exclusions Based on Medication

SPs are excluded from the Cardiovascular Fitness component if they are taking certain medications. The list of medications was determined by a working group of physicians from NCHS and the Cooper Institute for Aerobic Research. The final categories of medications include calcium channel blockers, antidysrhythmic medications, beta-blockers, nitrates, nitroglycerin, and digitalis. Appendix D lists the medications requiring SPs to be excluded from treadmill testing. This list is updated every 3 months by consultants from the Cooper Institute for Aerobic Research and NCHS so that the medication list is current for new medications that become available in the marketplace. SPs are asked about medications during both the household interview and during the Physician Component Examination.

4.3.1.1.1   Medications Reported during the Household Interview Questionnaire

At the beginning of each MEC session, MEC physicians review the list of medications that SPs reported to the Household interviewer during the Household Interview Questionnaire. They compare the list against the protocol list of exclusion medications and if SPs reported taking any one of the medications during the Household Questionnaire, they are excluded from the CV Fitness component. Physicians record the exclusion as a "Safety Exclusion." The system blocks the SP from CV Fitness and sets the Component status for CV Fitness to "Not Done" with the comment "Safety Exclusion." SPs are not asked the CV safety exclusion questions in the physician examination and do not go to the CV Fitness room. If SPs do not report taking any exclusion medications during the Household Interview Questionnaire, they are not excluded during this part of the physician examination review.

4.3.1.1.2   Medications Reported during MEC Physician's Examination

To assure that SPs have not started on any exclusion class medications since the household questionnaire, physicians ask SPs about current medications as part of the CV safety exclusion process. If SPs are taking medications on the exclusion list, the system excludes them from the CV Fitness component and records the CV Fitness component status as "Not Done" with the comment "Safety Exclusion." SPs are blocked from the CV Fitness Examination.

4.3.1.2   Exclusions Based on Medical Conditions and Pregnancy

Sample Persons more than 12 weeks pregnant are excluded from the CV Fitness component. Pregnancy is determined by SP self-report during either the Household Interview or the MEC examination, and by urine sample during the MEC examination using the Biomerica Nimbus Plus®. If any of the medical conditions are documented during the Household Questionnaire, SPs are excluded from the CV component before they enter the MEC. The system automatically records the component status as "Not Done" and adds a comment of "Safety Exclusion." The SP does not go to the Cardiovascular Fitness Component room in the MEC to have this exclusion recorded. During the MEC examination, the urine pregnancy test is done on all female SPs aged 8-59 years regardless of their self-report of pregnancy during the household questionnaire. SPs who self-report pregnancy during the household questionnaire or during the MEC shared exclusion questions, or whose urine test reveals a positive for pregnancy result, are excluded from treadmill testing for reasons of pregnancy. The exclusion is coded as "Safety Exclusion" with a comment reason of "SP is pregnant."

4.3.1.3   Exclusions Based on Heart Rate and Blood Pressure

The resting heart rate and blood pressure measurements taken during the physician's examination are used as the baseline measurements reviewed for exclusion from the treadmill test. SPs are automatically excluded from the CV Fitness component submaximal treadmill testing if <u>any one</u> criterion is met:

- Heart rate is greater than 100 beats per minute.

- Systolic blood pressure is greater than 180 mm Hg.

- Diastolic blood pressure is greater than 100 mm Hg.

- Irregular beat greater than 3 per minute.

If any of the specified conditions are present, the system excludes the SP from the treadmill test. The CV Fitness Component Status defaults to "Not Done" with the comment "Safety Exclusion."

4.4 Sexually Transmitted Diseases (STD), Human Immunodeficiency Virus (HIV) and Bacterial Vaginosis (BV)

SPs that consent have blood drawn for STD and HIV testing. Female SPs who consent to self-collect vaginal swabs have the swabs tested for Human Papilloma Virus (HPV), Trichomonas, and Bacterial Vaginosis (BV). The specific tests are determined by age categories:

- All SPs Ages 14-17   Chlamydia, gonorrhea and herpes type 2

- All SPs Ages 18-39   Chlamydia, gonorrhea, herpes type 2, HIV and syphilis

- All SPs Ages 40-49   Herpes type 2, HIV and syphilis

- Female SPs ages 14-49 Human Papilloma Virus (HPV), Trichomonas, and Bacterial Vaginosis (BV)

- Female SPs ages 50-59 HPV

SPs consent to these tests during the Household Interview, but may change their mind prior to the actual examination. Some SPs agree during the home interview, but decide not to be tested when they arrive at the MEC. Other SPs do not agree to be tested during the home interview, but change their mind and want to be tested when they arrive for the MEC examination. In either case, the MEC examination is responsive to the decision of the SP. The physicians' role in STD, HIV and BV testing is to discuss these tests with SPs. The objective of the physician STD and HIV pretest discussion is to educate eligible participants about the STD, HIV and BV testing and to explain the mechanism for getting their personal test results. The confidential nature of the test result reports is explained.

4.4.1 Guidelines Affecting STD, HIV and BV Test Result Reporting

Two guidelines affect the confidential reporting of STD and HIV test results to participants in NHANES. First, NHANES is not subject to state laws that require reporting STD results to state health departments. Second, adolescents in the United States can consent to the confidential diagnosis and treatment of STDs. Medical care for these conditions can be provided to adolescents without parental consent or knowledge. Therefore, there is no legal obligation to disclose findings to anyone other than the participant (CDC, 1993 Sexually Transmitted Diseases Treatment Guideline, MMWR 42 RR-14).

STD, HIV and BV test results are confidential and are **not disclosed to anyone,** including the participant's doctor, insurer, family or friends, except at the SP's specific request, and **only** after the SP properly provides the password selected during the examination. Everyone working with the NHANES signs a legal document making them subject to the Privacy Act, the Public Health Service, and other laws.

Because of the medical, social, and emotional consequences of positive STD and HIV tests, disclosure of results are always handled in a sensitive, respectful, and confidential manner. SPs can only obtain their results when they call the toll-free telephone number provided to them during the MEC examination. STD and HIV results are the only NHANES SP health examination results that are provided verbally. All other findings from the health examination are reported to persons in a written report that is mailed to them. The methods for reporting results of STD testing differ slightly for adolescents and adults. These methods are described in the following sections.

4.4.1.1 Procedures for Reporting STD, HIV and BV Results

During the Physician's Examination, eligible participants are informed about the STD and HIV tests conducted during the MEC examination. To assure that the STD results are only provided to the SP for whom the results are specified, SPs are asked to provide their own password. Physicians record the password in the ISIS at the time of the Physician Component Examination. Physicians inform participants that they must call a toll-free number in order to get their individual STD results. SPs use their personally selected password to confirm their identity when they call for their results. The physician encourages SPs to keep their password to themselves and not share the information with anyone. Physicians also encourage SPs to call for their results after the designated date. This self-initiated request for test results is the most foolproof method of ensuring that test results will go only to the tested individual. All SPs receive a reminder notice (Exhibit 4-1, Reminder form to get STD and HIV results) that includes the toll-free number, the date after which the results will be available, and their password.

Adult participants (aged 18 and over) receive their reminder notice from the coordinator as they leave the MEC. The reminder notice is in an envelope that is handed directly to the SP.

Minors (SPs 14-18 years of age) receive the same reminder notice, but instead of receiving it at checkout from the coordinator, the physician personally places the form in a sealed envelope marked with a number that was previously placed on the SP's examination gown. (When SPs change into an examination gown at the beginning of the session, they are given a numbered basket in which to store clothing. The assistant coordinator marks the number of the basket on their gown for subsequent identification). The physician gives the envelope to the assistant coordinator who places it in the SP's numbered basket. The physician reminds the SP to retrieve the envelope from the basket when changing clothes to leave the MEC.

4.4.2 Informing SPs of STD, HIV and BV Results

SPs call the National Center for Health Statistics personnel for STD, HIV and BV reports. When SPs call to obtain their test results, they provide their password. Test results are not provided unless the caller correctly states the password. Under no circumstances are STD test results put in writing with a respondent's name, address, or any other personal identifiers. Test results are only communicated by telephone specifically and solely to the SP.

Exhibit 4-1. Reminder form to get STD and HIV results

National Health and Nutrition Examination Survey
STD AND HIV CALLBACK REMINDER

How to get results for sexually transmitted diseases and HIV

Call toll free: **1-888-301-2360**

When: **anytime after 8/3/1999**

Hours: **Monday – Friday, 8:30 am – 6:00 pm Eastern Time**

When calling for results, you will need to provide the following information:

Sample Number: 955543

Password: Picture

We will only give results to the person tested.

Participants who do **not** call for their report are sent a letter reminding them to call the toll-free number to receive their special test results. If they do not call the survey, staff from NCHS contact them by phone and tell them their results, whether positive or negative. If a health problem is identified, the participant is informed and referred for treatment in their area.

4.5   Vaginal Swabs

Women within the ages of 14-49 are being asked to self-collect vaginal swabs for Human Papillomavirus (HPV), Trichomonas, and Bacterial Vaginosis (BV). Women within the ages of 50-59 are asked to do a vaginal swab for HPV. The swabs are self-collected by the women in the privacy of the bathroom after receiving instructions from the physician. The next sections instruct the physician in the vaginal swab protocol.

4.5.1   Instructing the SP for Vaginal Swabs

The physician will explain the HPV assessment (along with BV and trichomonas) after discussing the tests for sexually transmitted diseases and HIV, and getting the password the participant will use to obtain her results. The following is the suggested physician script.

Instructions for SPs 14-49 Years Old

"Additionally we ask all girls and women your age to participate in a test for human Papillomavirus, bacterial vaginosis, and Trichomonas. You may not have heard about these conditions. Human Papillomavirus and Trichomonas are sexually transmitted and many women who are infected do not have any symptoms. Bacterial vaginosis occurs when some of your body's naturally occurring bacteria, or cells, starts to grow too much. This kind of overgrowth may not cause symptoms, that is, you may have BV and not know it. We have learned this condition is more likely to occur in women who are sexually active, but it can also occur in those who have never had sex. Here is some additional information about these diseases. You will find a sheet like this in your packet when you leave. [Show Reproductive Health/Sexually Transmitted Diseases Chart]

We will test for all three of these using vaginal fluid. I will explain how to collect a vaginal specimen yourself. Here is a kit that contains three swabs; each swab is much smaller than a tampon. You will do this in the bathroom where you will have complete privacy. I recommend that you wash your hands before starting and after completing the collection. Also, because you will be inserting a swab into your vagina, you may want to undress partially before starting. Once you are ready to begin, first twist the top off the clear soft plastic tube marked with a green dot on top. Do not discard the top. Place the top on a clean surface. Remove the swab from the plastic tube. Hold the stick at the end and do not touch the foam part of the swab. Hold the lips of the vagina open with one hand. Insert the swab fully into the vagina (like a tampon) with your other hand. Turn the foam swab against the walls of your vagina as you count to 'ten.' Carefully remove the swab without touching the skin or hair outside of the vagina. Place the swab into the soft plastic tube and replace the cover onto the tube. For the second swab collection, use the swab from the red-capped tube. Remove the swab from the hard plastic tube, keeping it attached to the lid. Hold the stick at the middle and do not touch the cotton part of the swab. Insert the swab into the vagina (like a tampon) and turn the cotton swab against the walls of your vagina as you count to 'ten.' Carefully remove the swab without touching the skin or hair outside of the vagina and return the swab into the hard plastic tube. Repeat the collection procedure for the third swab in the clear plastic tube (the one without the green dot). Remove the swab and hold the plastic stick at the middle. Do not touch the soft part of the swab with your hand. Repeat the collection steps and, when you are done, put the swab back into the plastic tube and replace the cover. When you are done, you can give the three tubes to the staff person who will be waiting outside the bathroom." There are written instructions in English and Spanish inside the package if you need a reference.

Instructions for women in the third trimester vary in that the SP is instructed to insert the swab half-way into the vaginal area by holding the swab at about halfway from the end of the swab.

Collection Instructions for Women 50-59 Years

"I will explain how to collect a vaginal specimen yourself. Here is a kit that contains one swab. The swab is much smaller than a tampon. You will do this in the bathroom where you will have complete privacy. I recommend that you wash your hands before starting and after completing the collection. Also, because you will be inserting a swab into your vagina, you may want to undress partially before starting. Once you are ready to begin, twist the top off the clear soft plastic tube, and remove the swab from the tube. Do not discard the top. Place the top on a clean surface. Hold the plastic stick at the end and do not touch the foam part of the swab. Hold the lips of the vagina open with one hand. Insert the swab fully into the vagina (like a tampon) with your other hand. Turn the swab against the walls of your vagina as you count to 'ten.' Carefully remove the swab without touching the skin or hair outside of the vagina. Place the swab into the plastic tube and replace the cover onto the tube. When you are done, you can give the tube to the staff person who will be waiting outside the bathroom." There are written instructions in English and Spanish inside the package if you need a reference.

"Do you have any questions about this test?"

"How do you feel about taking part in this test?"

(If participant indicates she is uncomfortable, you can probe "you seem unsure about doing this, what are you thinking about?" Remember the participant has the right to refuse this test.

If the participant refuses this test, explain, "This will not affect your participation in the rest of the study.") If the participant agrees to the test, explain:

"Like the blood and urine tests that are being done, these results are very private, and we will give these results only to you. We will not put the results in the report that is mailed to your home. We will give you a toll-free number to call in four weeks, and results will be reported only after you provide the password which you gave me a few minutes ago *<password provided during STD/HIV pre-test counseling>* "

Persons 18-49:

"When you leave, you will have a piece of paper in your packet with a toll-free number, the dates to call, and the password you just gave me. Please be sure to call for your STD and BV test results during those dates."

Persons 50-59:

"When you leave, you will have a piece of paper in your packet with a toll-free number, the dates to call, and the password you just gave me. Please be sure to call for your HPV test results during those dates."

Youth under 18 years:

"Here is a piece of paper with a toll-free number, the dates to call, and the password you just gave me. Please be sure to call for your STD and BV results during those dates."

4.6   Prostate Specific Antigen Testing

Men who are 40 years old and above are asked have their blood tested for Prostate Specific Antigen. The physician explains why this test is important, and reviews when the results will be received and what they mean. It is important that the physician fully explain that for PSA, a positive test does not mean that the SP has cancer, or that a negative result does not mean that the SP does not have cancer. The suggested script for the physician to use to gain agreement for PSA testing follows.

4.6.1   Physician Script for PSA

"I would like to provide you with some information on the blood test for Prostate Specific Antigen, or PSA. This test is commonly used by doctors along with a digital rectal exam for early detection of prostate cancer. Prostate cancer is a major public health problem among men, especially those with increasing age and in certain racial/ethnic groups. This testing will help us to do national-level planning to control this problem.

We will not do a rectal examination, but would like to test your blood for PSA to help us determine what the levels or concentrations are in men in the United States. Before we proceed, here are some facts you should know:

The PSA test measures a protein produced by the prostate gland. When prostate cancer is present, the PSA tends to rise. It is important to note that an elevated PSA does not necessarily mean cancer is present. Other problems such as prostate enlargement or an infection of the prostate may cause the PSA test result to be high.

Another fact to consider is that a normal PSA test does not guarantee that prostate cancer is not present. Certain medications and supplements are also known to affect the PSA test value.

You will receive the result of your PSA test in the Final Report of Findings sent to you home 12-16 weeks after the exam. If your PSA level is high, you will receive a letter from the survey program about your PSA level in approximately three weeks. You should discuss your PSA results with your doctor. If you have an elevated PSA test, your doctor or health care provider will want to do other tests to see whether prostate cancer is present or not present.

Are you willing to have your blood tested for PSA?"

If the SP answers yes, then ask the exclusion questions referred to below. If any one question is answered yes, explain to the SP that the test could not be accurately done, and explain why. If the SP does not want to have the PSA test done, mark the section as not done, refused. This will block the lab from shipping blood for PSA.

4.6.2   Introduction to Exclusion Questions

"Some medical procedures and prostate conditions will result in a high PSA. Because the survey is interested in learning about normal levels of PSA in the population, participants will be excluded if they have a condition or recent procedure that may affect the PSA result. Moreover, if you have had some of these conditions or procedures, a PSA test may not be useful detect if you currently have prostate cancer. I am now going to ask you some questions about your prostate health."

Ask the Questions in the ISIS Application Related to These Topics

- Digital rectal exam in the past week

- Prostate biopsy in the past month

- Cystoscopy in the past month

- History of prostate cancer

- History of prostate surgery, including prostatic enlargement

- History of radiation treatment for prostate cancer

- History of medication for prostate cancer

4.7 Data Entry Screens

The following sections instruct physicians about how to carry out the data entry for the physician component. The ISIS screens are displayed as a visual reference.

4.7.1 Reviewing SP Medications from Household Interview

At the beginning of each session, prior to starting the physician's examination, physicians review the medications reported by the SP at the Household Interview for exclusions to the Cardiovascular Fitness component. During the Household Interview, the interviewers ask SPs to get all their medication bottles for the interviewer to examine. The interviewer enters names of the medications in the ISIS system and this information is later uploaded to the ISIS Mobile Examination Center (MEC) system and is accessible for the physician to review during the physician examination. Physicians must access the medications list to review the medications SPs are taking. Exhibit 4-2, CV Medication Review, is the screen for this review.

Exhibit 4-2. Cardiovascular Medication Review

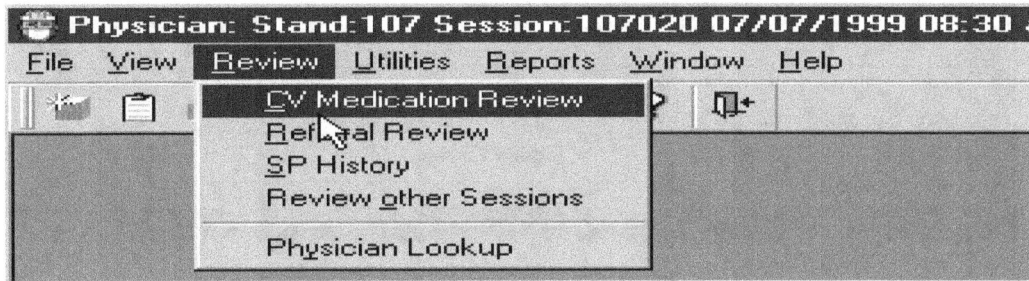

- From the Toolbar, select "Review," then "Cardiovascular Medication Review."

- Click on CV Medication Review

- This will bring up the "CV Review for Exclusion Medication."

Exhibit 4-3. CV review for exclusion medication, screen 1

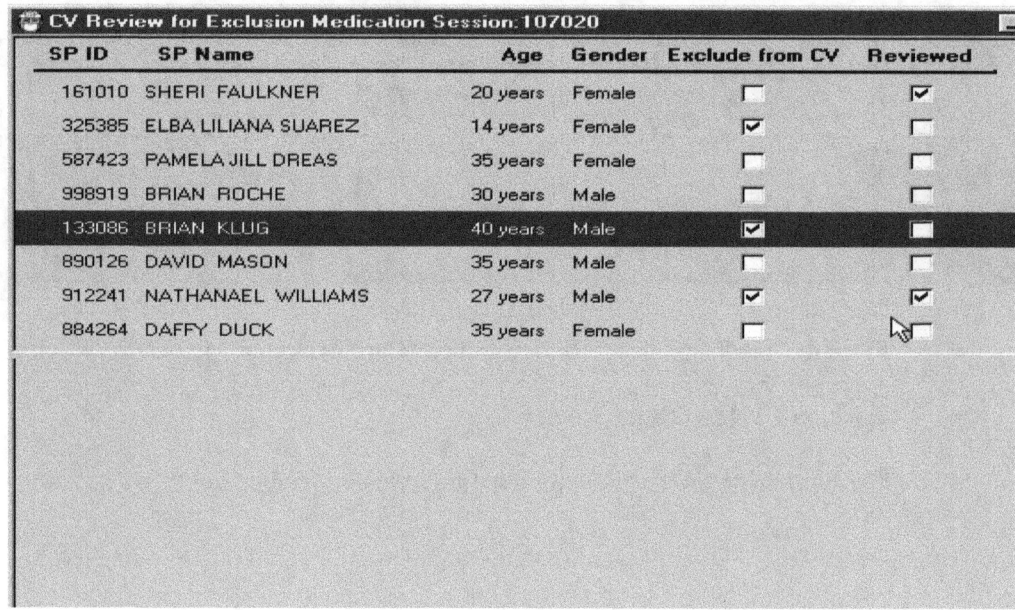

- The "CV Review for Exclusion Medication" screen is displayed.

- The names of all SP's eligible for CV Fitness are listed in the display box.

- Click on a SP's name to highlight that name and to have the medications for that SP displayed in the lower part of the box.

- All medications or medical conditions reported by the SP and taken at the time of the Household Interview are listed.

- Check the medications listed for each SP with the list of exclusion medications provided in Appendix D. If the SP reported taking any medication on the exclusion medication list, check the *Exclude from CV box*.

- This excludes the SP from CV Fitness.

Exhibit 4-4. CV review for medication exclusion, screen 2

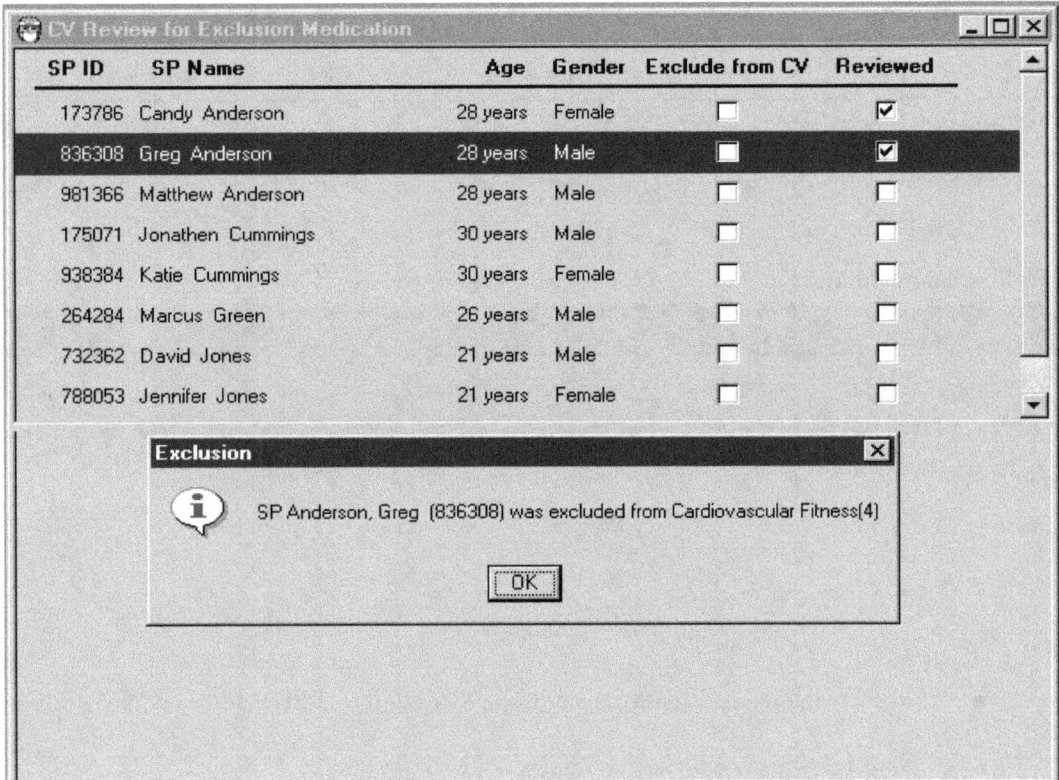

- A message is displayed: "SP <name> was excluded from Cardiovascular Fitness." Click OK to confirm this message.

- SPs are excluded from the CV Fitness examination and from being asked the CV Safety exclusion questions in the Physician's Examination.

- Go to the next SP and review any medications for exclusions from CV Fitness. If the SP is not taking any of the exclusion medications, click the "Reviewed" box for that SP. The SP will remain eligible for the CV Fitness Examination.

Exhibit 4-5. CV review for exclusion medication, screen 3

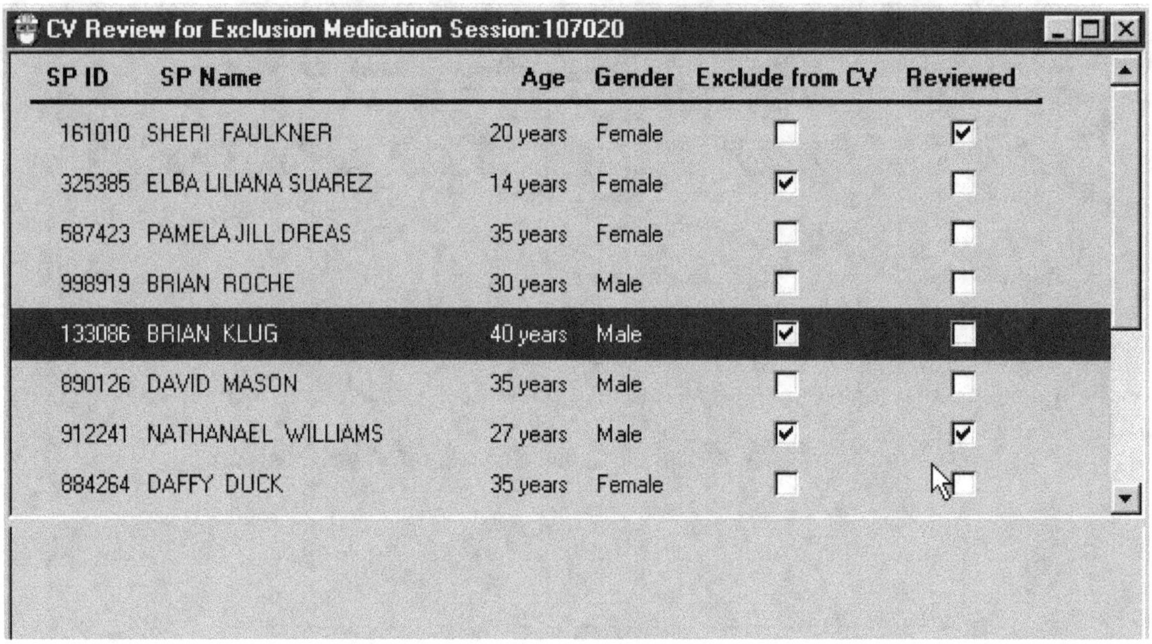

SP ID	SP Name	Age	Gender	Exclude from CV	Reviewed
161010	SHERI FAULKNER	20 years	Female	☐	☑
325385	ELBA LILIANA SUAREZ	14 years	Female	☑	☐
587423	PAMELA JILL DREAS	35 years	Female	☐	☐
998919	BRIAN ROCHE	30 years	Male	☐	☐
133086	BRIAN KLUG	40 years	Male	☑	☐
890126	DAVID MASON	35 years	Male	☐	☐
912241	NATHANAEL WILLIAMS	27 years	Male	☑	☑
884264	DAFFY DUCK	35 years	Female	☐	☐

CV Review for Exclusion Medication Session:107020

- Review the medication for each of the SPs eligible for CV Fitness during this session.

- Scroll down as necessary to review each SP on the list.

- After reviewing every SP, close the CV Review for Exclusion Medication Screen.

- Each SP should have a check mark in the *"Reviewed"* box. For SPs who were excluded from CV Fitness because of medications listed during the household interview, there should be a check mark in the *"Exclude from CV"* box.

4.7.2   **Reviewing SP History**

Medical conditions for all SPs in the session can be reviewed in the Physician's Examination under "SP History."

Exhibit 4-6. Review menu to select SP History

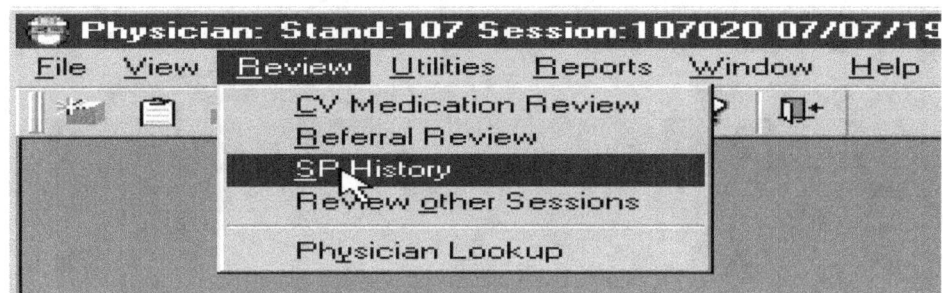

■   To access "SP History," select "Review" from the Toolbar and then choose "SP History."

■   The "SP History" box is displayed.

Exhibit 4-7. SP History selections

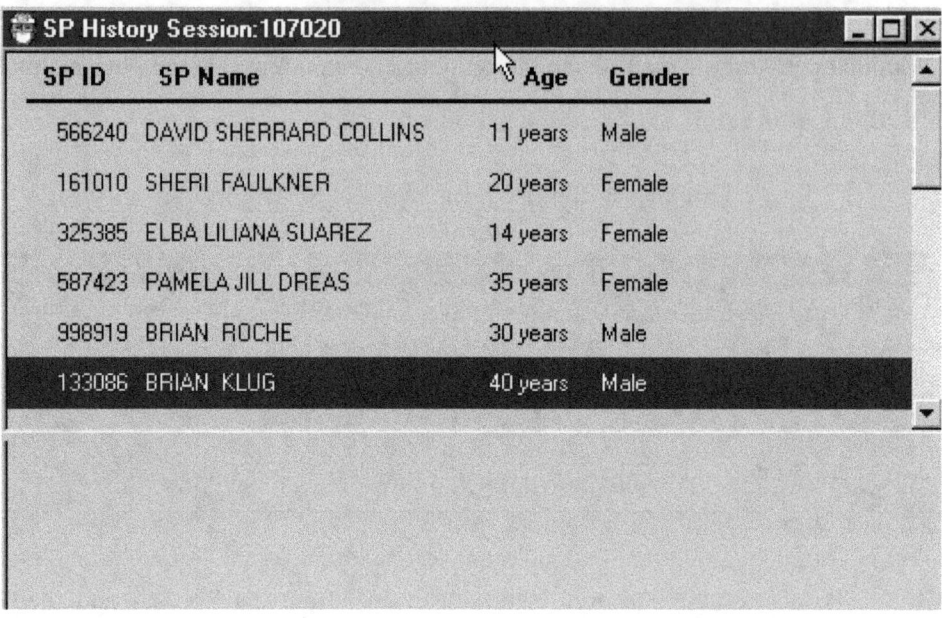

- A list of all SPs in the session is displayed in the "SP History" box.

- Each SP's ID number, name, age, and gender is displayed.

- Highlight the name of the SP to view the medical conditions, medications, and self-reported pregnancy history.

4.7.3   Child Heart Rate, Pulse

Heart rate (0-4 years of age) or pulse (5-7 years of age) is counted for 30 seconds and the number of beats in a 30-second period is entered in the heart rate field. The system calculates this rate and displays the number of beats in 60 seconds on the screen. The 60-second heart rates are stored in the database.

Exhibit 4-8. Child heart rate/pulse

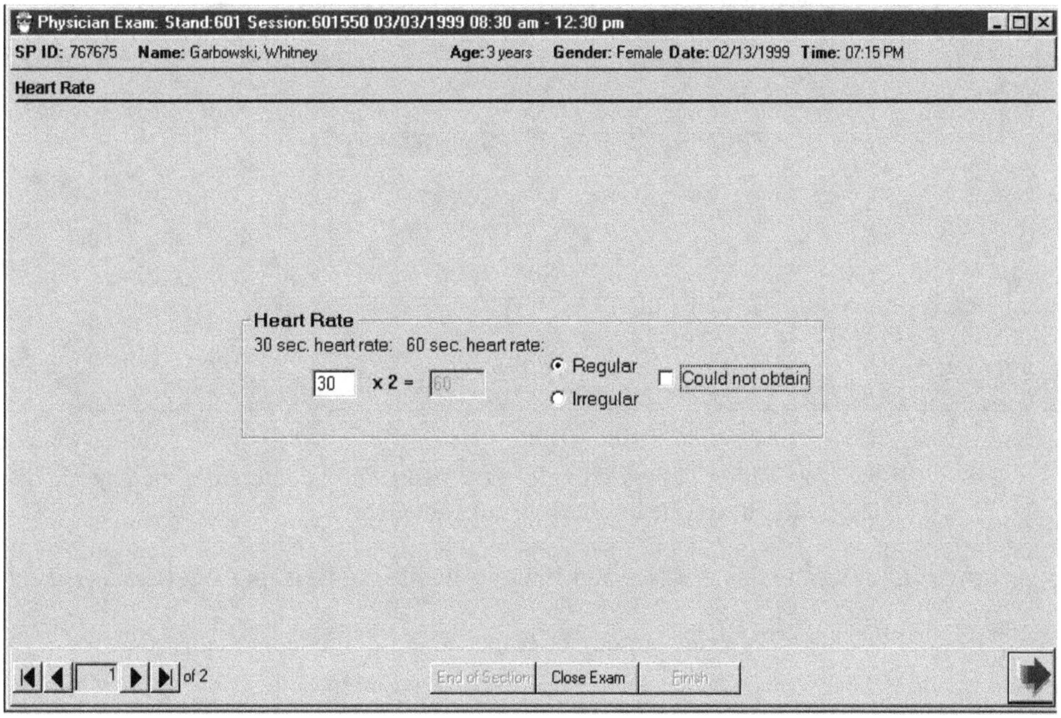

- Enter the 30-second heart rate or pulse in the field. The system calculates the 60-second heart rate and displays it in the *60-second heart rate field*.

- When taking the heart rate and pulse, note whether it is regular or irregular. The default is regular. If the heart rate is irregular, click the *irregular field option* box.

Exhibit 4-9. Child heart rate: Required data entry

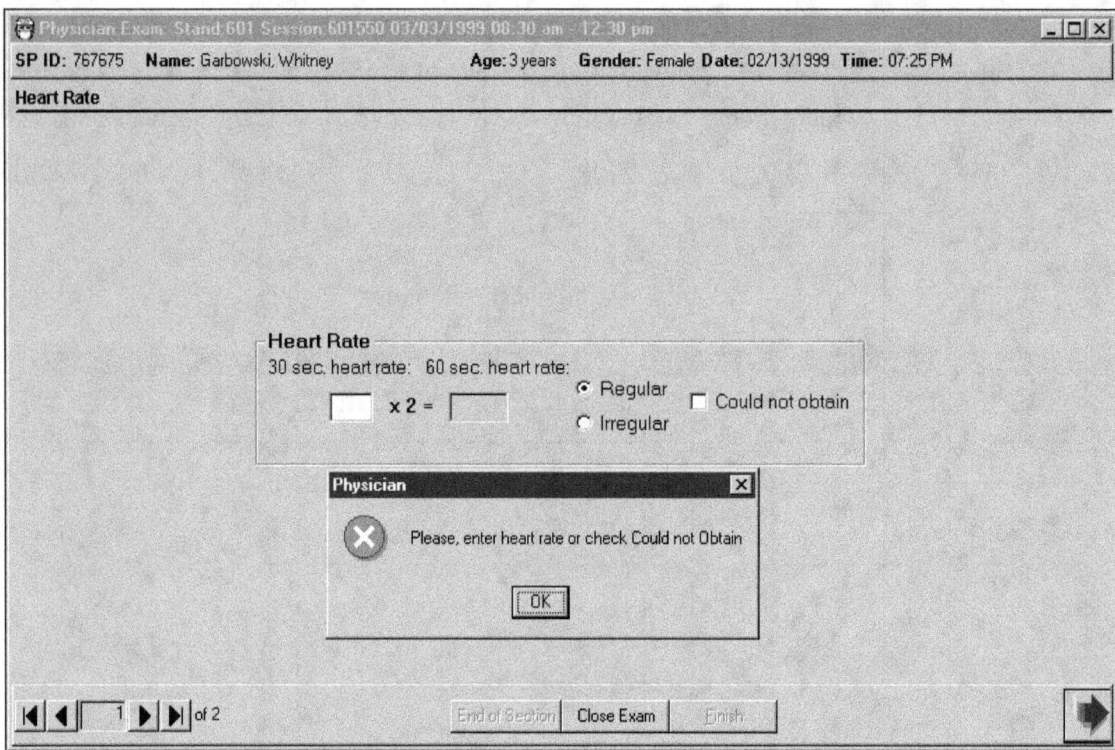

- If the next button is pressed before the heart rate is entered, a message is displayed: "Please enter heart rate or check 'Could not Obtain'."

- Click OK to this message and enter the number of beats in the *30-sec. heart rate* field.

- Click the Next arrow button to advance to the Component Status screen.

Exhibit 4-10. Component status for child heart rate/pulse

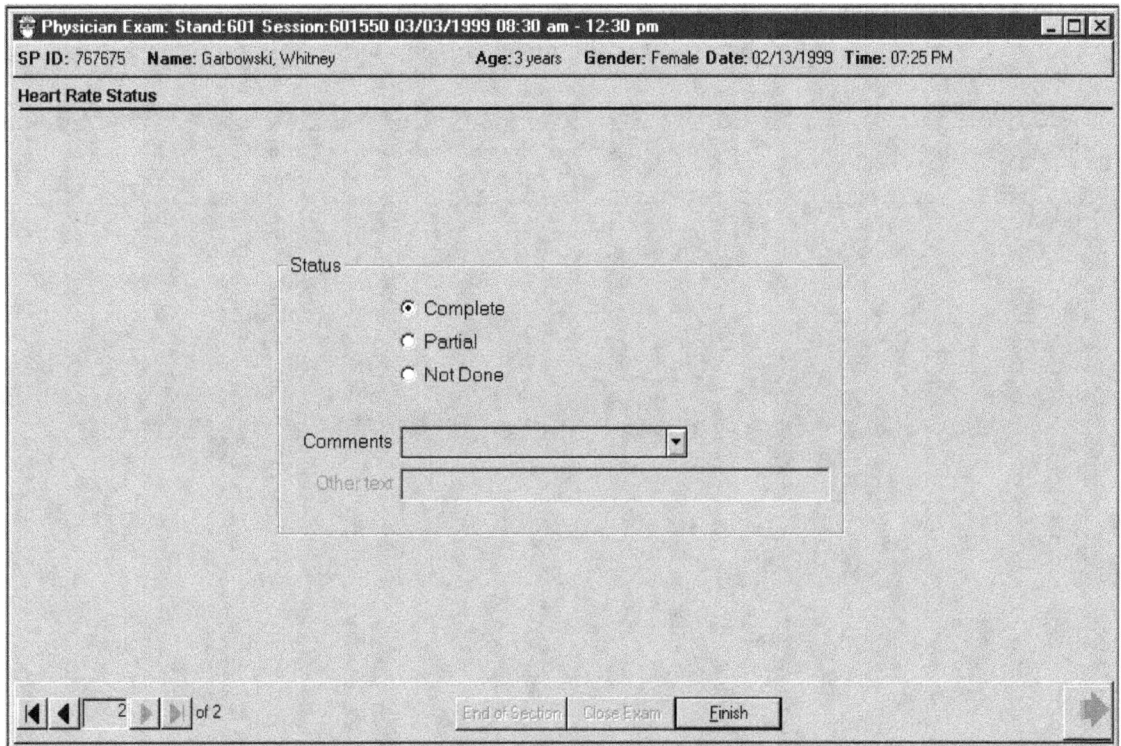

- If the heart rate was entered, the component status defaults to "complete."

- If the heart rate was not done, the status defaults to partial.

- Select an appropriate comment from the drop-down list.

- Select the Finish button to close the examination.

4.7.4   **Blood Pressure Data Entry**

Exhibit 4-11. Default blood pressure screen

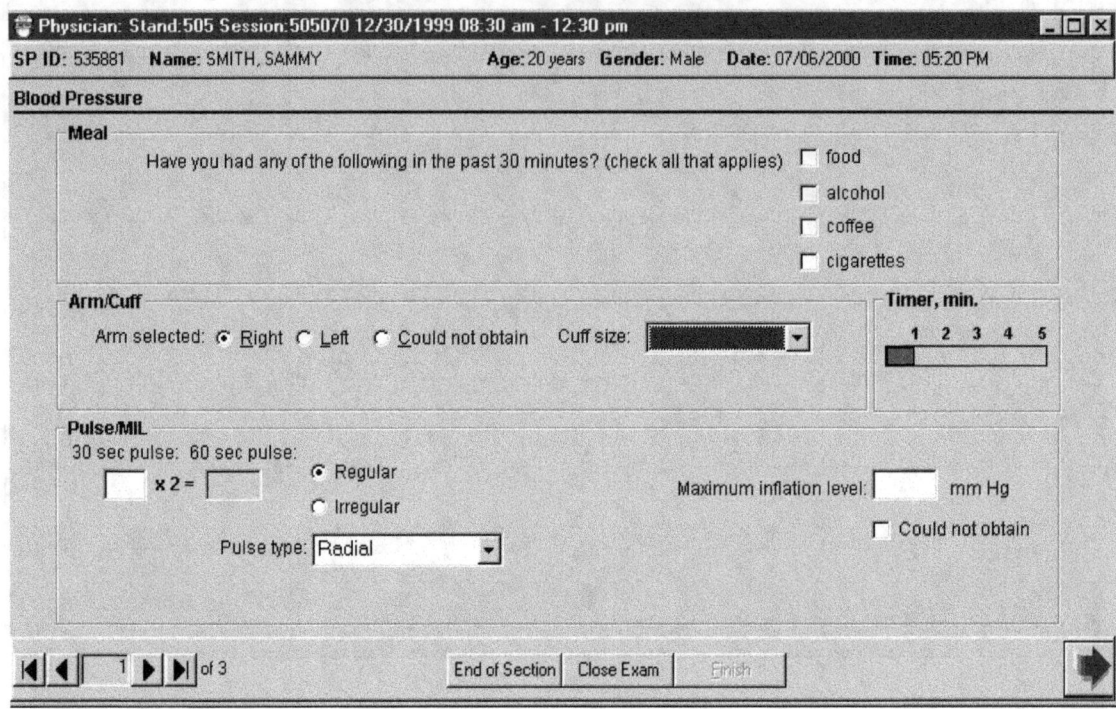

- A timer on the right side of the screen starts a 5-minute count when this screen is opened. The timer is used to help determine when the pulse, MIL, and blood pressure measurements are to be made.

- Determine if the SP has had food, alcohol, coffee, or cigarettes in the last 30 minutes. Check all that apply. Answering "Yes" does not exclude SPs from any of the Physician Examination.

- The pulse should not be taken until the SP has been resting quietly for <u>at least</u> 3 minutes. The SP should be seated quietly during this time to allow the heart rate and blood pressure measurements to stabilize to a standard resting state.

- The MIL should not be taken until the SP has been resting quietly for <u>at least</u> 4 minutes.

- The blood pressure should not be taken until the SP has been resting for <u>at least</u> 5 minutes of rest.

- The default for "Arm/cuff" is the right arm. If the left arm is used, click on left.

- If "Could not Obtain" is selected, the cuff size, MIL, and blood pressure fields are disabled.

Exhibit 4-12. Blood pressure cuff size

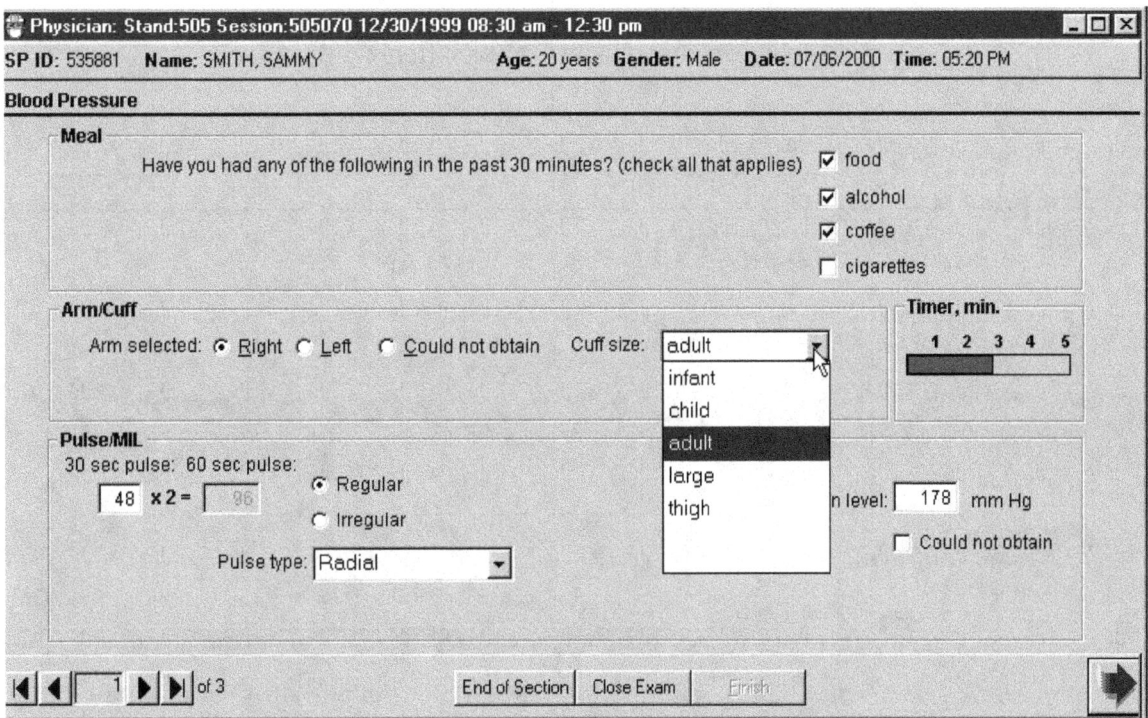

- Check which arm is being used for the BP. The default is the right arm.

- Select cuff size from the drop-down menu. The sizes of cuffs are child/adult, large adult, and adult thigh.

- If the cuff size is not selected before the Next button is pressed, a message is displayed with a reminder to select cuff size.

- The default site for taking the pulse is radial. If the radial pulse is not palpable, try the brachial. If a brachial pulse is obtained, select and record brachial from the drop-down menu of the *Pulse Type* field.

- Enter the 30-second pulse in the *30-sec pulse* field. The system will automatically calculate the 60-second heart rate and display it on the screen.

- Note whether the heart rate was regular or irregular. If the heart rate was irregular, click the box indicating irregular.

- The default pulse type is radial. If the pulse type was brachial, use the drop down menu to change the pulse type to brachial.

4.7.5   Exclusion from CV Fitness Based on Pulse and Irregular Beats

Exhibit 4-13. Irregular rhythm exclusion from CV Fitness

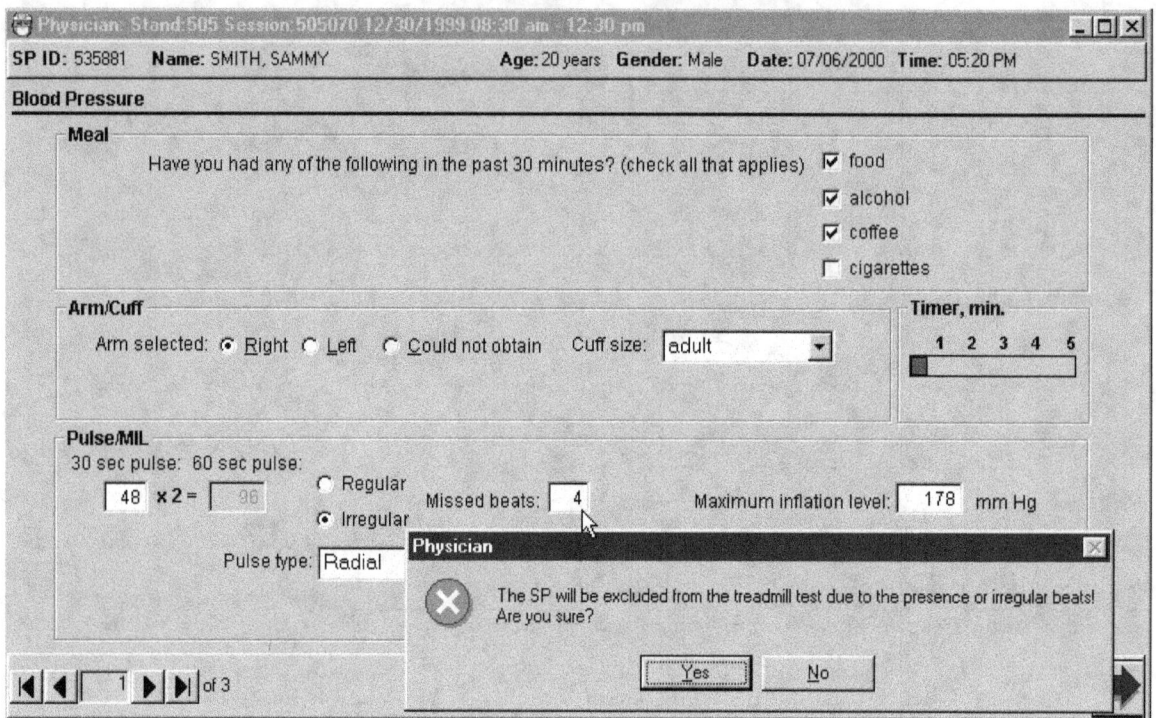

- If the pulse is irregular, SPs are excluded from the treadmill test (CV Fitness component). A message is displayed: "The SP will be excluded from the treadmill test due to presence of irregular beats. Are you sure?" If this is correct information, click OK to this message.

- If the SP is 12-49 years of age, a field will open up requiring entry of the number of missed beats in 60 seconds.

- Count the pulse a second time and enter the number of missed beats for 60 seconds. If the number of missed beats for 60 seconds is greater than 3, the SP is excluded from the treadmill test.

- The system will display a message: "The SP is excluded from the treadmill test due to the presence of irregular beats. Are you sure?" If this is correct, click OK to this message.

- The SP is excluded from the CV safety exclusion questions and from the treadmill test.

Exhibit 4-14. Heart rate exclusion from CV Fitness

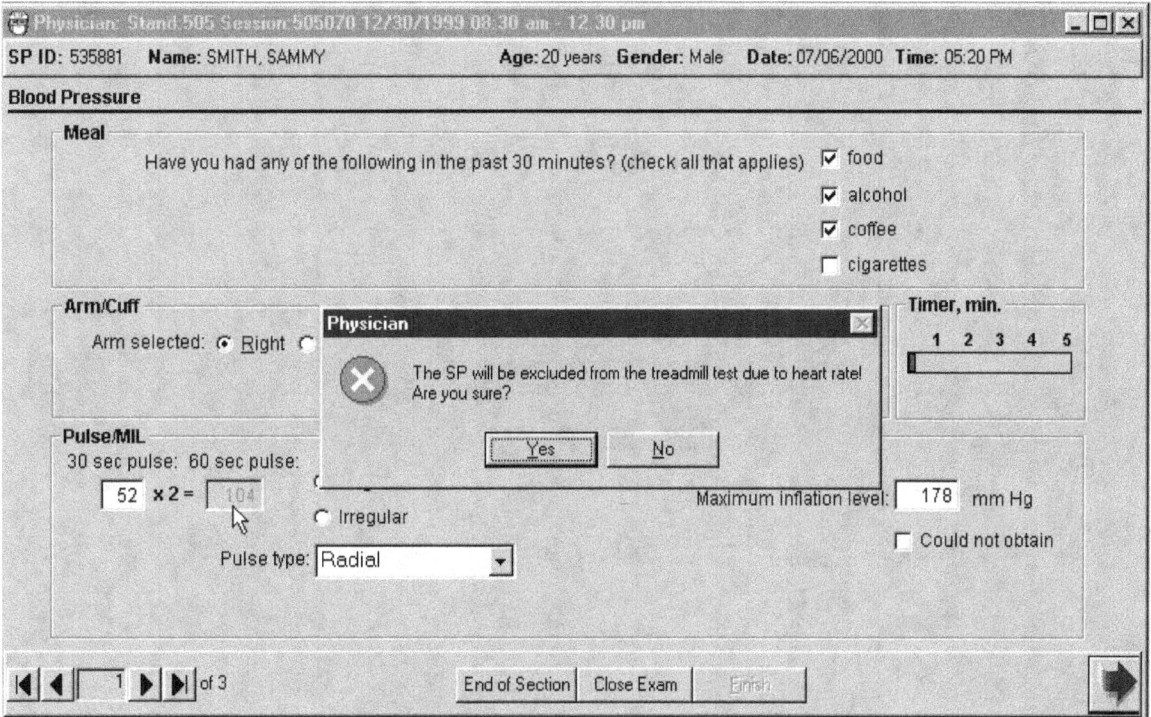

- If the pulse is greater than 100 beats per minute, SPs are excluded from the treadmill test (CV Fitness component). A message is displayed: "The SP is excluded from the treadmill test due to heart rate. Are you sure?" If this is correct, click OK to this message.

- The system will display a message: "The SP will be excluded from the treadmill test due to the heart rate. Are you sure?" If this is correct, click OK to this message.

- The SP is excluded from the CV safety exclusion questions and from the treadmill test.

Exhibit 4-15. Required pulse entry

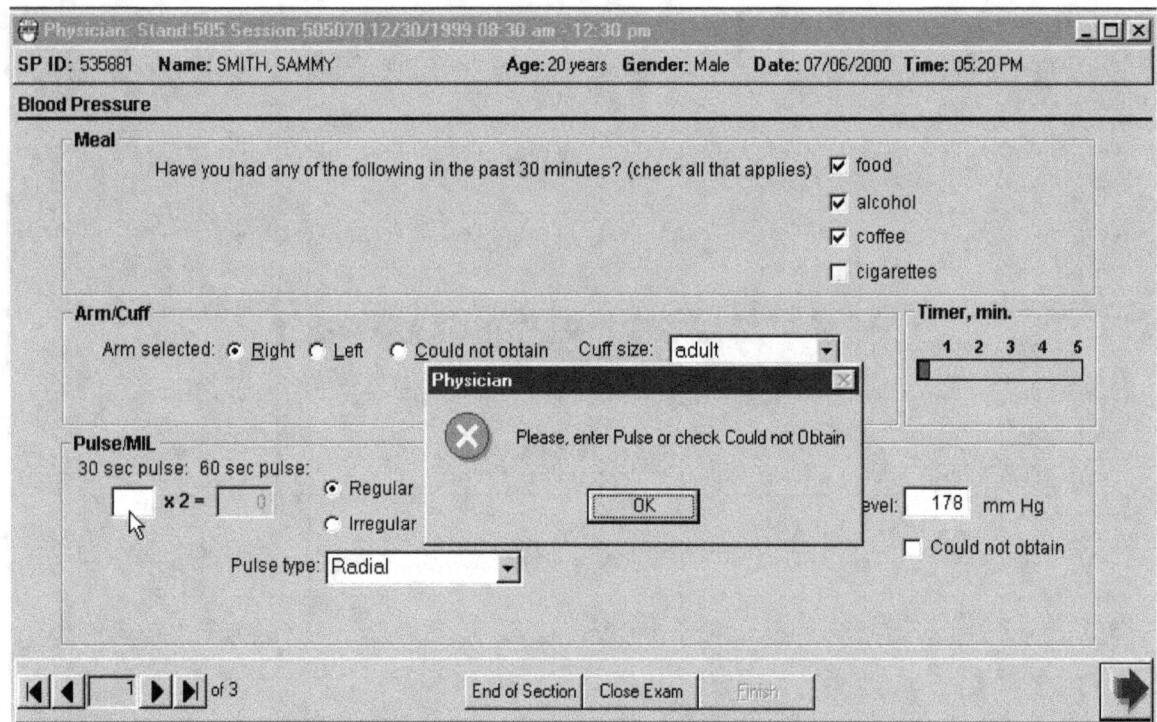

- If the physician tries to exit from this screen before recording the pulse measurement a system message is displayed: "Please, enter Pulse or check 'Could not Obtain'."

- Click OK to this message and record the 30-sec pulse in the *30-sec pulse* field.

Exhibit 4-16. Could not obtain pulse exclusion from CV Fitness

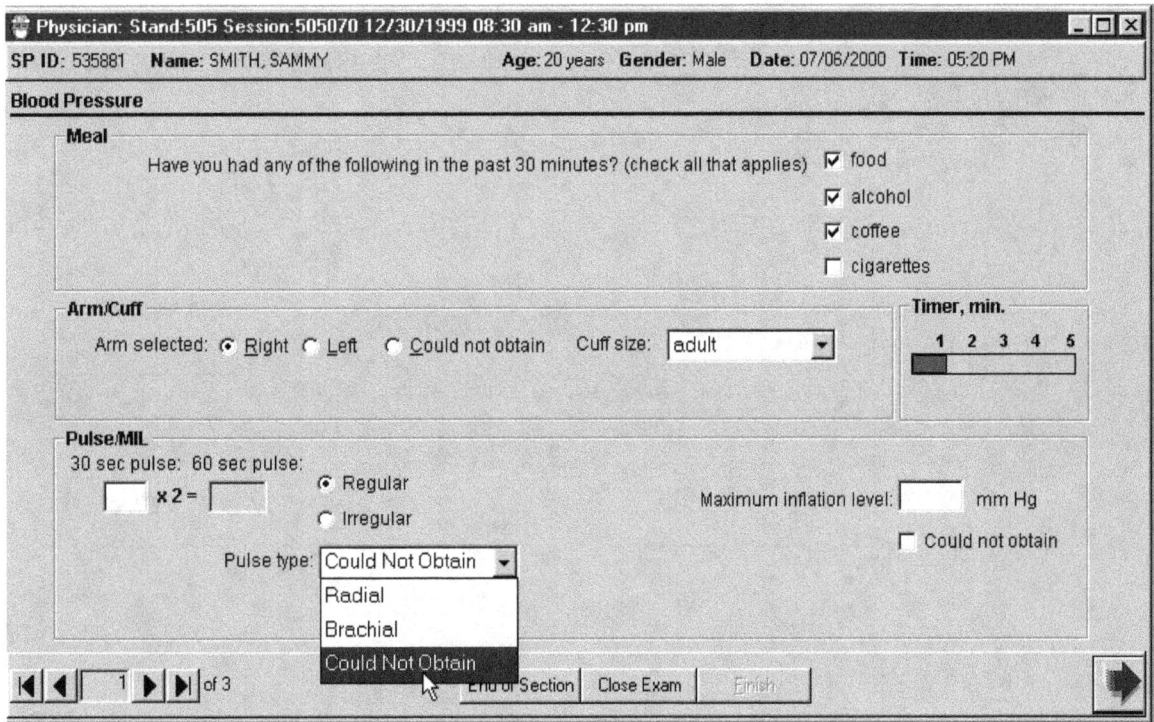

- If you are unable to obtain a pulse, select "Could not Obtain" (CNO) from the drop-down menu for the *Pulse Type* field. The SP is excluded from the treadmill test. The safety exclusion questions for CV Fitness will not be enabled.

- A message is displayed: "SP <name of SP> was excluded from Cardiovascular Fitness."

- Click OK to this message.

- The SP is excluded from the CV safety exclusion questions in the Physician's Examination. The CV Exclusion Status defaults to "Not Done" with the comment "safety exclusion."

- The SP is excluded from the CV Fitness component. The Component Status for CV Fitness defaults to "Not Done" with the comment "Safety Exclusion."

- If the pulse is not obtained, an attempt should be made to get the BP measurement using the stethoscope. See blood pressure screens for data entry.

Exhibit 4-17. Out of range maximum inflation level

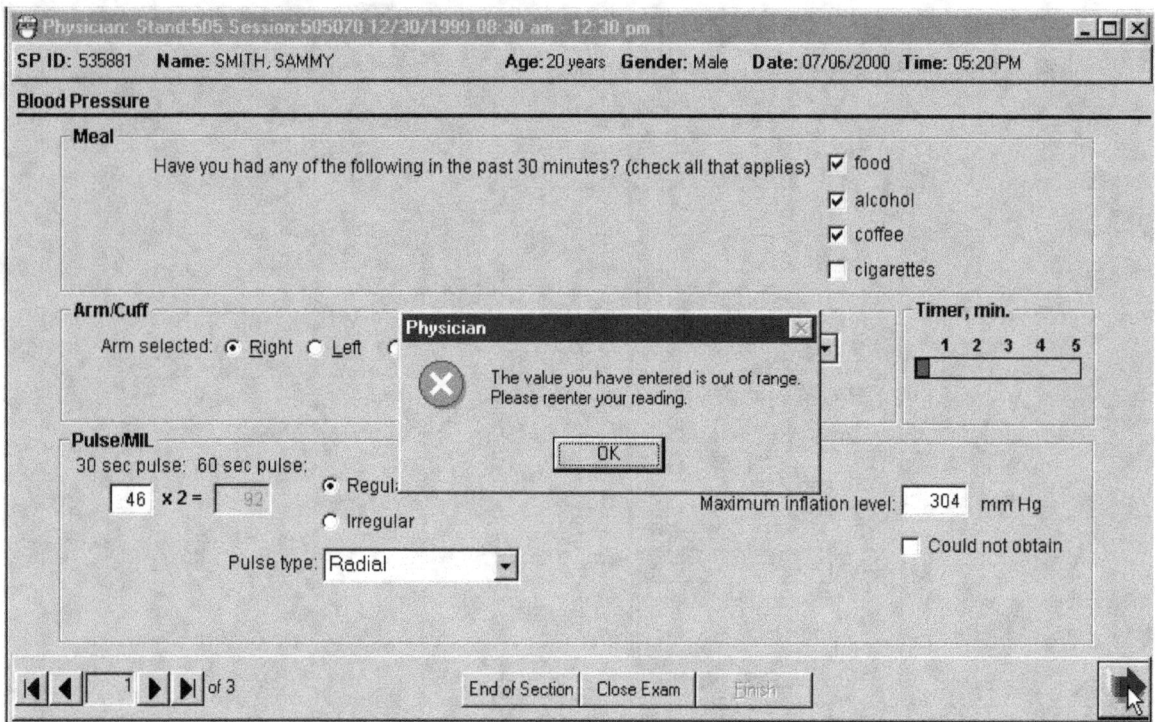

- Get the maximum inflation level (MIL) and enter this in the *Maximum-Inflation-Level* data entry field. If a number greater than 300 is entered a message is displayed: "The value you entered is out of range. Please reenter your reading." The mercury manometer does not register numbers greater than 300.

Exhibit 4-18. MIL data entry required

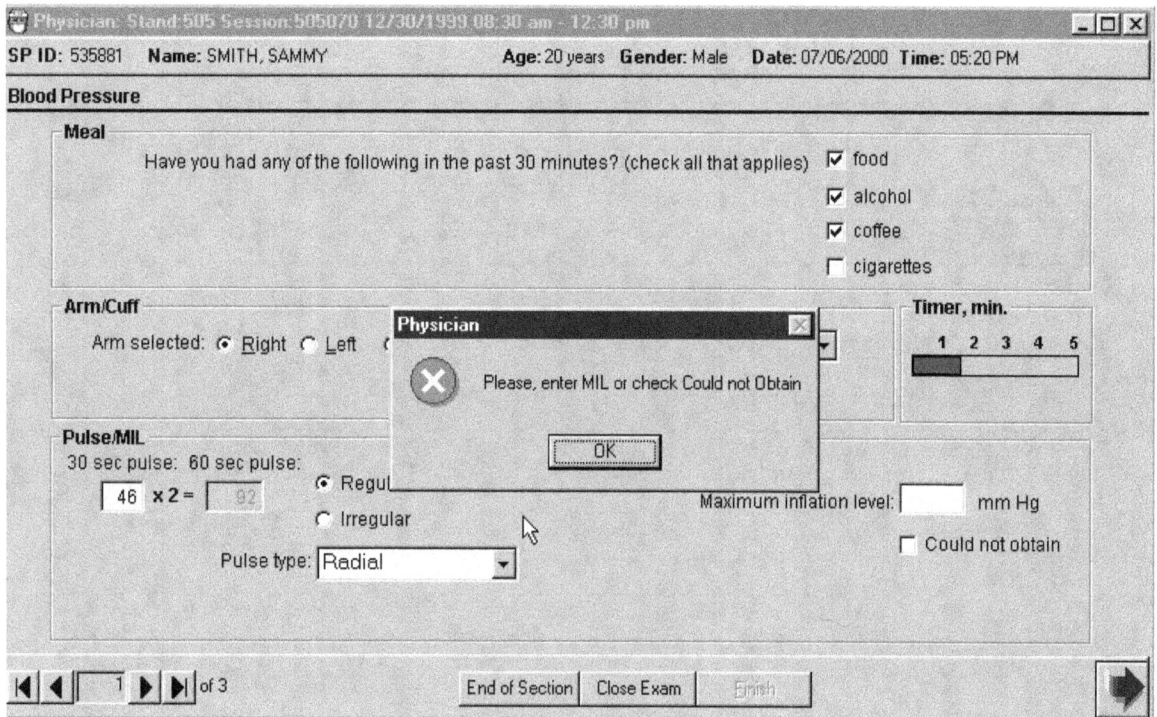

- If the Next button is entered before the MIL is entered, the system will display a message: "Please enter MIL or check "Could not Obtain." If "Could not Obtain" is selected for MIL, an attempt should be made to get a blood pressure measurement.

4.7.6   **Blood Pressure Measurement Screens**

Exhibit 4-19. Default blood pressure data entry screen

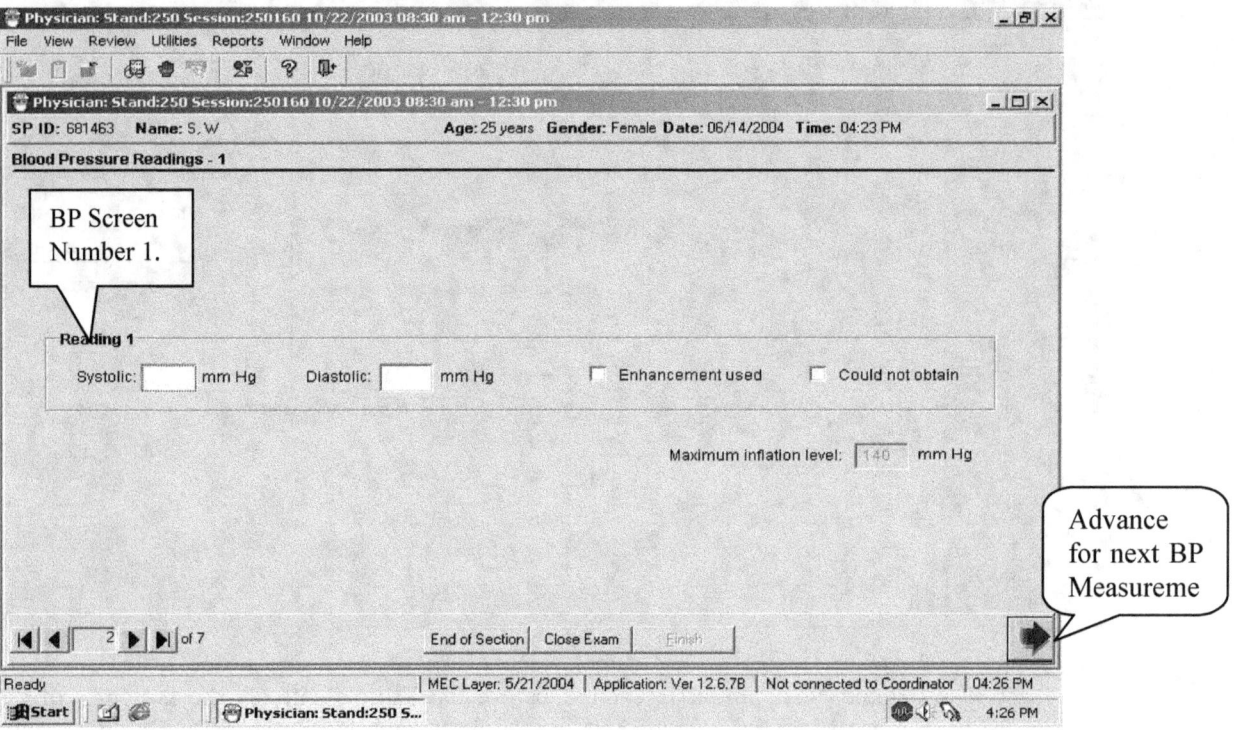

- Blood pressures are measured 3 times with a 30-second pause between each successive measurement.

- If you are unable to get a blood pressure measurement, check "Could not Obtain" for that measurement.

- If the blood pressure is difficult to hear, enhancement methods may, and should, be used. See Section 4.2.3.11 for a description of these methods. If the enhancements are used, click on the enhancement button for that measurement.

- *Each BP measurement is recorded on a* new screen. *Advance the screen after each successive BP measurement. Do not go back to review previous BPs before taking the next measurement.*

Exhibit 4-20. BP Screen 2

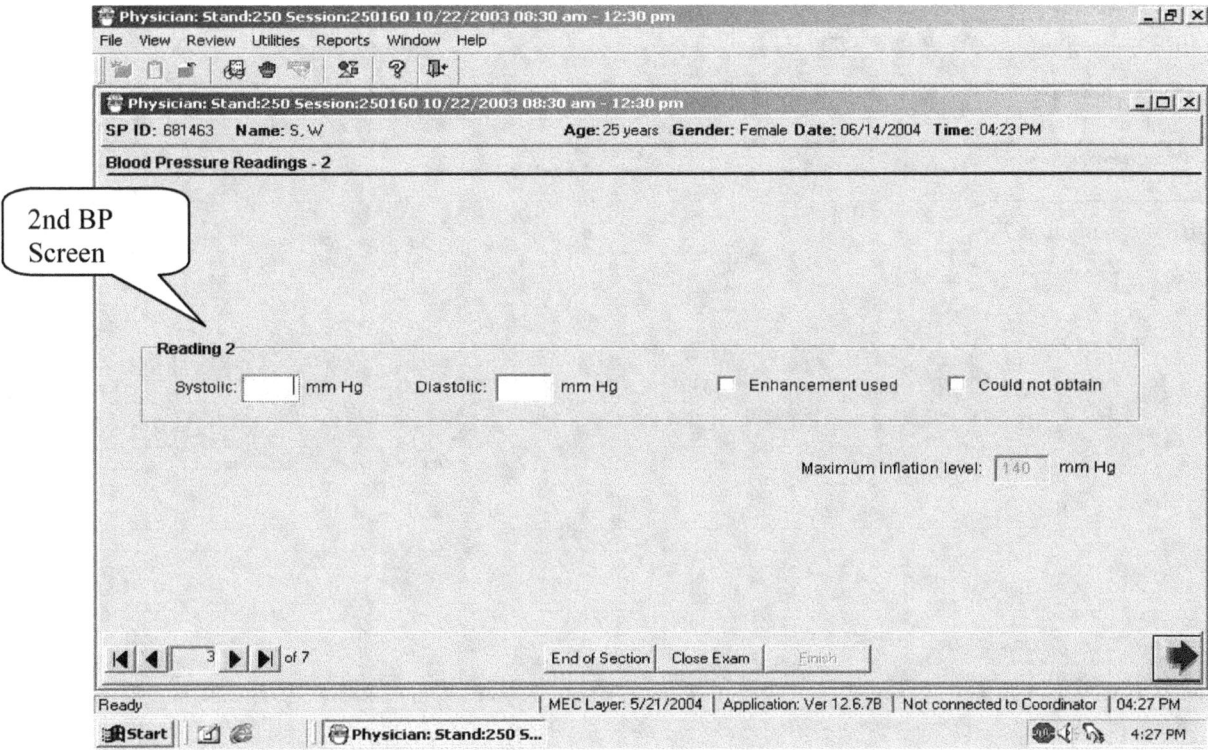

- Take the second BP using the same techniques as BP 1.

- Record the 2nd BP, and advance the screen.

Exhibit 4-21. Blood Pressure 3

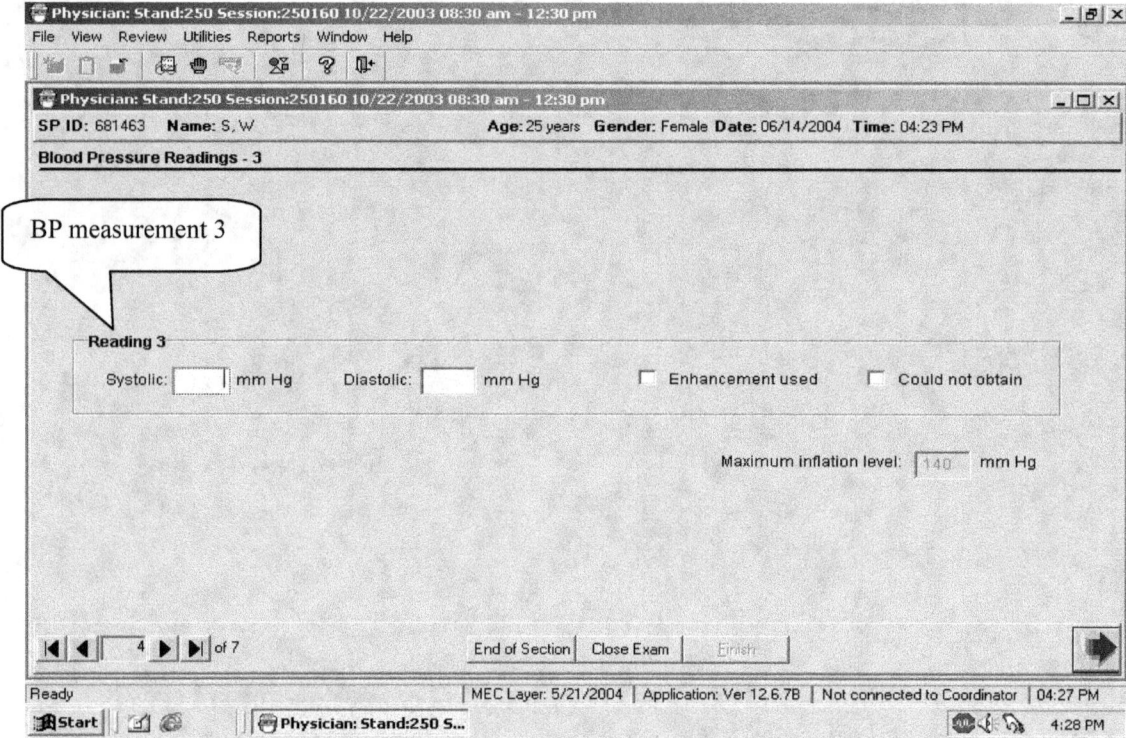

- Take the third BP using the same techniques as BPs 1 & 2.

- Record the 2nd BP, and advance the screen.

Exhibit 4-22. Blood Pressure 4

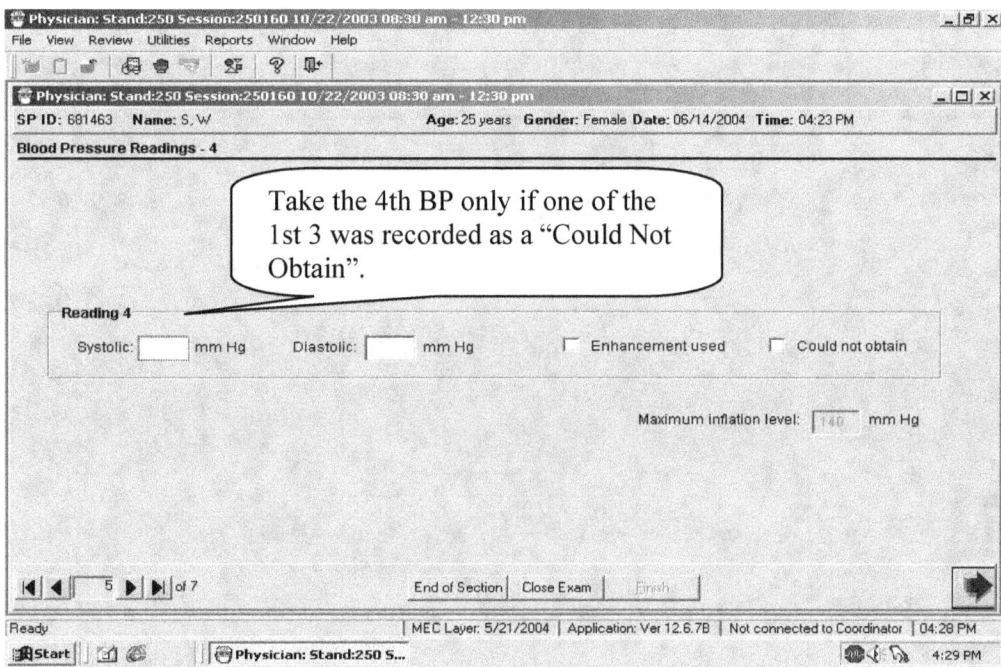

Exhibit 4-22. Blood Pressure 4

- If any of the first three measurements are checked as *"Could not Obtain,"* the BP section of the application will open up another field to allow a fourth measurement.

- Take the fourth measurement and record the results.

- **The maximum number of times the cuff should be inflated for blood pressure measurements is five including all MIL measurements.**

Exhibit 4-23. Even-numbered end digits for blood pressure measurement

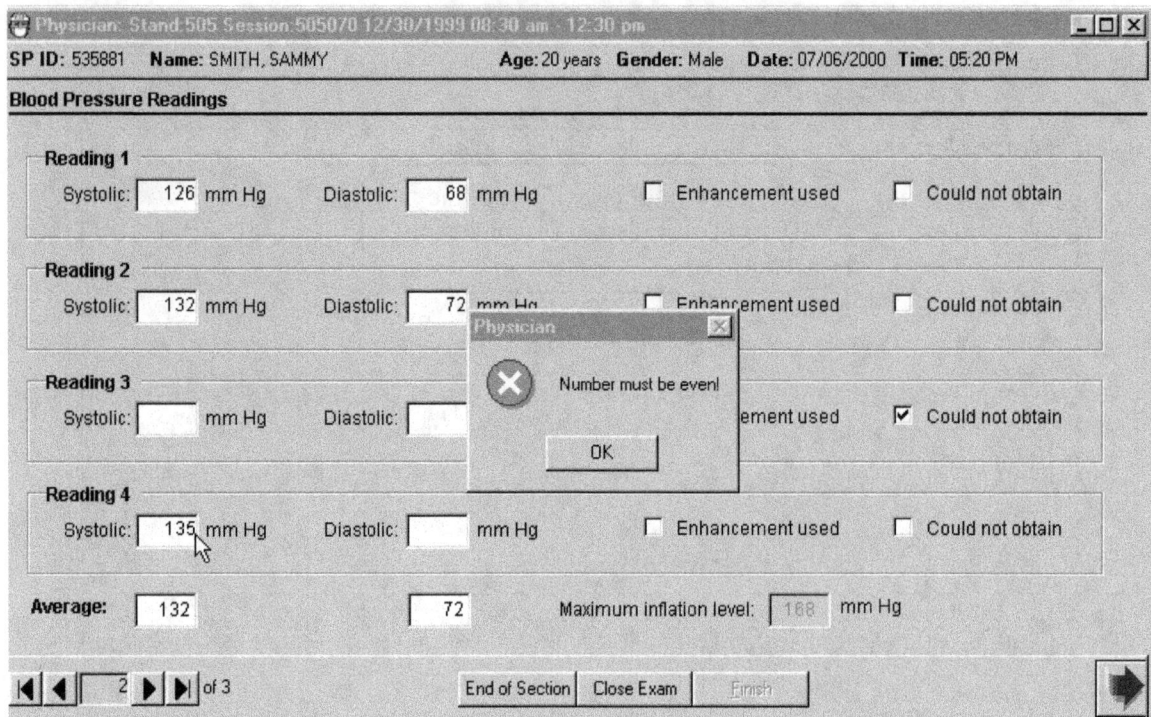

- The increment of the mercury manometer markings are in 2-millimeter intervals. All end digit BP measurements should be recorded as even numbered digits. If an odd number is entered as the end digit for either the systolic or diastolic measurement, a message is displayed: "Number must be even!"

- Click OK to this message. Re-enter the correct measurement and continue with data entry or measurement.

Exhibit 4-24. Systolic blood pressure greater than maximum inflation level

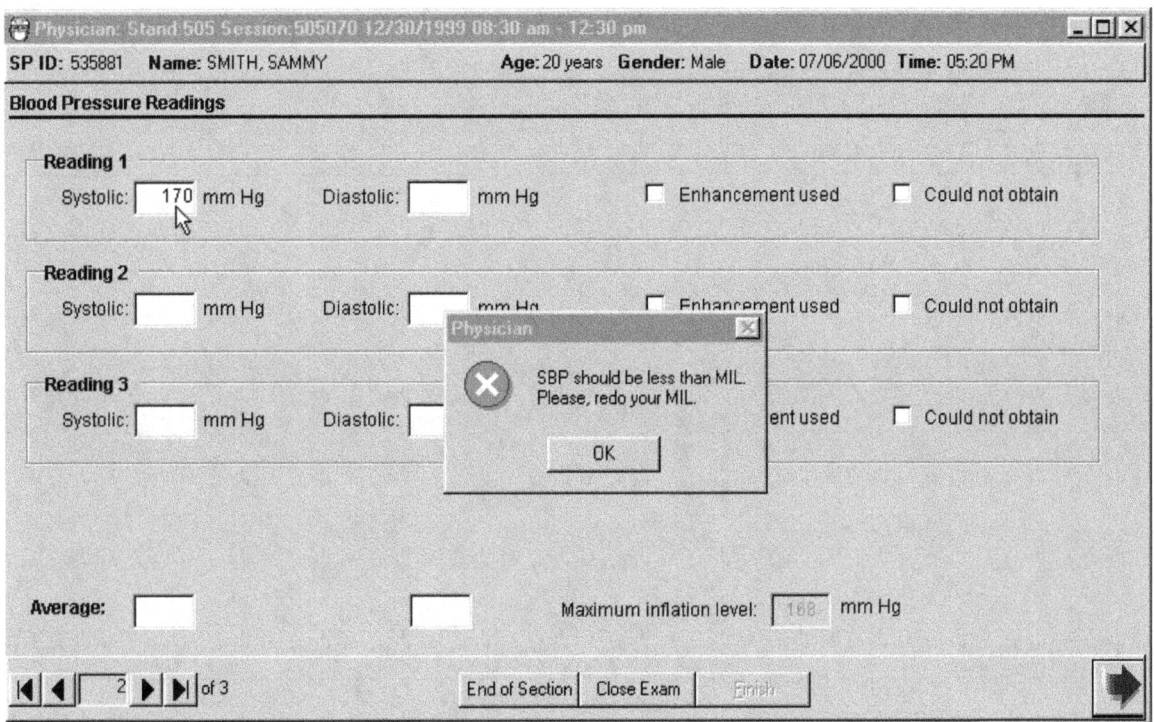

- IF the Systolic BP entered is greater than the MIL, a message is displayed: "SBP should be less than MIL. Please, redo your MIL".

- Redo the MIL and record. The maximum number of times the cuff can be inflated is five.

Exhibit 4-25. Averaging systolic blood pressure

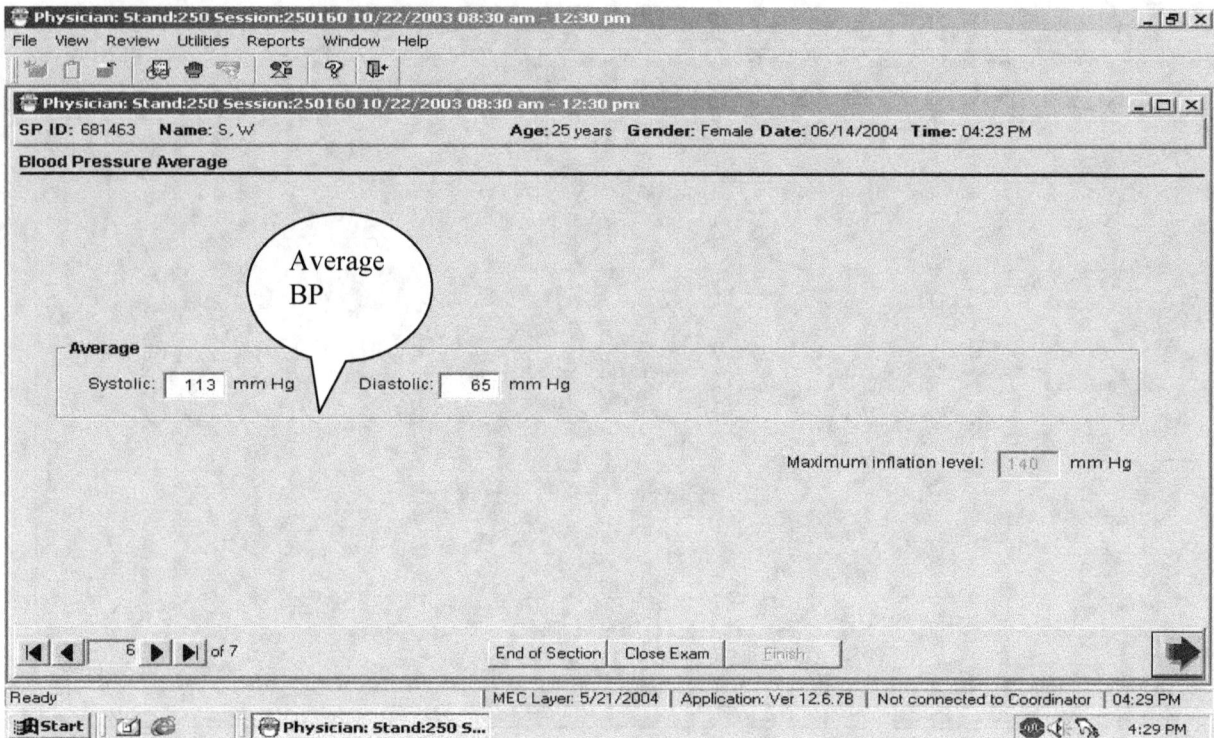

- There must be a MIL recorded for every SP.

- Ideally, every SP has three blood pressure measurements recorded.

- When three systolic blood pressure readings are recorded, the systolic average is calculated by the system as the average of the <u>last two systolic measurements</u>.

- When only one systolic blood pressure reading can be obtained, the one systolic reading is calculated by the system as the average.

- When only two systolic blood pressure readings can be obtained, the first systolic reading is discarded and the second systolic blood pressure measurement is calculated by the system as the systolic average.

- If all diastolic readings are zero, the average diastolic BP is calculated by the system as zero (0).

- If there is one diastolic reading of zero and one or more readings with a diastolic above zero (0), the system uses only the nonzero diastolic readings to calculate the average diastolic BP.

- If two out of three diastolic readings are zero (0), the system uses the one nonzero diastolic reading to calculate the average diastolic BP.

- When the average BP appears, tell the SP his/her BP.

Exhibit 4-26. Edit allowable systolic and diastolic blood pressure

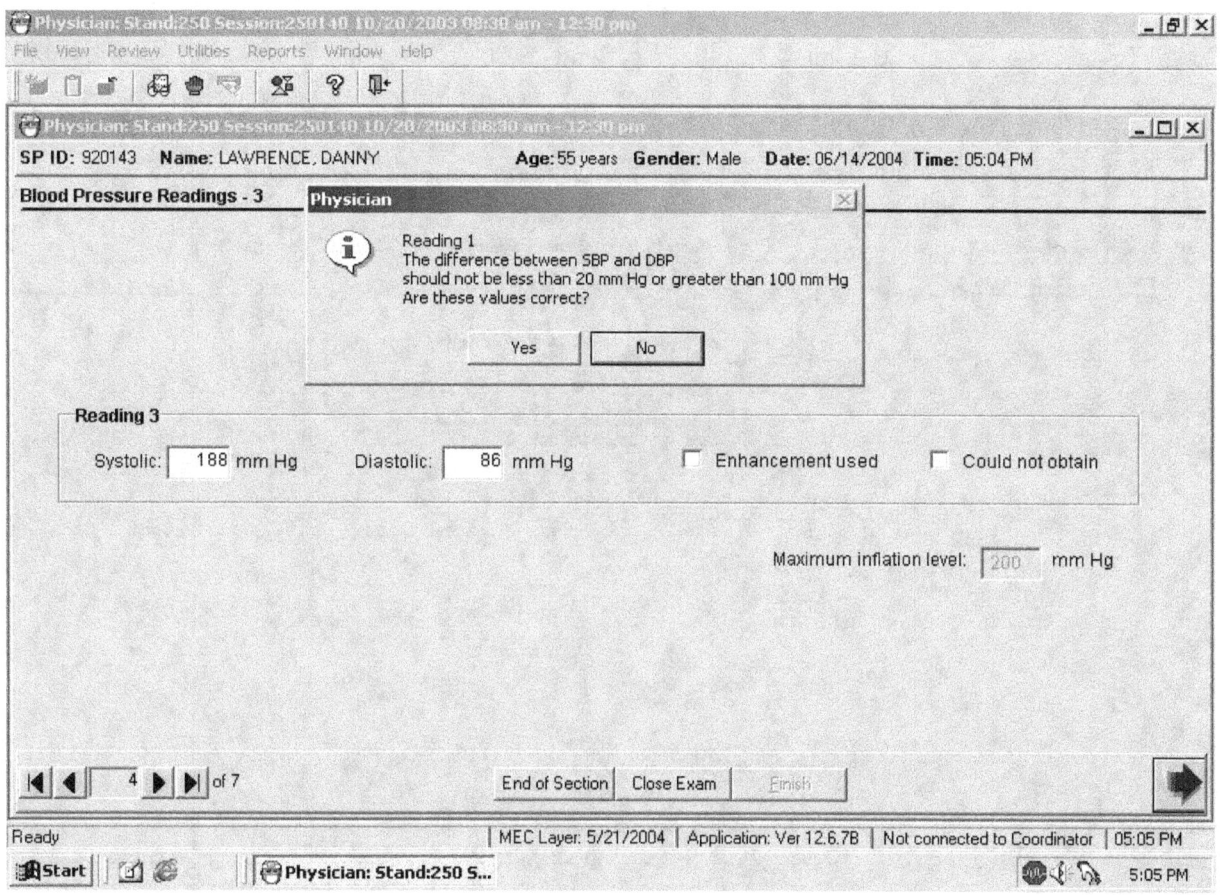

- If the systolic and diastolic BP are less than 20 mm Hq or more than 100 mm Hq, the application edits asks for verification of accuracy.

- If the measurements are correct, click yes.

- If the measures are incorrect, click no, and reenter the measurements.

4.7.7   Blood Pressure Edit Limits

Exhibit 4-27. Edit range limits for blood pressure

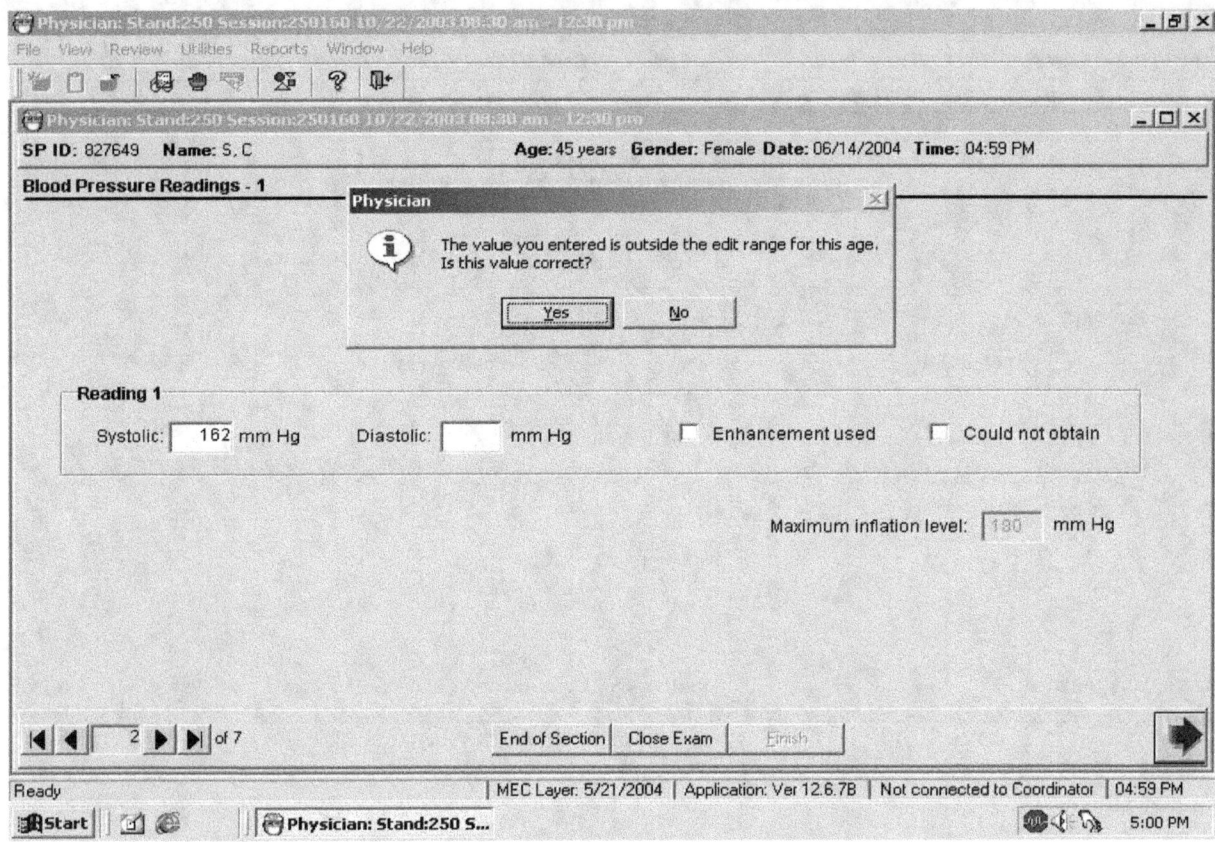

- If a systolic or diastolic value is outside the edit range for that SP, (age specific) the system displays a message: "The value you entered is outside the range for this age. Is this value correct?"

- If the value entered is correct, click yes, and proceed with the data entry.

- If the response is not correct, click on No and reenter the value, then proceed with the examination.

4.7.8 Blood Pressure Component Status and Comments

Exhibit 4-28. Comments in blood pressure component

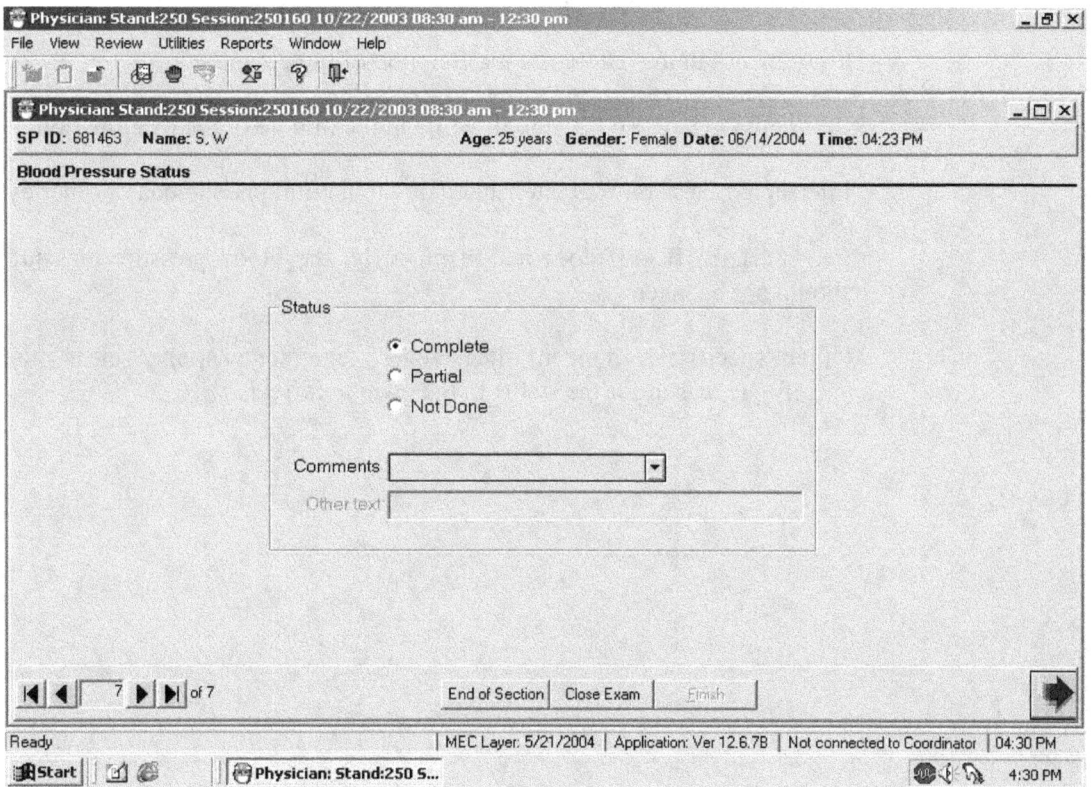

- If all the measurements were entered, the system sets the default last screen for the component status to "Complete."

- If one or more of the measurements were not recorded, the system sets the component status to "Partial."

- If the Component Status is partial, select the appropriate comment from the drop-down menu.

- The comments in the menu are:

  - Safety exclusion: SP is excluded due to a situation that may cause them harm or discomfort such as applying or inflating a cuff on an arm with visible edema, lesions, or other conditions.

  - SP refusal: SP refuses all or part of the examination.

  - No time: SP is unable to complete the examination due to time restrictions.

- Physical limitation: SP has a physical limitation that prevents examination completion.

- Communication problem: Physician is unable to communicate instructions for the examination adequately.

- Equipment failure: There is a malfunction of the equipment.

- SP ill/emergency: SP became ill while in the middle of the examination.

- Interrupted: Session was interrupted due to natural phenomena or other event.

- Poor cuff fit: If cuff does not fit properly, the blood pressure measurements should not be taken.

- Other, specific: If none of the standard comments apply, select other and specify the reason for the status in the open text field.

4.7.9   Exclusion from CV Fitness Based on Systolic Blood Pressure

Exhibit 4-29. Systolic blood pressure exclusion from CV Fitness

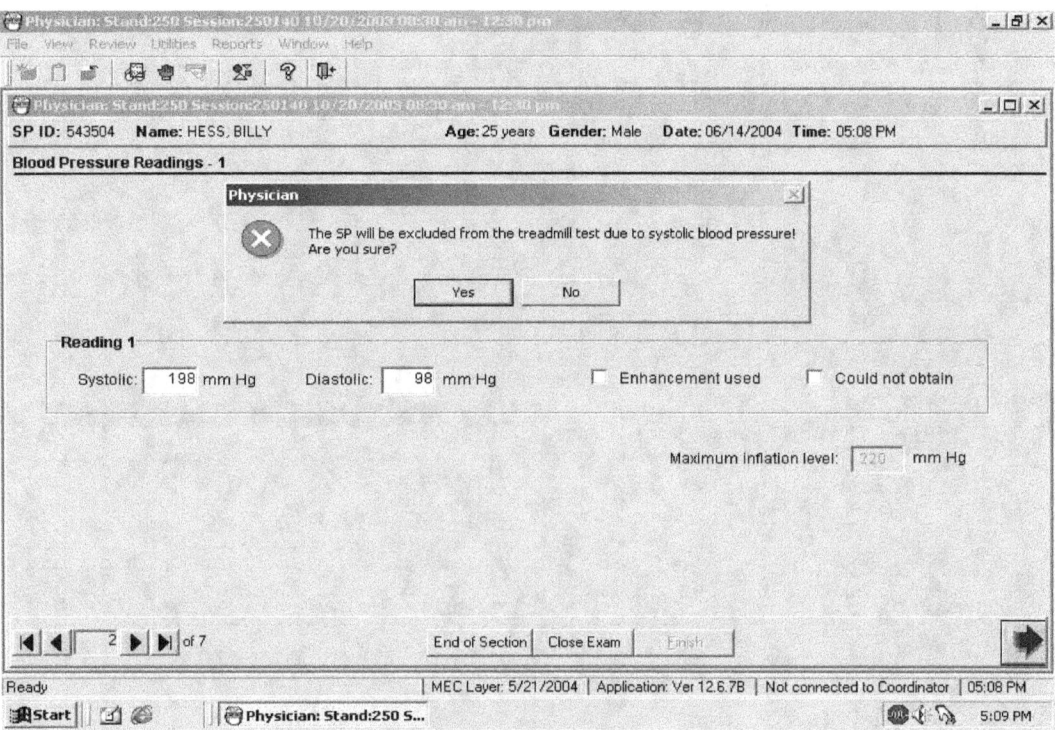

- If the Systolic BP is greater than 180 mm Hg, the SP is excluded from the treadmill test and from the safety exclusion questions in the Physicians' examination

- A message is displayed: "The SP will be excluded from the treadmill test due to systolic blood pressure! Are you sure?"

- Click "Yes" if the value entered was correct.

- The component status in CV Fitness defaults to "Not Done" with the comment "Safety Exclusion."

- The SP is also excluded from the safety exclusion questions for CV Fitness and the CV Fitness component.

4.7.10   Exclusion from CV Fitness Based on Diastolic Blood Pressure

Exhibit 4-30. Diastolic blood pressure exclusion from CV Fitness

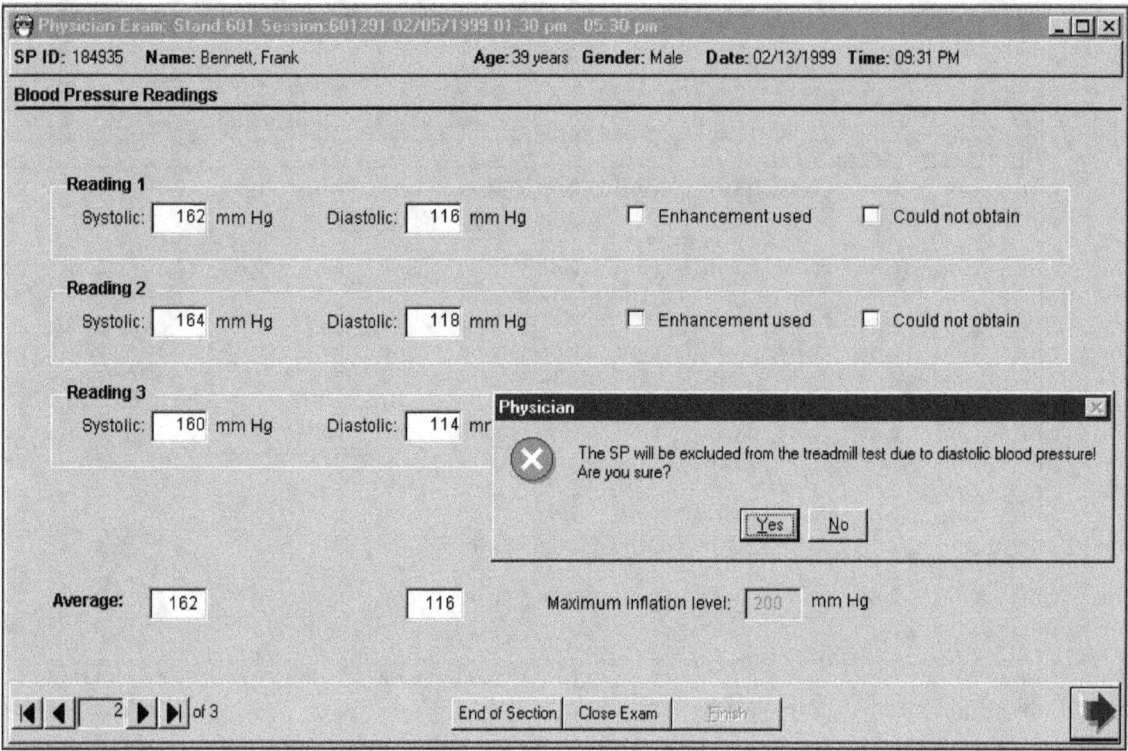

- If the Diastolic Blood Pressure is greater than 100 mm Hg, the SP is excluded from the treadmill test and the safety exclusion questions in the Physicians' Examination

- A message is displayed: "The SP is excluded from the treadmill test due to diastolic blood pressure! Are you sure?"

- Click "Yes" if the value entered was correct.

Exhibit 4-31. Exclusion message for CV Fitness

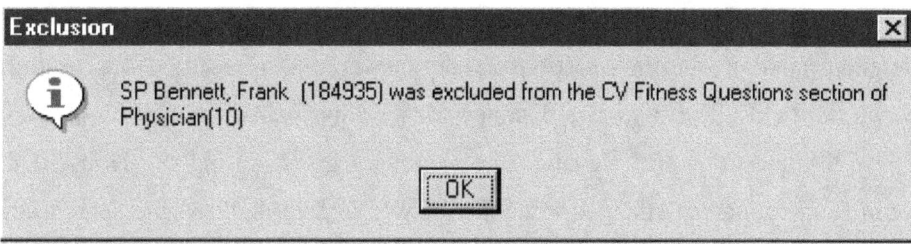

- This message is displayed after the data are recorded if the SP was excluded.

- The SP is excluded from the safety exclusion questions for CV Fitness and the CV Fitness component.

Exhibit 4-32. Exclusion status for Cardiovascular Fitness component

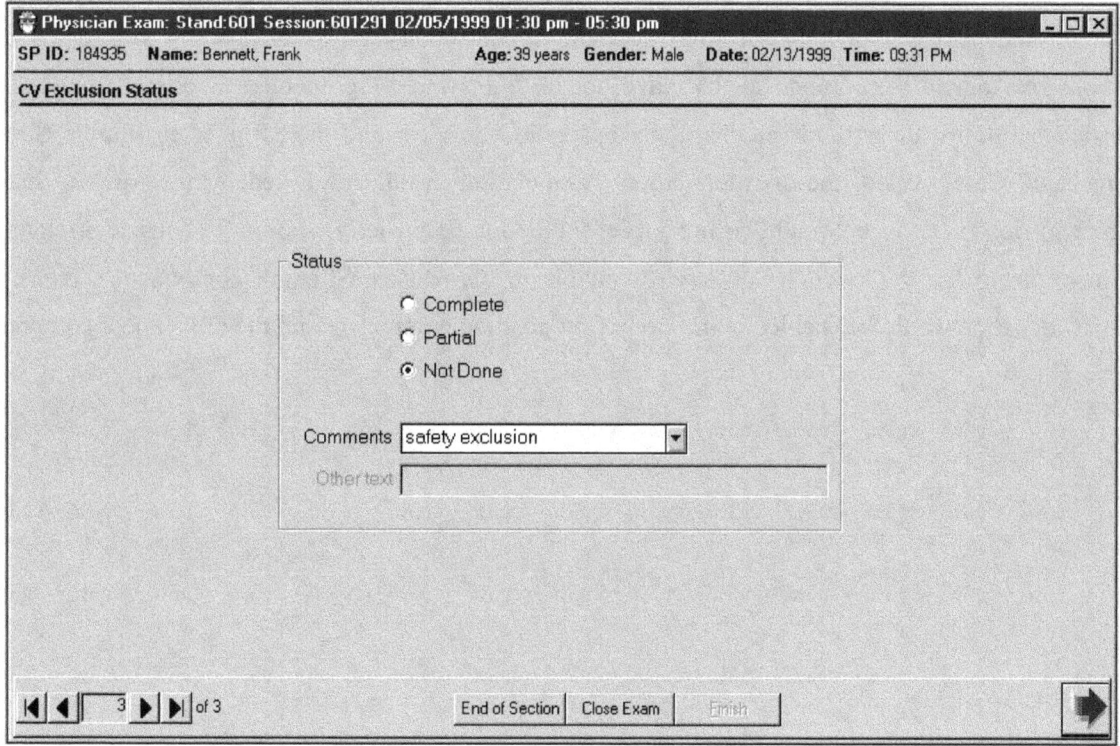

- The CV Fitness Exclusion Status in the **Physician Examination Component** defaults to "Not Done" with the comment "Safety Exclusion."

- The Status in **CV Fitness Component** defaults to "Not Done" with the comment "Safety Exclusion."

4.7.11   Shared Exclusion Questions

If the shared exclusion questions were answered during the Household Interview, the answers appear in the fields. The fields are disabled for the Physician Examination, as well as any other component where the questions are relevant. The responses given during the Household Interview or during any component cannot be changed after the answer is recorded and the screen advanced. If the shared exclusion questions were not answered during the Household Interview, they are enabled and are asked during the MEC examination in the first examination where shared exclusions are asked. Each question is asked only once, even when the question is relevant for more than one component. Some examinations do not require all the shared exclusions to be asked. In this situation, there may be some questions answered in one examination and then disabled in the remaining examinations. Shared exclusion questions are component specific. Answers provided during previous components appear on the screen for the next examiner to see, but the field for data entry is disabled. Only shared exclusion questions relevant to the component that have not been answered are enabled. Example: If the shared exclusion questions are not answered in the Household Interview and the SP goes to Muscle Strength before Body Composition, the questions about "amputation" would be asked by the Muscle Strength technician. However, since "weight" is not a relevant Shared Exclusion Question for Muscle Strength, the ISIS does not make the "weight" question available in the Muscle Strength component screens. The "weight" question would be enabled in the Body Composition component and the CV Fitness component.

Exhibit 4-33. Shared exclusions

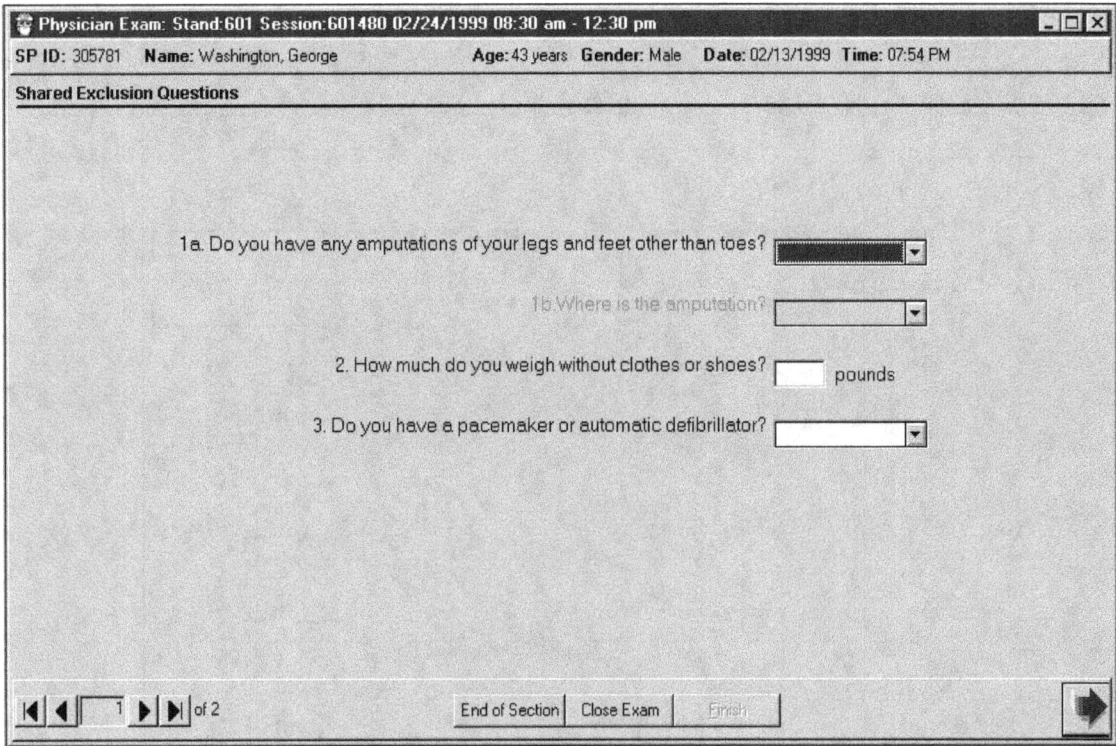

- If the shared exclusion questions are answered in the Household Examination, the questions will appear answered and disabled. These responses cannot be changed in the MEC.

- If the responses excluded the SP from CV Fitness, the SP would be blocked from the safety exclusion questions by the coordinator system and the SP would not be sent to the CV Fitness examination.

- The component status for CV Fitness for this SP would be set to Not Done with a comment specific to the reason for exclusion (safety exclusion, physical limitation, etc.).

Exhibit 4-34. Shared exclusion: Amputation(s)

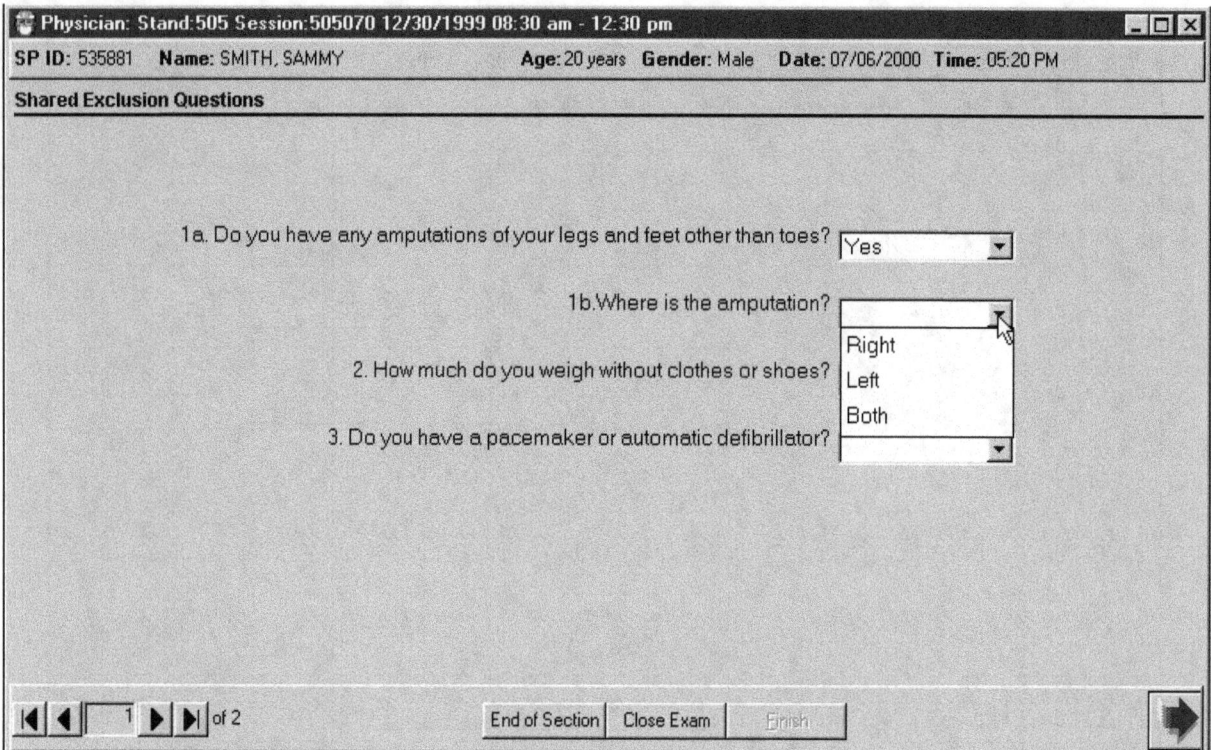

- If the answer to "Do you have any amputations of your fingers and toes?" is no, the next question is disabled and the SP remains eligible for the examination.

- If the answer is yes, determine the location of the amputation. The choices are right, left, or both.

Exhibit 4-35. Shared exclusion: Message

- If the answer is right, left, or both, the SP is excluded from CV Fitness due to a physical limitation. The system displays a message: "SP <SP name> was excluded from Cardiovascular Fitness."

- The SP is excluded from the remaining safety exclusion questions for CV Fitness and from the CV Fitness test.

Exhibit 4-36. Shared exclusion: Equipment weight limitation

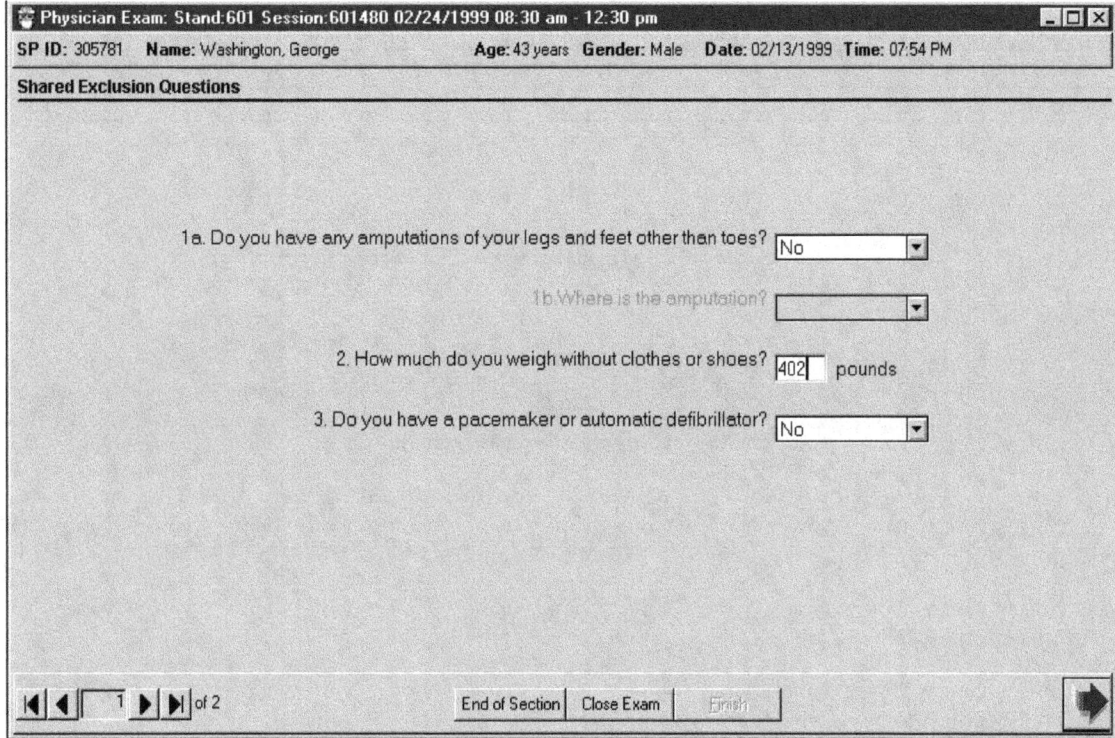

- If the answer to the question "How much do you weigh without clothes or shoes?" is less than 350 pounds, the question is disabled and the SP remains eligible for the CV Fitness examination.

- If the response is greater than 350 pounds, the SP is excluded from CV Fitness due to weight limitation on the treadmill equipment.

- The component status for CV Fitness defaults to "Not Done" with the comment "weight limitation on equipment."

Exhibit 4-37. Shared exclusion: Pacemaker

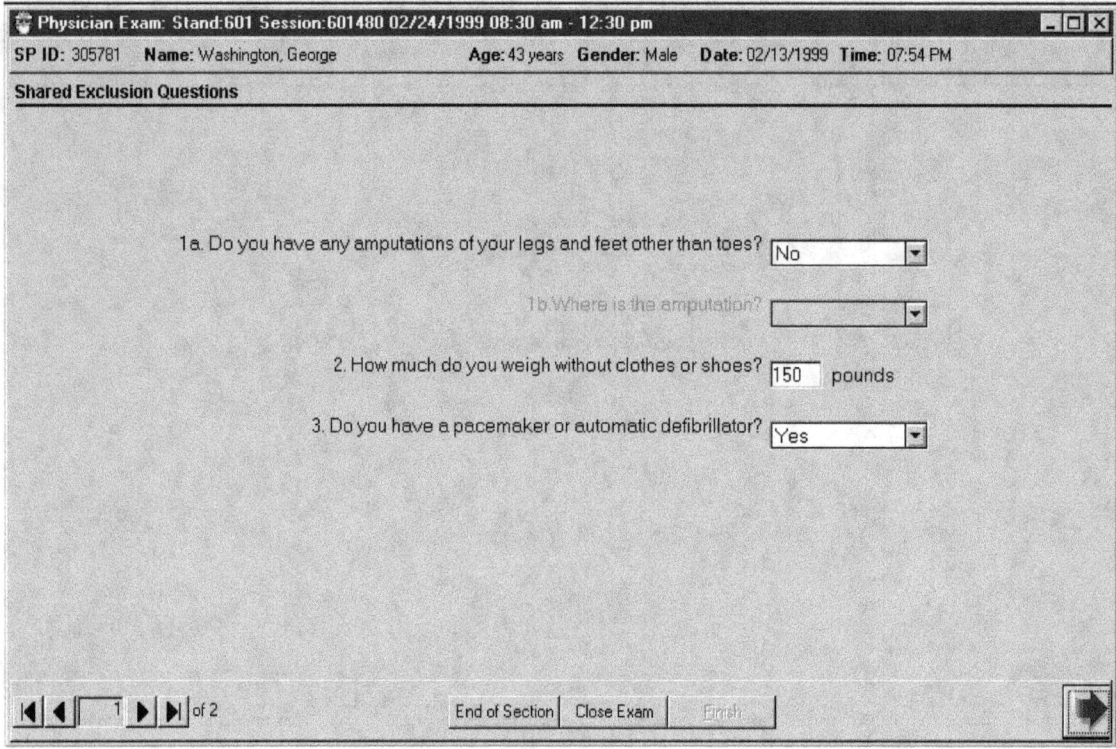

- If the response to the question "Do you have a pacemaker or automatic defibrillator?" is no, continue with the CV safety exclusion questions.

- If the response to the above question is yes, the SP is excluded from the CV safety exclusion questions and the CV fitness examination.

Exhibit 4-38. Shared exclusion questions: Required data entry

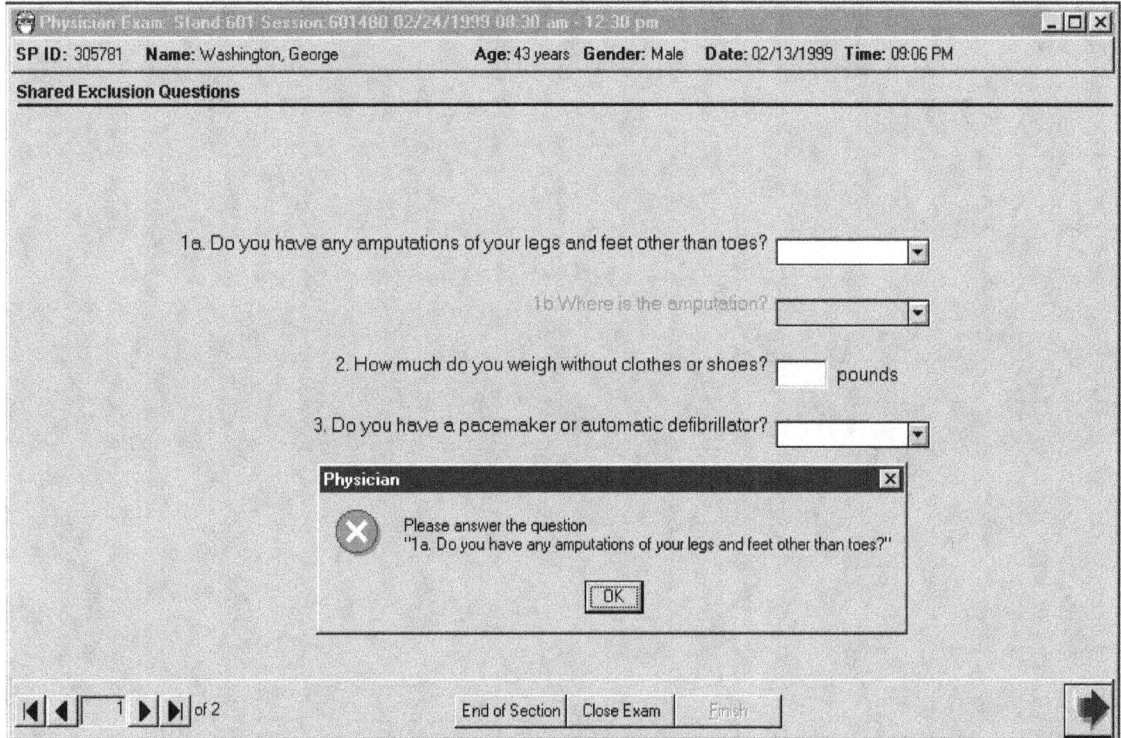

- If the Next button is pressed to go to the next screen, a message is displayed: "Please answer the question." The specific question that was not answered will also be part of this message.

- Click OK to this message and answer the question, then go to the next screen.

Exhibit 4-39. Component completion status for shared exclusions

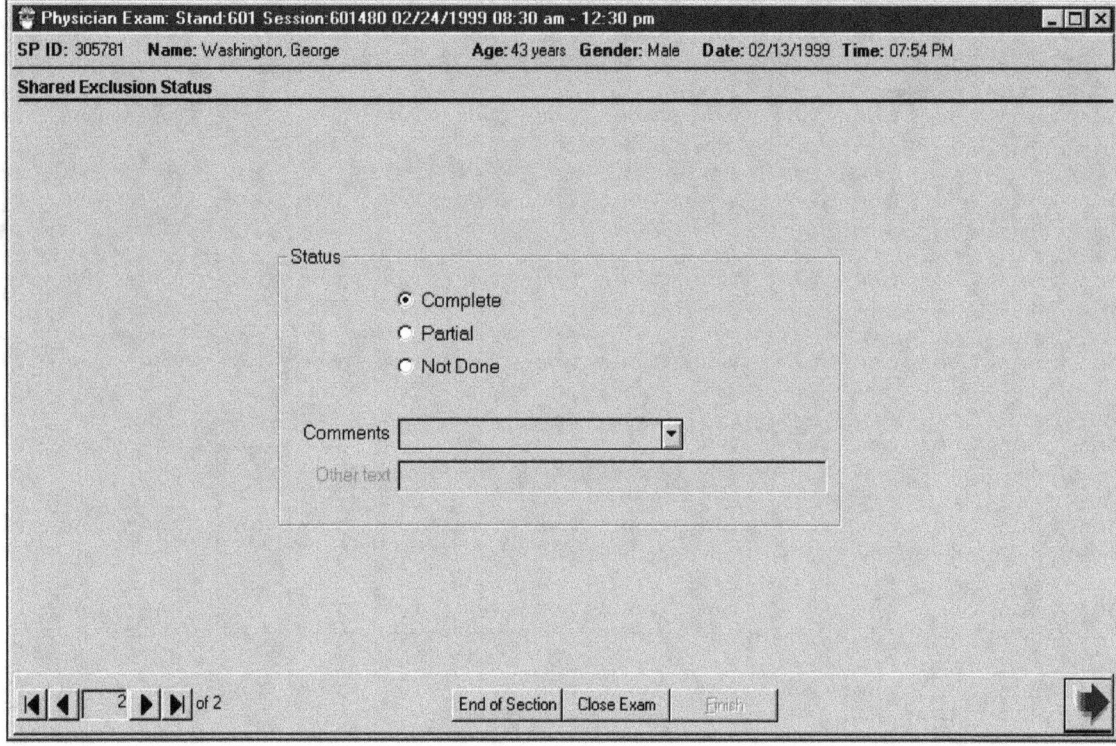

- If all the shared exclusion questions are answered, the component status for shared exclusions defaults to "Complete."

- If all questions were not answered the status defaults to partial. The examination is closed with the "Close Examination" button.

- If the SP was excluded by any of the shared exclusion questions the system displays a series of messages to indicate the other components that are blocked for this SP.

Exhibit 4-40. Body Composition exclusion message

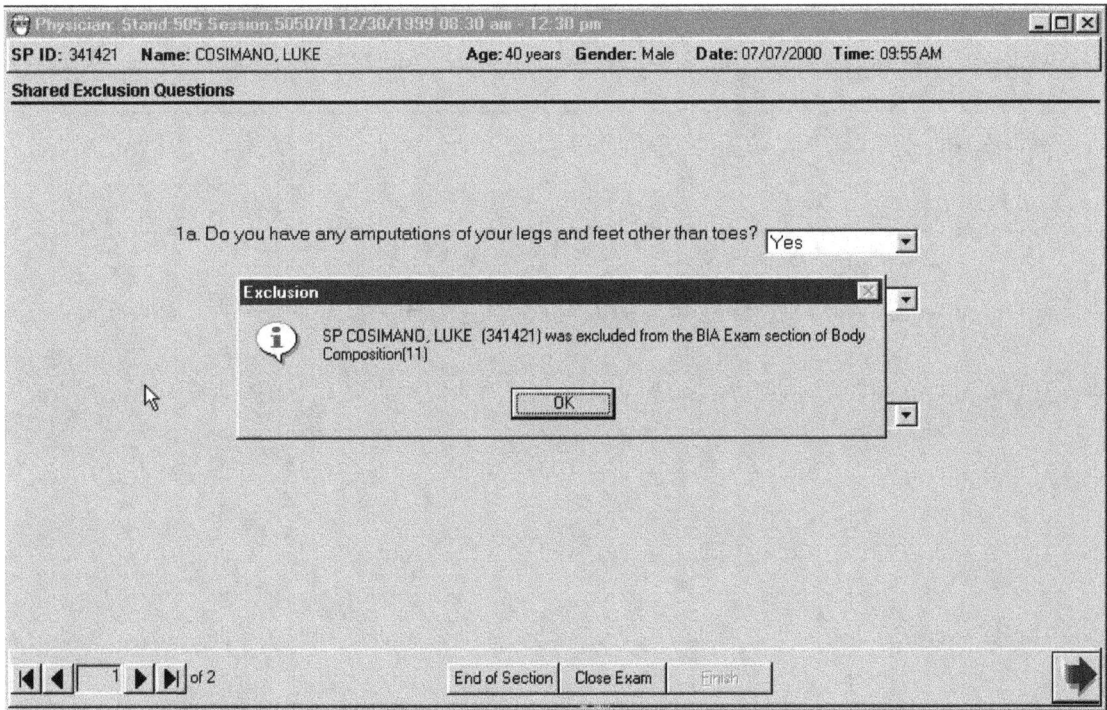

- The SP is excluded from the BIA section of Body Composition if the response to the question on amputations and pacemaker or defibrillator is yes.

- The SP is excluded from Body Composition if the weight is greater than 300 pounds.

Exhibit 4-41. Balance exclusion message

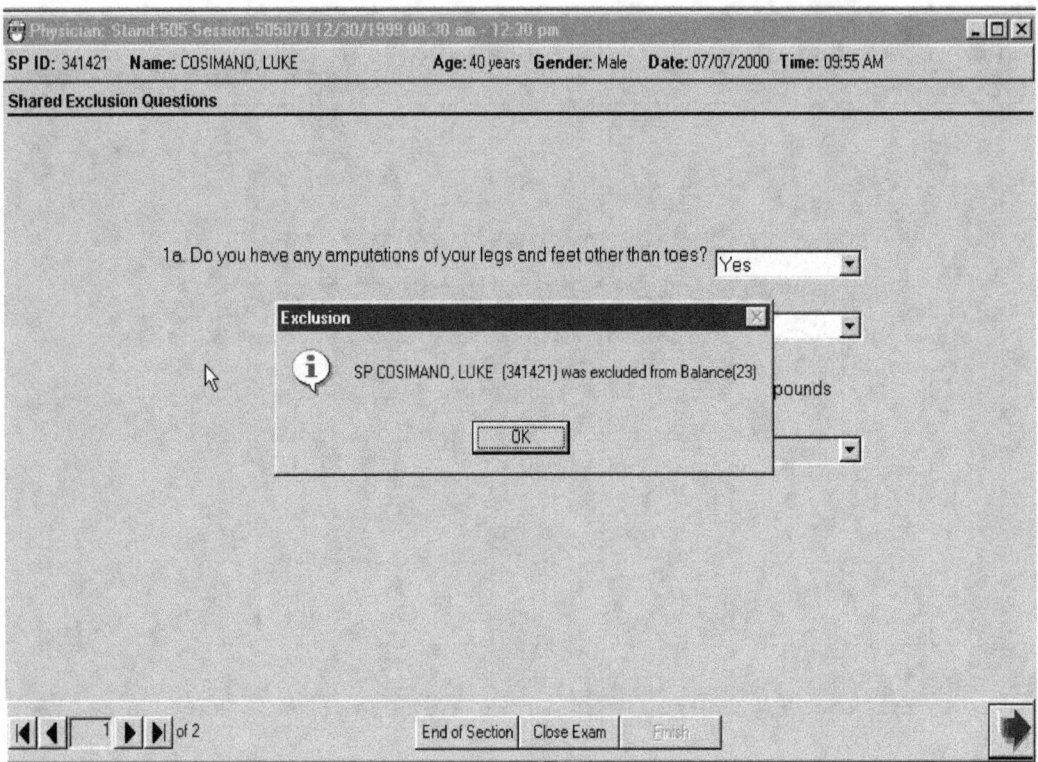

- The SP is excluded from Balance if the weight is greater than 250 pounds.

Exhibit 4-42. Shared exclusion: Pregnancy

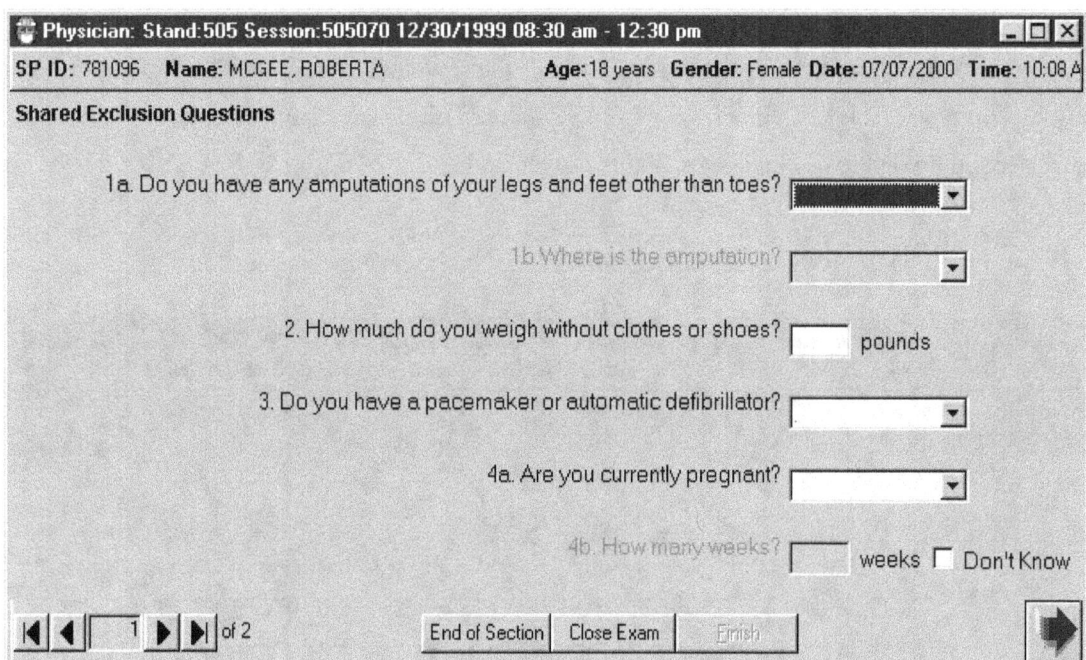

- If the SP is female, there are shared exclusion questions on self-reported pregnancy.

- If the response to the question "Are you currently pregnant?" is no, proceed with the CV Fitness safety exclusion questions.

- If the response to the pregnancy question is yes, ask "How many weeks?" If the response is <u>less than 12 weeks,</u> go to the CV Fitness safety exclusion questions.

- If the response to the term of pregnancy question is <u>greater than 12 weeks</u>, the SP is excluded from being asked the safety exclusion questions in the Physician's Examination and the CV Fitness examination.

- The component status for CV Fitness defaults to "Not Done" with the comment "SP pregnant."

4.7.12   CV Safety Exclusion Questions

The safety exclusion questions for cardiovascular fitness examination are asked during the Physician's Examination. SPs are excluded automatically if a "Yes" response is obtained for questions 1 through 8, 9F, 9G, and 10. If a SP is taking an exclusion medication in question 1, they are excluded. SPs who are taking anti-hypertensive medication are not excluded unless the medication they are taking for their high blood pressure is on the medication exclusion list.

When a SP is excluded based on the response to a question, the remaining questions on the screen are disabled and the SP will not need to answer the remaining questions. The CV Exclusion status defaults to complete. The CV Fitness component status defaults to "Not Done" with the appropriate comment depending on the question signaling the exclusion.

Exhibit 4-43. Medical conditions CV safety exclusion questions

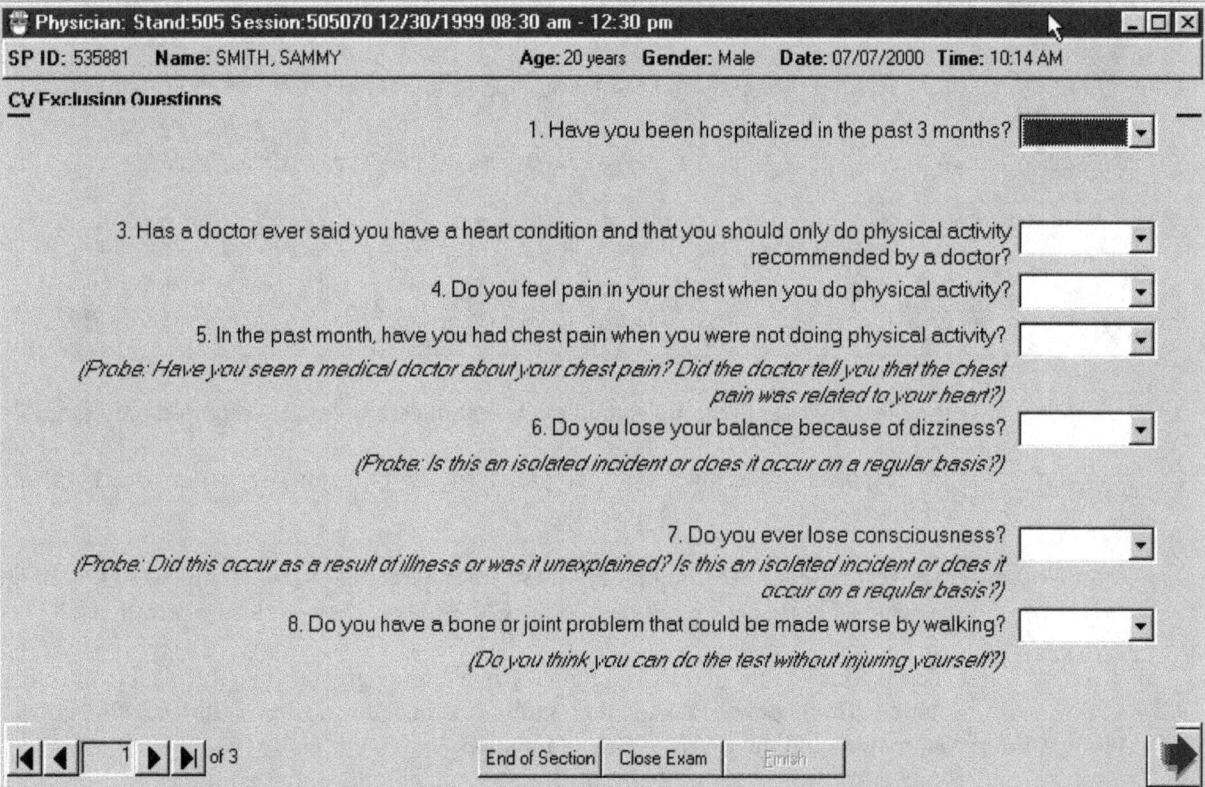

- The safety exclusion questions are read to the SP exactly as written.

- Read the entire question before accepting an answer.

- If the SP interrupts and answers the question before you have completed reading the question, tell him/her that you are required to read the entire question before accepting an answer.

Exhibit 4-44. CV safety exclusion: Hospitalizations

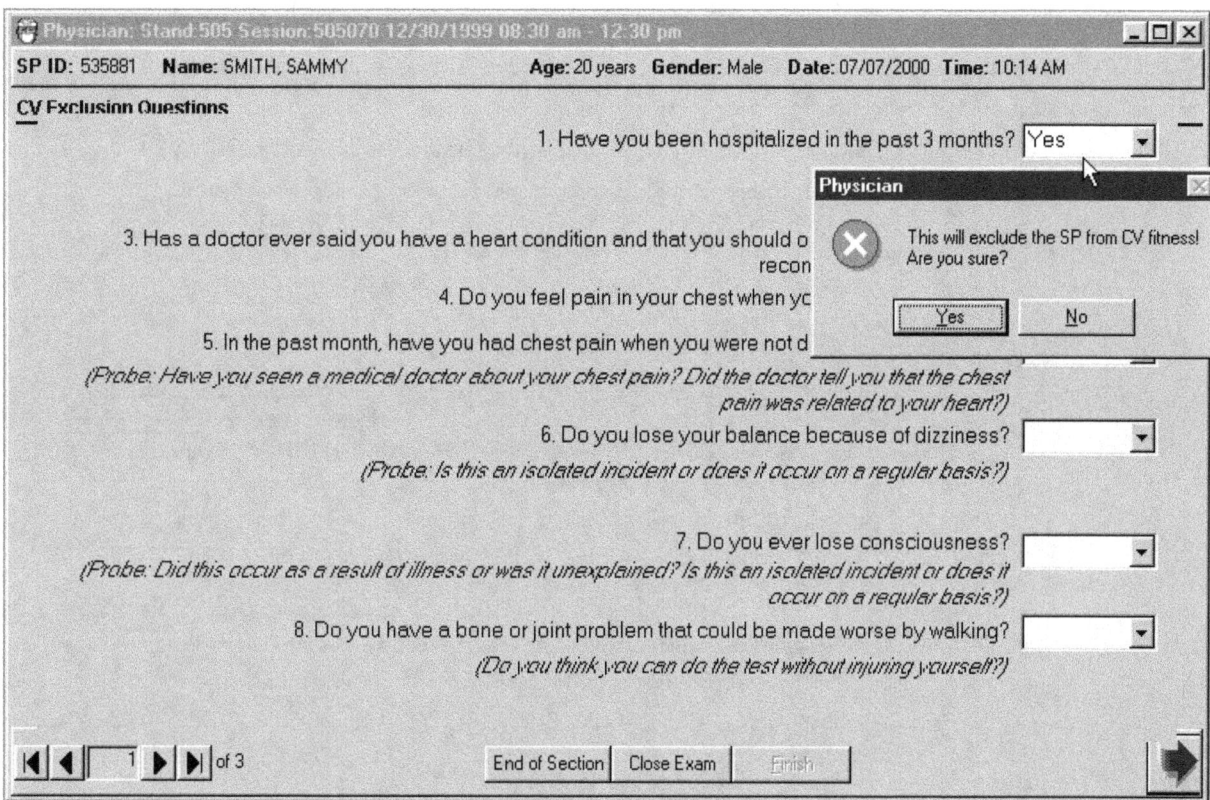

- If the response to the first question "Have you been hospitalized in the past 3 months?" is "No," proceed to question 2.

- If the response is "Yes," the SP is excluded from CV Fitness

- If the response is "Don't Know," the SP is excluded and remaining questions are disabled.

- When the Next button is pressed to go to the next screen, the system advances to the CV exclusion screen and the CV exclusion status defaults to complete. The CV Fitness examination component status defaults to "Not Done," with the comment "Safety Exclusion."

Exhibit 4-45. CV safety exclusion: Adolescent school activity

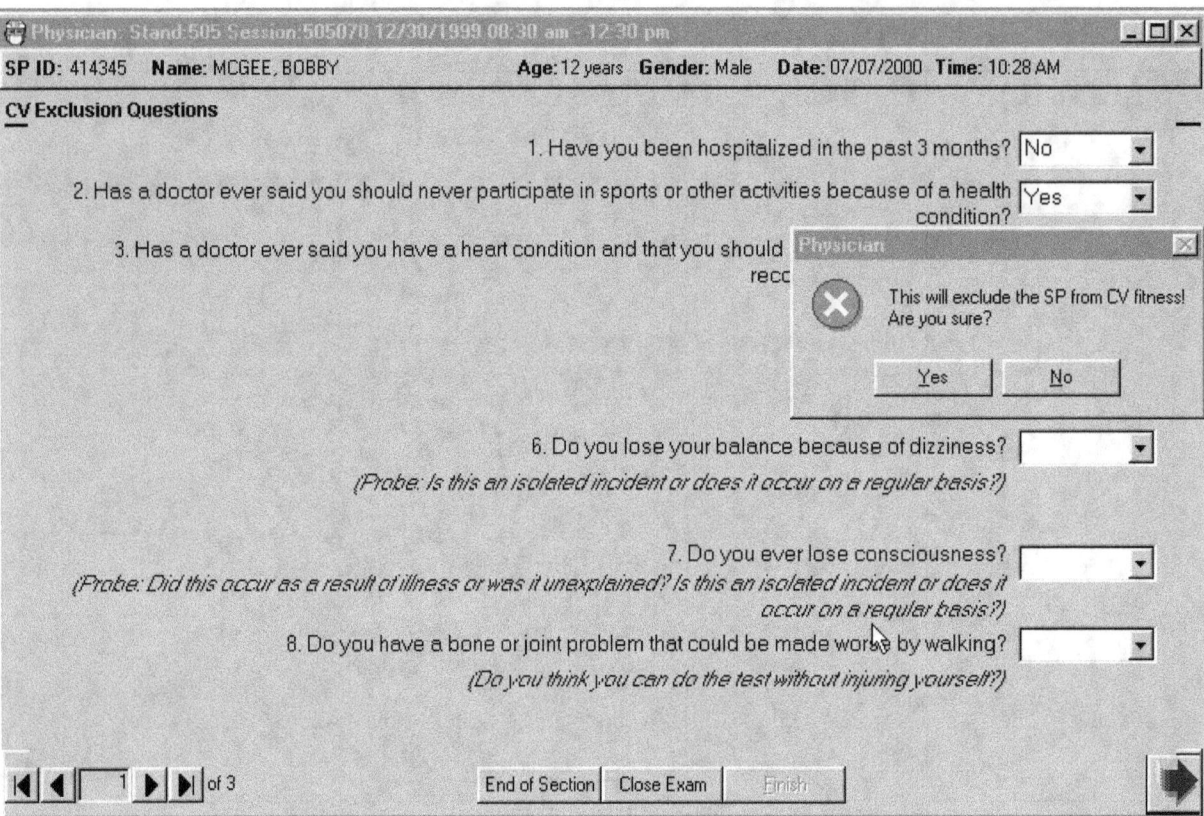

- Question 2 is asked of SPs 12-19 years of age. "Has a doctor ever said you should not participate in sports or other activities because of a heart condition?"

- If the response to this question is "No," proceed to the next question.

- If the response is "Yes," or "Don't Know," the SP is excluded from the CV Fitness examination and the remaining questions are disabled.

- A message is displayed: "This will exclude the SP from CV Fitness! Are you sure?" If the response is correct, click "Yes" to the message.

- The CV Exclusion status defaults to "Complete" and the CV Fitness component status defaults to "Not Done" with the comment "Safety Exclusion."

Exhibit 4-46. CV safety exclusion questions: Heart condition

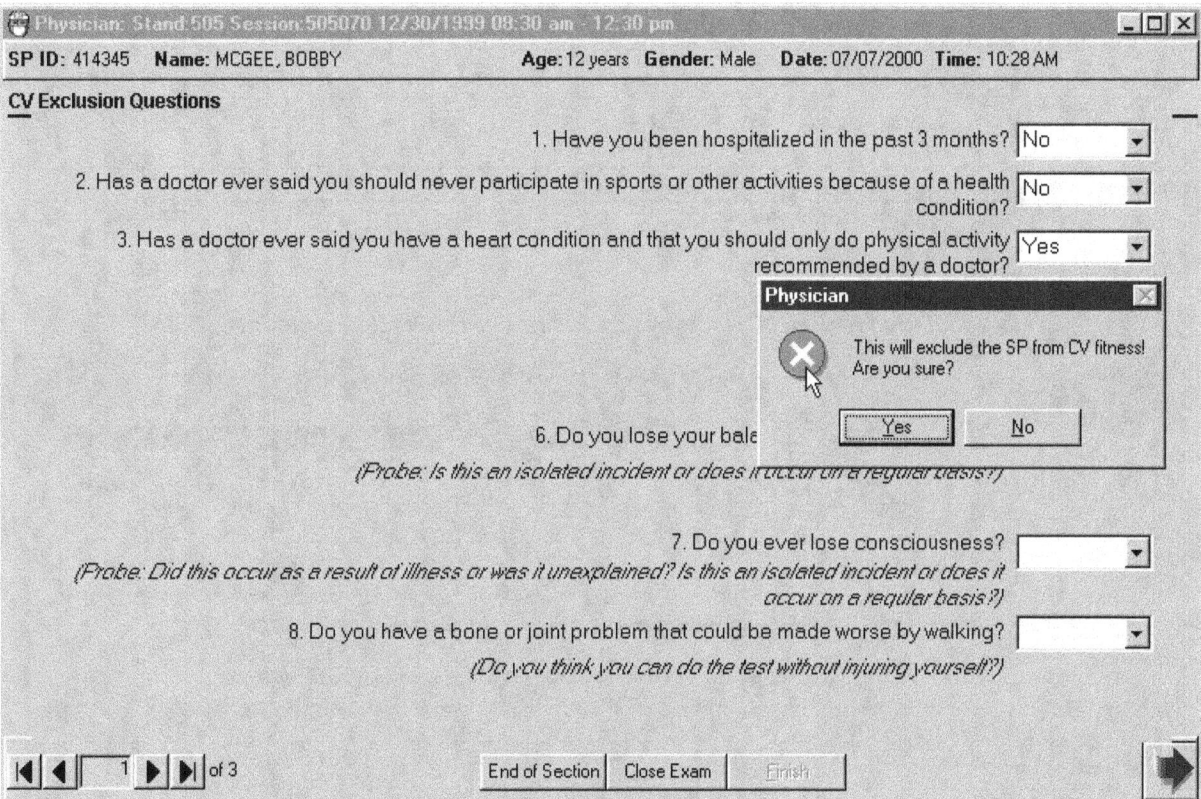

- Question 3: "Has a doctor ever said you have a heart condition and that you should only do physical activity recommended by a doctor."

- If the response to this question is "No," proceed to the next question.

- If the response is "Yes" or "Don't Know," the SP is excluded from the CV Fitness examination and the remaining questions are disabled.

- A message is displayed: "This will exclude the SP from CV Fitness! Are you sure?" If the response was correct, click "Yes" to the message.

- The CV exclusion status defaults to "Complete" and the CV Fitness component status defaults to "Not Done" with the comment "Safety Exclusion."

Exhibit 4-47. CV safety exclusion questions: Chest pain

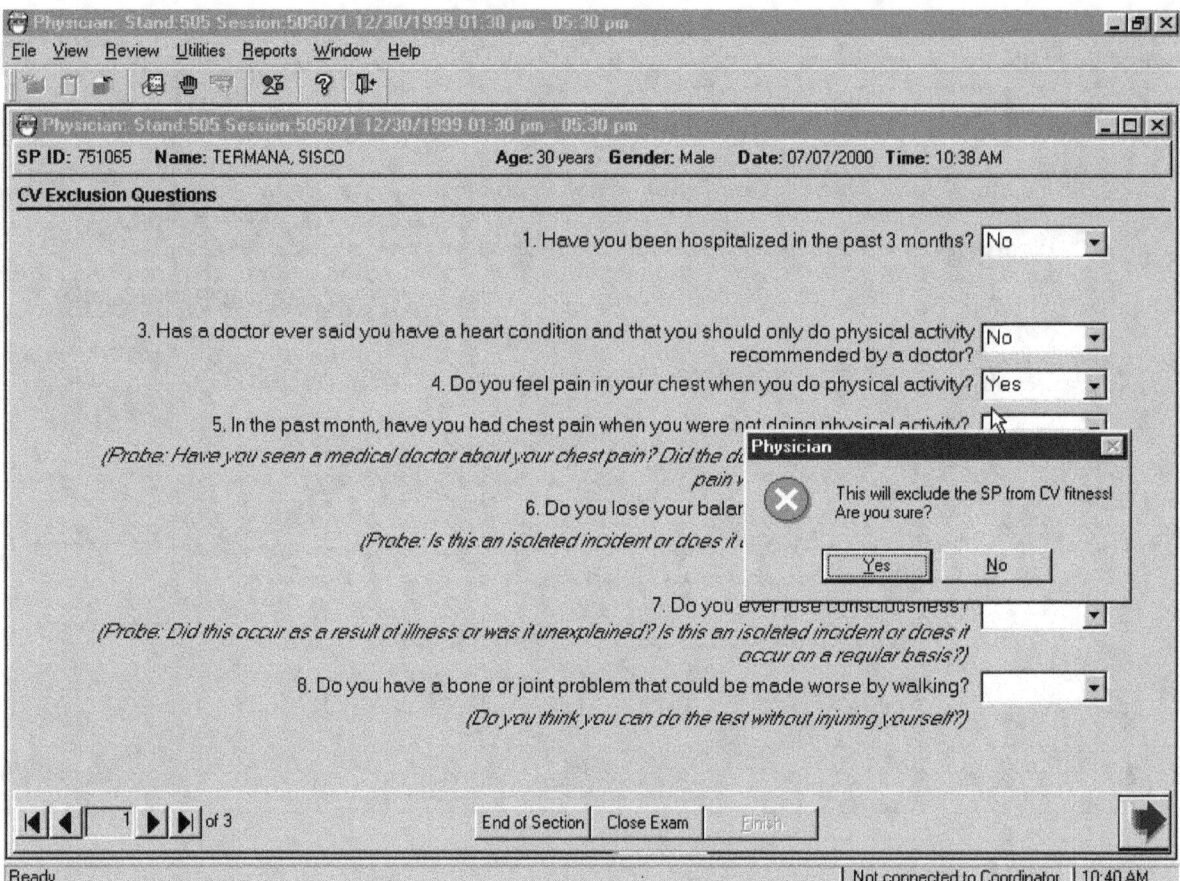

- Question 4 is asked of SPs 20-49 years of age: "Do you feel pain in your chest when you do physical activity?"

- If the response to this question is "No," proceed to the next question.

- If the response is "Yes" or "Don't Know," the SP is excluded from the CV Fitness examination and the remaining questions are disabled.

- A message is displayed: "This will exclude the SP from CV Fitness! Are you sure?" If the response was correct, click "Yes" to the message.

- The CV exclusion status defaults to "Complete" and the CV Fitness component status defaults to "Not Done" with the comment "Safety Exclusion."

Exhibit 4-48. CV safety exclusion questions: Chest pain at rest

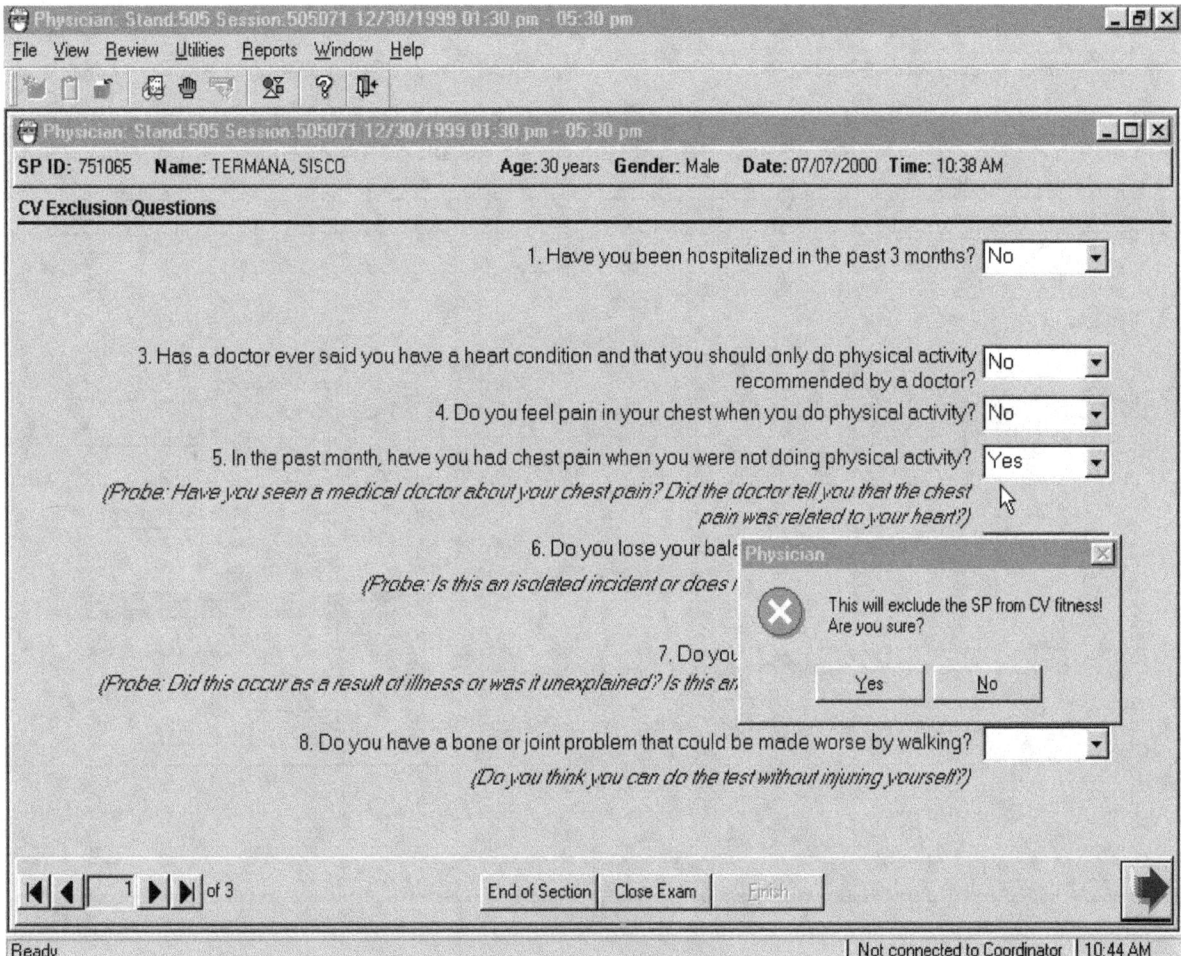

- Question 5 is asked of SPs 20-49 years of age: In the past month, have you had chest pain when you were not doing physical activity?"

- If the SP does not know how to respond to this question, ask one or both of the following probes:

  - Probe 1   "Have you seen a medical doctor about your chest pain?"

  - Probe 2   "Did the doctor tell you that the chest pain was related to your heart?"

- If the response to this question is "No," proceed to the next question.

- If the response is "Yes" or "Don't Know," the SP is excluded from the CV Fitness examination and the remaining questions are disabled.

- A message is displayed: "This will exclude the SP from CV Fitness! Are you sure?" If the response was correct, click "Yes" to the message.

- The CV Exclusion status defaults to "Complete" and the CV Fitness component status defaults to "Not Done" with the comment "Safety Exclusion."

Exhibit 4-49. CV safety exclusion question: Dizziness

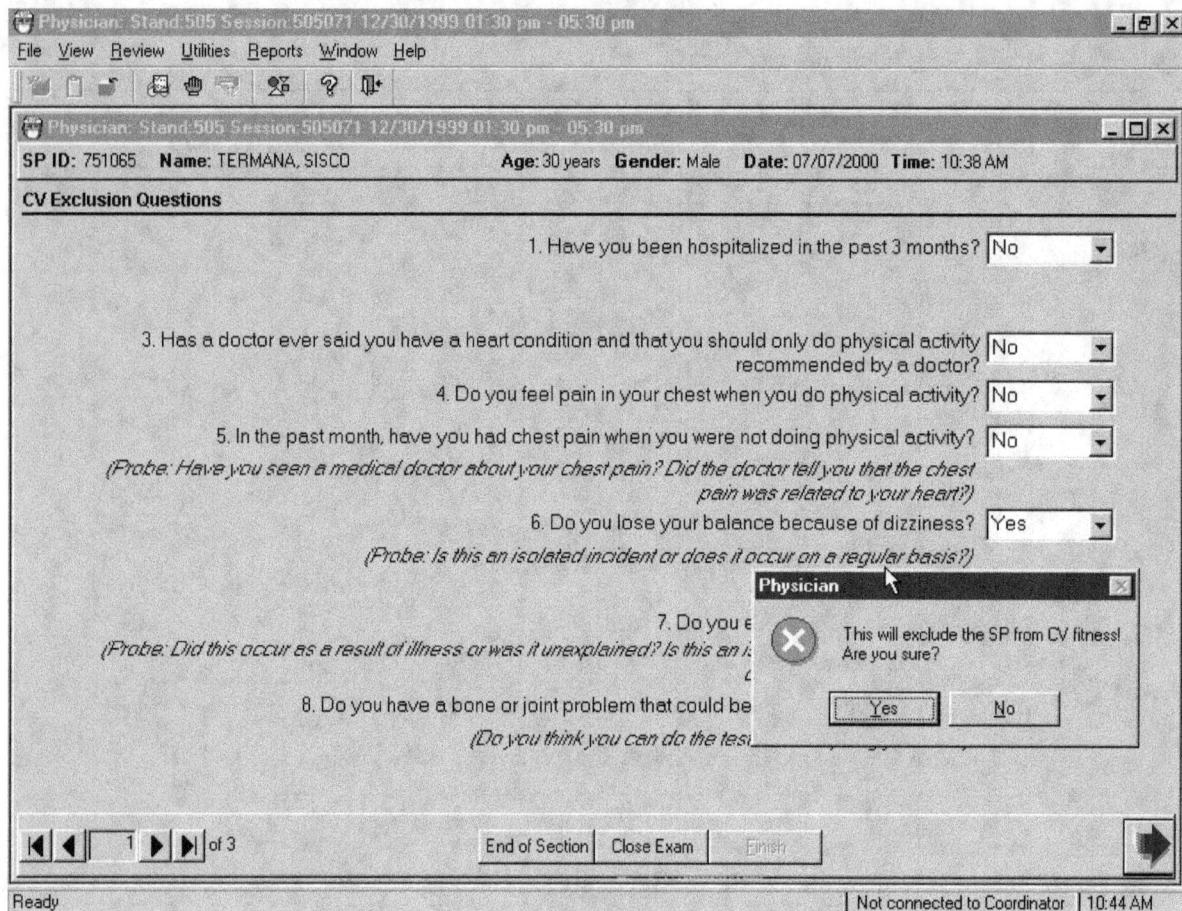

- Ask question 6: "Do you lose your balance because of dizziness?"

- If the SP does not know how to respond to this question, ask the following probe:

  - Probe: "Is this an isolated incident or does it occur on a regular basis?"

- The key point to this probe is to determine whether this is a regular occurrence.

- If the response to this question is "No," proceed to the next question.

- If the response is "Yes" or "Don't Know," the SP is excluded from the CV Fitness examination and the remaining questions are disabled.

- A message is displayed: "This will exclude the SP from CV Fitness! Are you sure?" If the response was correct, click "Yes" to the message.

- The CV Exclusion status defaults to "Complete" and the CV Fitness component status defaults to "Not Done" with the comment "Safety Exclusion."

Exhibit 4-50. CV safety exclusion questions (loss of consciousness)

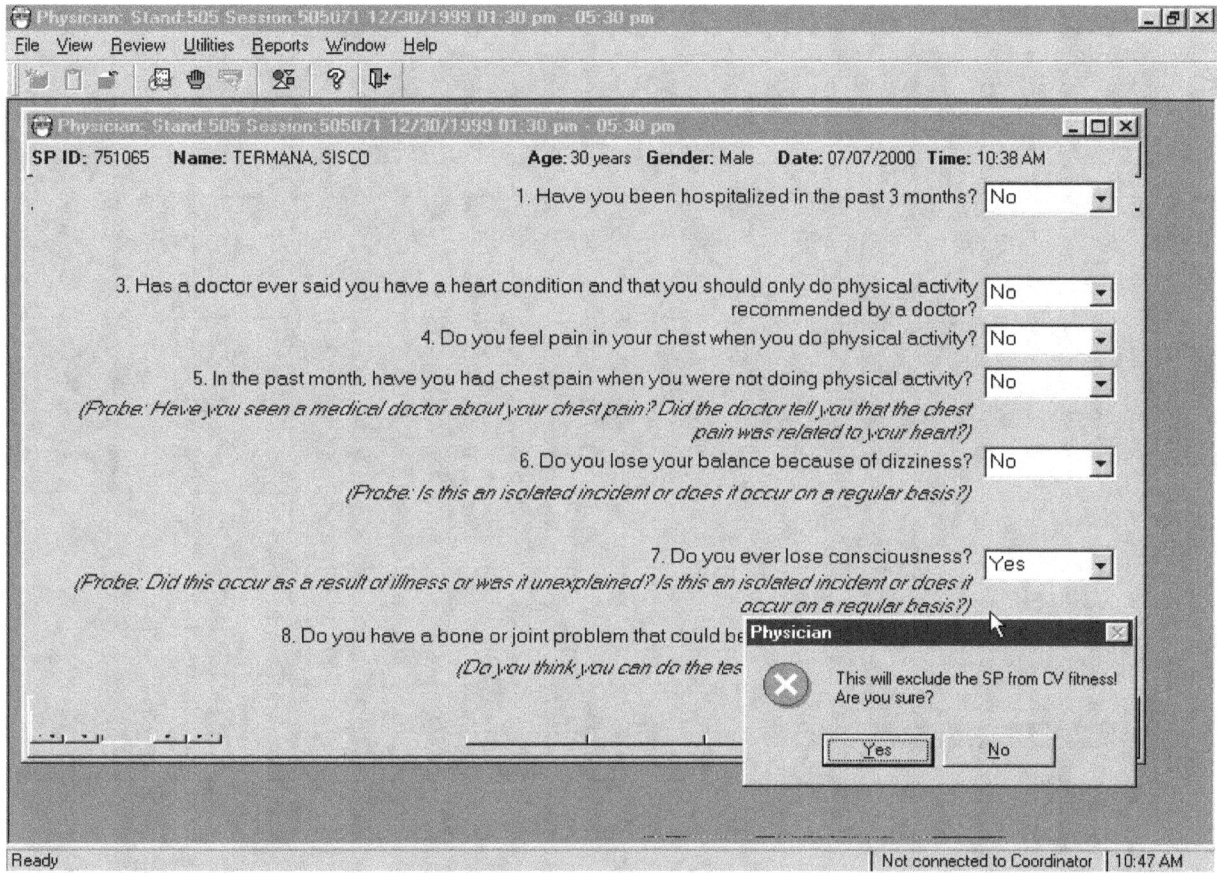

- Ask question 7: "Do you ever lose consciousness?"

- If the SP does not know how to respond to this question, ask the following probe:

  - Probe: "Did this occur as a result of illness or was it unexplained?"

  - Probe: "Is this an isolated incident or does it occur on a regular basis?"

- Use the probes only when necessary. The key point to this probe is to determine whether this is a regular occurrence and whether or not it was unexplained.

- If the response to this question is "No," proceed to the next question.

- If the response is "Yes" or "Don't Know," the SP is excluded from the CV Fitness examination and the remaining questions are disabled.

- A message is displayed: "This will exclude the SP from CV Fitness! Are you sure?" If the response was correct, click "Yes" to the message.

- The CV Exclusion status defaults to "Complete" and the CV Fitness component status defaults to "Not Done" with the comment "Safety Exclusion."

Exhibit 4-51. CV safety exclusion question: Bone/joint problem

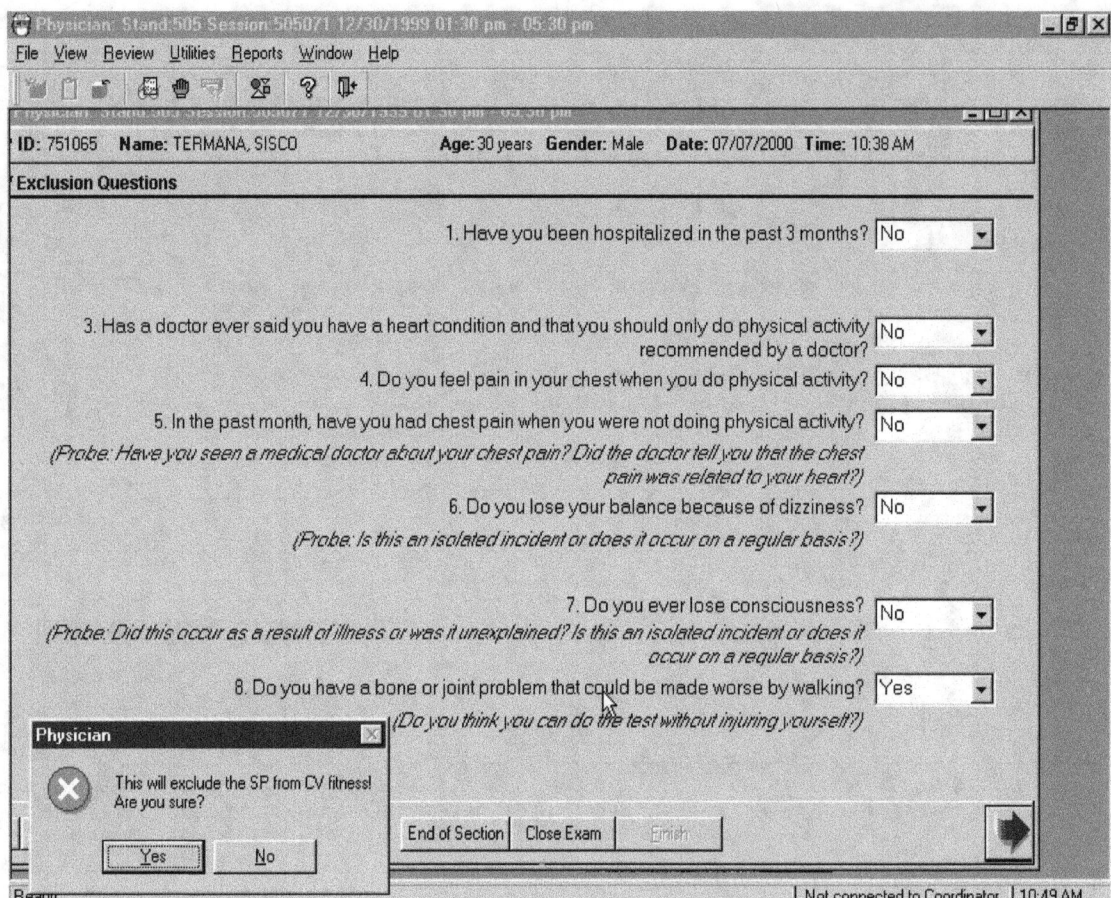

- Ask question 8: "Do you have a bone or joint problem that could be made worse by walking?"

- If the SP does not know how to respond to this question, ask the following probe:

  - Probe: "Do you think you can do the test without injuring yourself."

- Use the probes only when necessary. The key point to this probe is to determine whether this is a regular occurrence and whether or not it was unexplained.

- If the response to this question is "No," proceed to the next question.

- If the response is "Yes" or "Don't Know," the SP is excluded from the CV Fitness examination and the remaining questions are disabled.

- A message is displayed: "This will exclude the SP from CV Fitness! Are you sure?" If the response was correct, click "Yes" to the message.

- The CV Exclusion status defaults to "Complete" and the CV Fitness component status defaults to "Not Done" with the comment "Safety Exclusion."

Exhibit 4-52. CV safety exclusion questions: Prescription medications

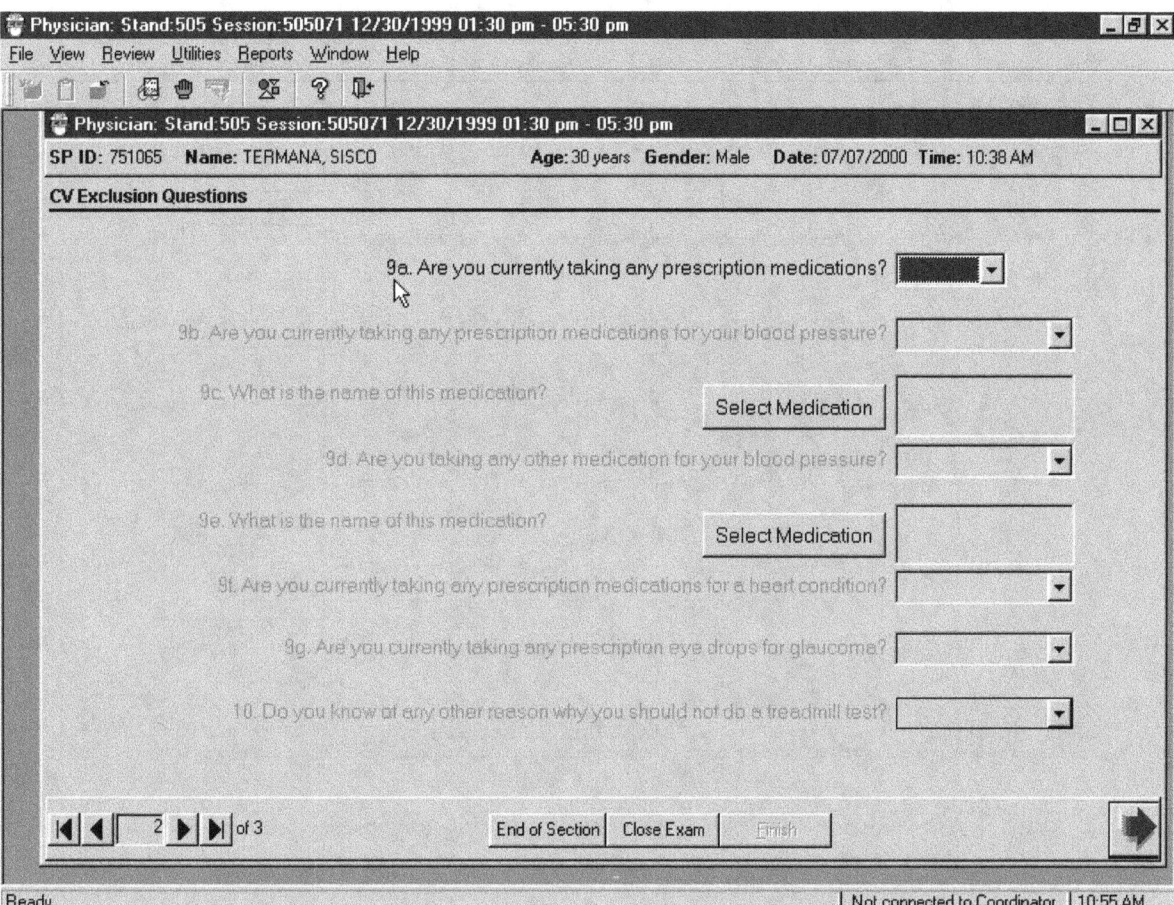

- Ask question 9A. "Are you currently taking any prescription medications?"

- If the response to this question is "No," proceed to Question 10.

- If the response is "Yes," go to Question 9B.

- If the response is "Don't Know," the SP is excluded from the CV Fitness examination and the remaining questions are disabled.

- A message is displayed: "This will exclude the SP from CV Fitness! Are you sure?" If the response was correct, click "Yes" to the message.

- The CV Exclusion status defaults to "Complete" and the CV Fitness component status defaults to "Not Done" with the comment "Safety Exclusion."

Exhibit 4-53. CV safety exclusion questions (prescription medications)

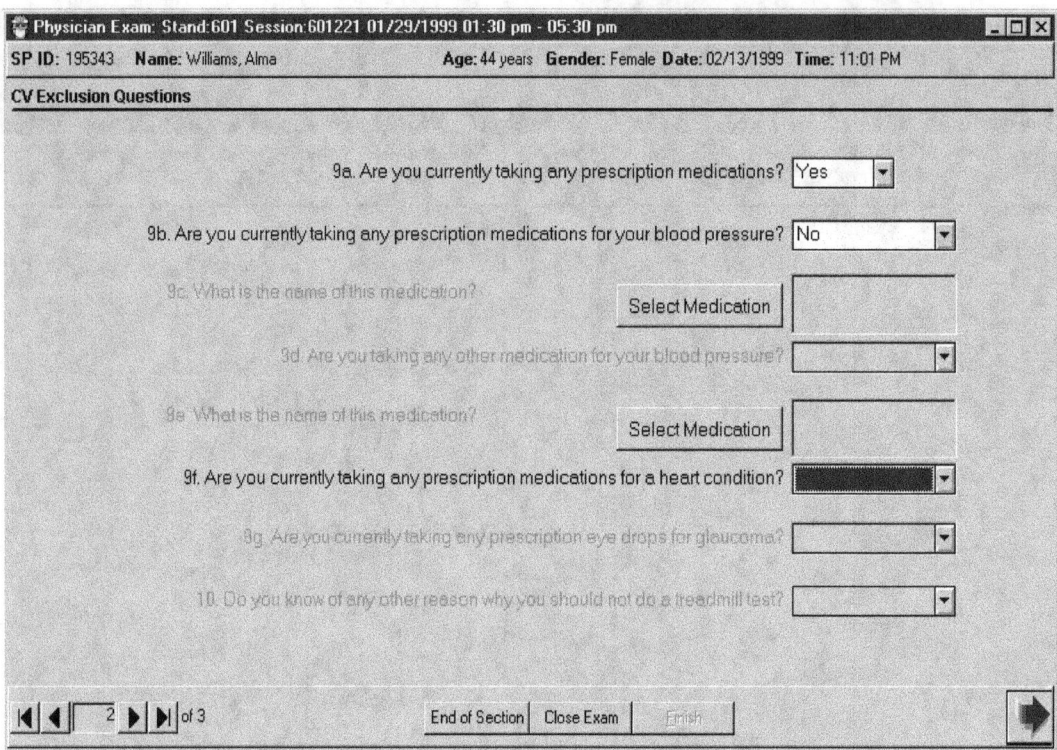

- Ask question 9b: "Are you currently taking any prescription medications for your blood pressure?"

- If the response to this question is "No," proceed to Question 9f.

- If the response is "Yes," go to Question 9c.

- If the response to 9b is "Don't Know," the SP is excluded from the CV Fitness examination and the remaining questions are disabled.

- A message is displayed: "This will exclude the SP from CV Fitness! Are you sure?" If the response was correct, click "Yes" to the message.

- The CV Exclusion status defaults to "Complete" and the CV Fitness component status defaults to "Not Done" with the comment "Safety Exclusion."

Exhibit 4-54. CV safety exclusion questions: Select medications

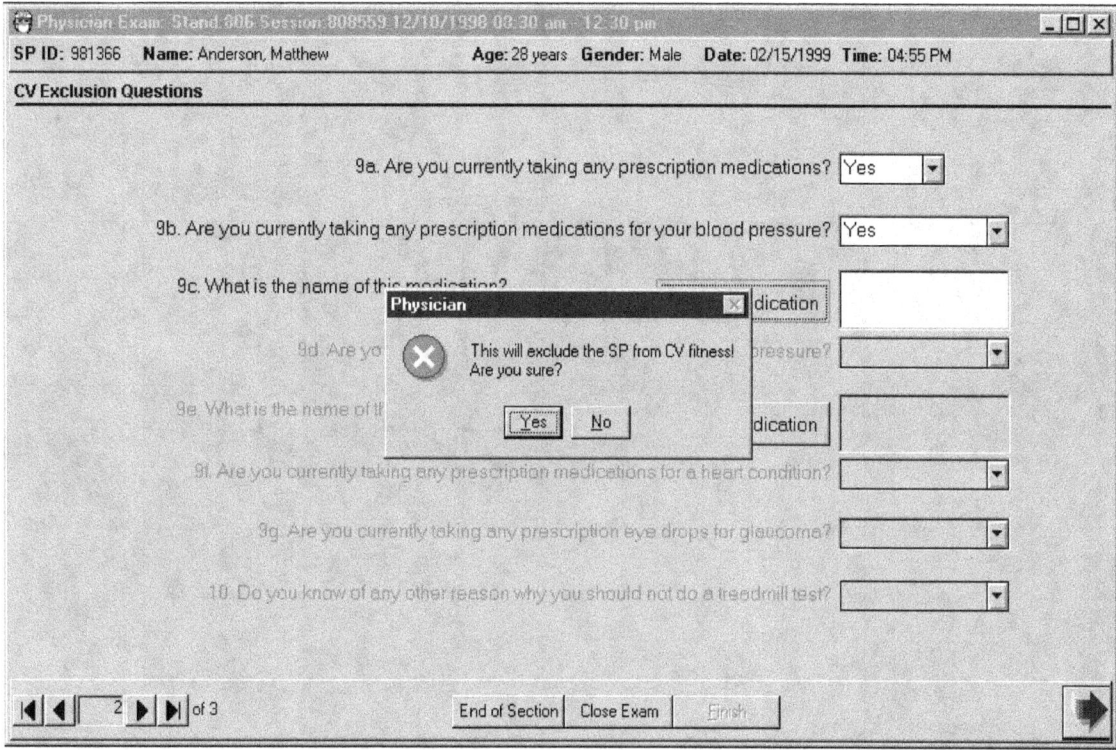

- If the response to 9b is "Don't Know," the SP is excluded from the CV Fitness examination and the remaining questions are disabled.

- A message is displayed: "This will exclude the SP from CV Fitness! Are you sure?" If the response was correct, click "Yes" to the message.

- The CV Exclusion status defaults to "Complete" and the CV Fitness component status defaults to "Not Done" with the comment "Safety Exclusion."

- If the response to 9b is "Yes," go to Question 9c.

- Question 9c: "What is the name of your medications?"

- On 9c, click on "Select Medication."

Exhibit 4-55. CV safety exclusion questions: Select medication box

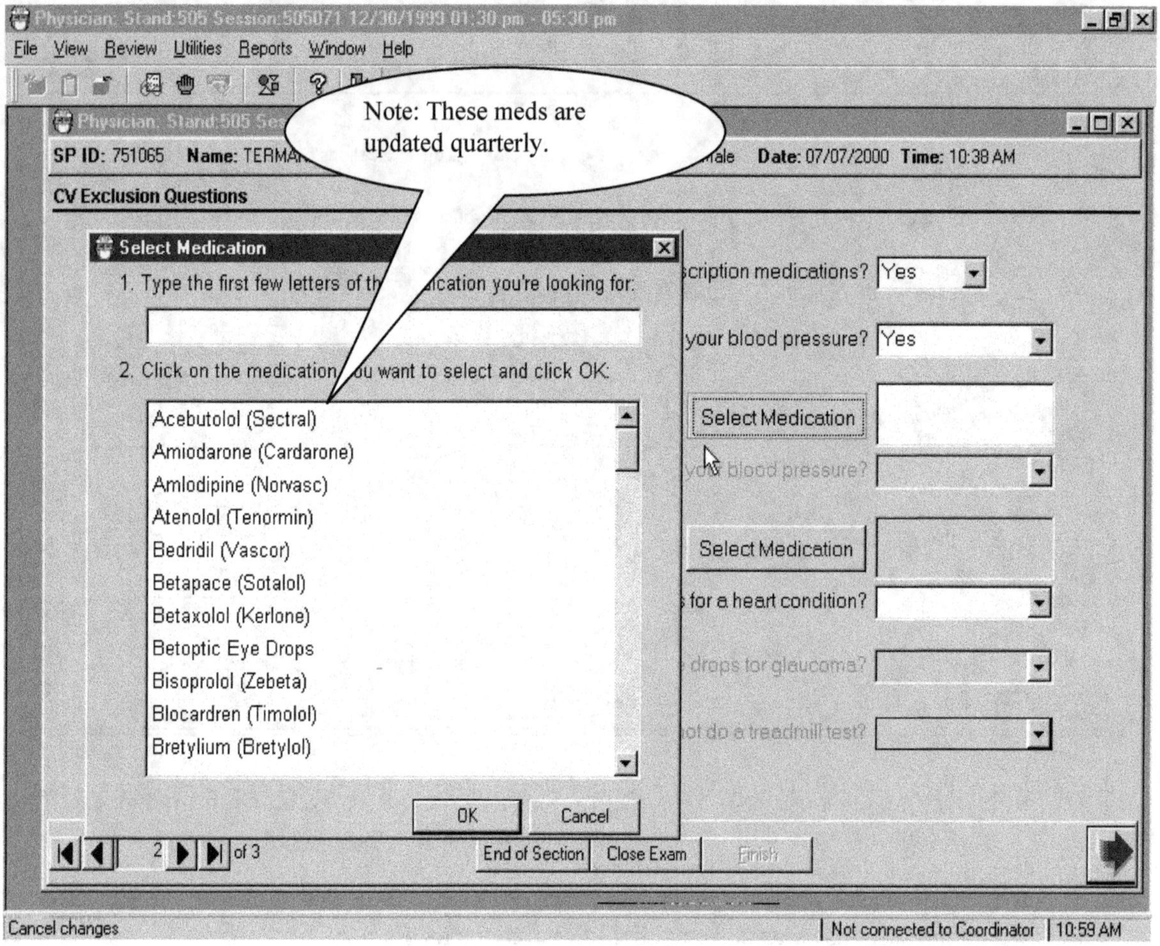

- When "select medication" is clicked, a pop-up box with the exclusion medications is displayed.

- Type in the name of the medication in the first field in the box or scroll through the list to find the name(s) of medications the SP is taking.

- Highlight the name of the medication and select OK to enter the name of the medication in the medication name field.

- If the medication is on the exclusion list, the rest of the questions are disabled.

- The SP is excluded from the CV Fitness Examination.

Exhibit 4-56. CV safety exclusion questions: Medications-exclusion warning

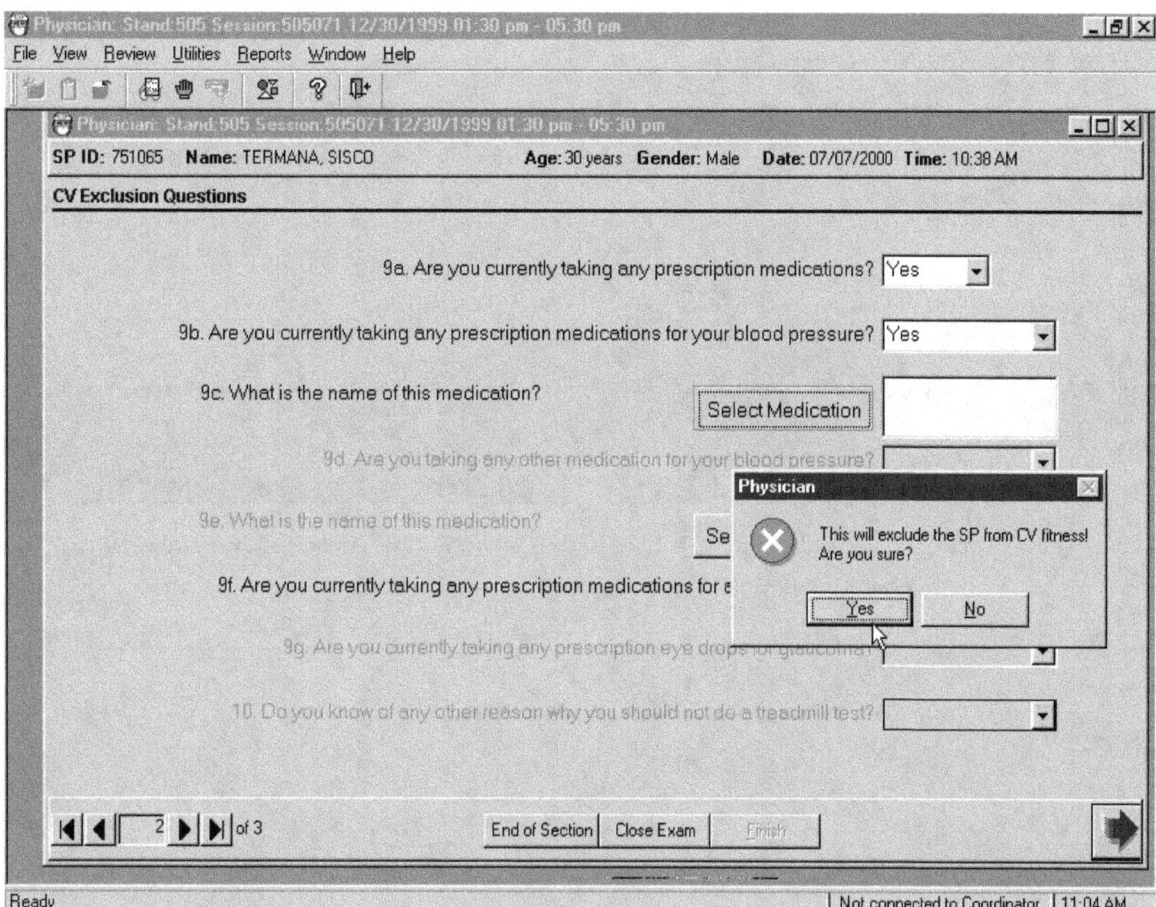

- The selected medications are displayed in the medication field.

- When a medication is selected from the pop-up box of exclusion medications, the SP is excluded for the CV Fitness examination.

- A warning message is displayed: "This will exclude SP from CV Fitness! Are you sure?"

- If the response was correct, click "Yes" to this message.

- Select the Next button to advance to the next screen.

Exhibit 4-57. CV safety exclusion questions: Exclusion confirmation

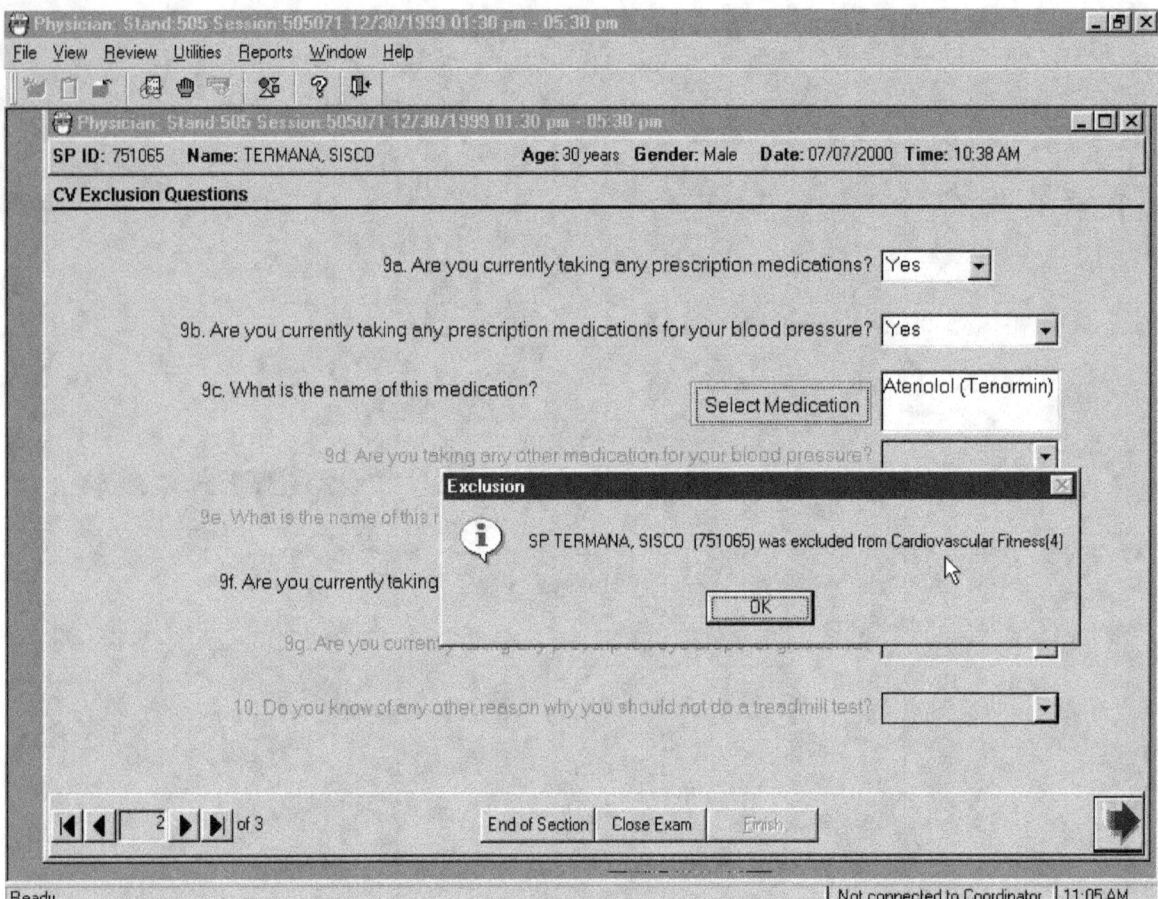

- When the Next button is pressed to advance to the next screen, a confirmation message is displayed: "SP <Name, ID> was excluded from Cardiovascular Fitness."

- The SP is excluded from the CV Fitness test and from the remainder of the CV exclusion questions.

- The remaining questions are disabled.

Exhibit 4-58. CV safety exclusion questions: Non-exclusion medications

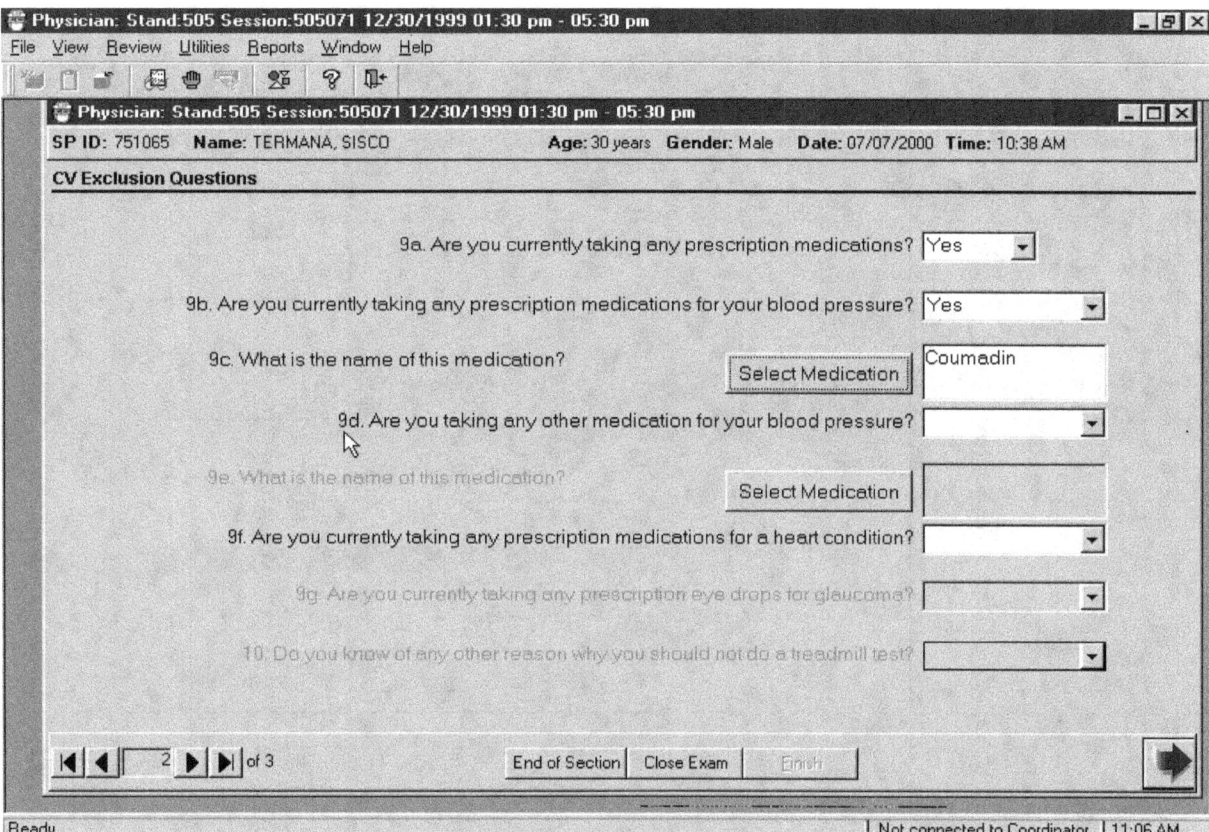

- If the medication listed in 9c is not on the exclusion list, go to Question 9d.

- Question 9d: "Are you taking any other medications for your blood pressure?"

- If the response is "Don't Know," the SP is excluded from CV Fitness.

- If the response is yes, go to 9d.

- If the response is "No," continue with the remaining questions.

Exhibit 4-59. CV safety exclusion questions: Second medication

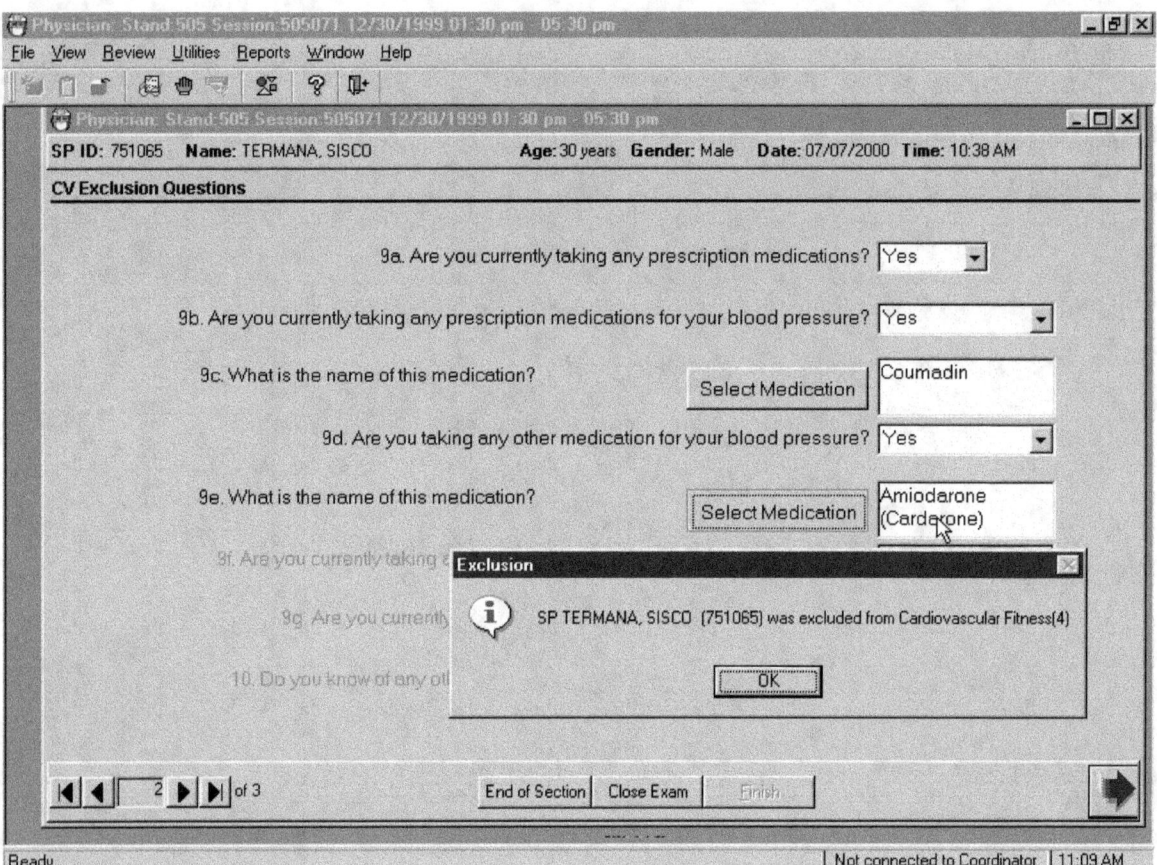

- Question 9d: "What is the name of this medication?"

- Press "Select Medication" and type the name of the medication or select the medication from the list. If the medication is on the exclusion list, the rest of the questions are disabled.

- The SP is excluded from the CV Fitness Examination.

- If the response to 9d is "No," continue with the remaining questions.

Exhibit 4-60. CV safety exclusion questions: Medications for heart condition

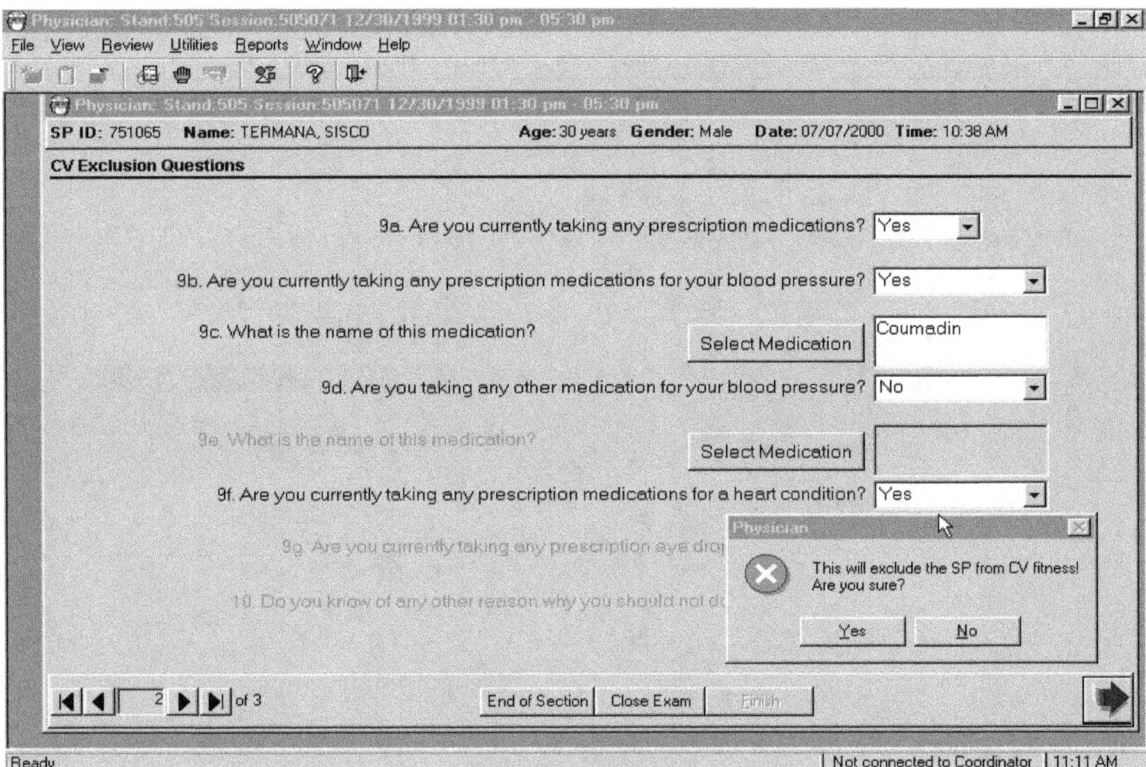

- Ask Question 9f: "Are you currently taking any prescription medications for a heart condition?"

- If the response to this question is "No," proceed to Question 10.

- If the response is "Yes" or "Don't Know," the SP is excluded from the CV Fitness examination and the remaining questions are disabled.

- A message is displayed: "This will exclude the SP from CV Fitness! Are you sure?" If the response was correct, click "Yes" to the message.

- The CV Exclusion status defaults to "Complete" and the CV Fitness component status defaults to "Not Done" with the comment "Safety Exclusion."

Exhibit 4-61. CV safety exclusion questions: Medications for glaucoma

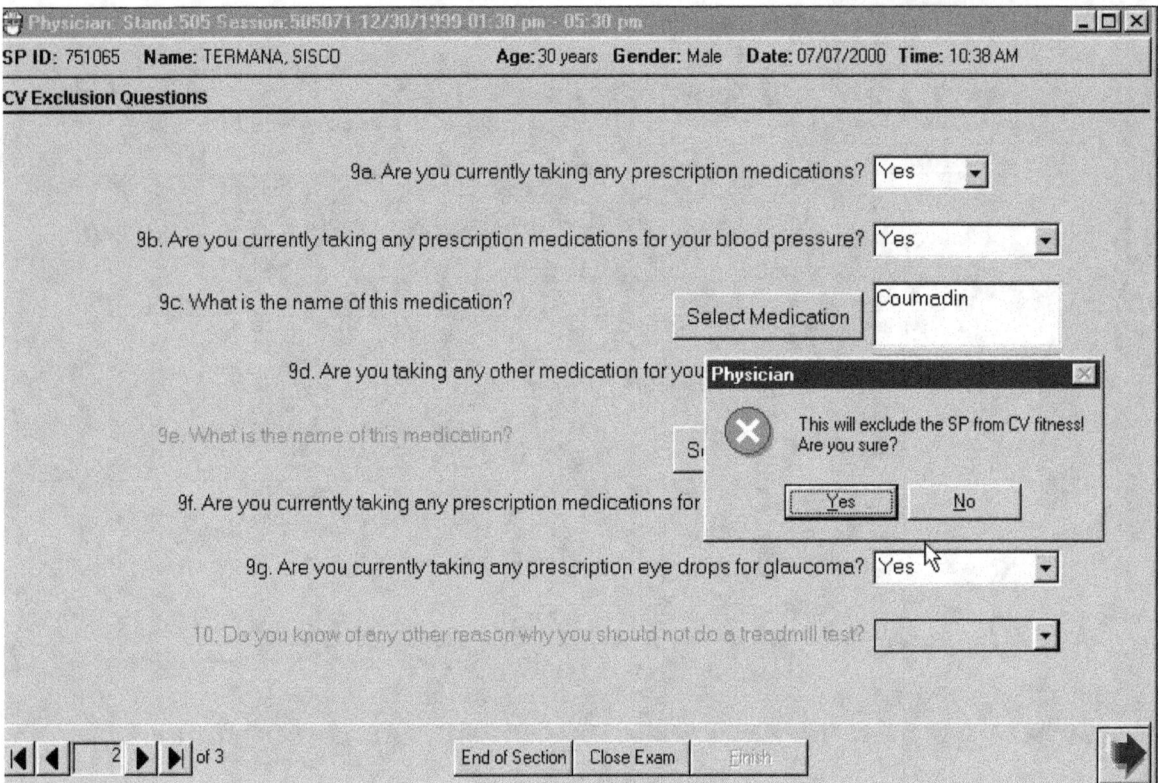

- Ask Question 9g: "Are you currently taking any prescription medications for glaucoma?"

- If the response to this question is "No," proceed to Question 10.

- If the response is "Yes" or "Don't Know," the SP is excluded from the CV Fitness examination and the remaining questions are disabled.

- A message is displayed: "This will exclude the SP from CV Fitness! Are you sure?" If the response was correct, click "Yes" to the message.

- The CV Exclusion status defaults to "Complete" and the CV Fitness component status defaults to "Not Done" with the comment "Safety Exclusion."

Exhibit 4-62. CV safety exclusion questions: Other reasons

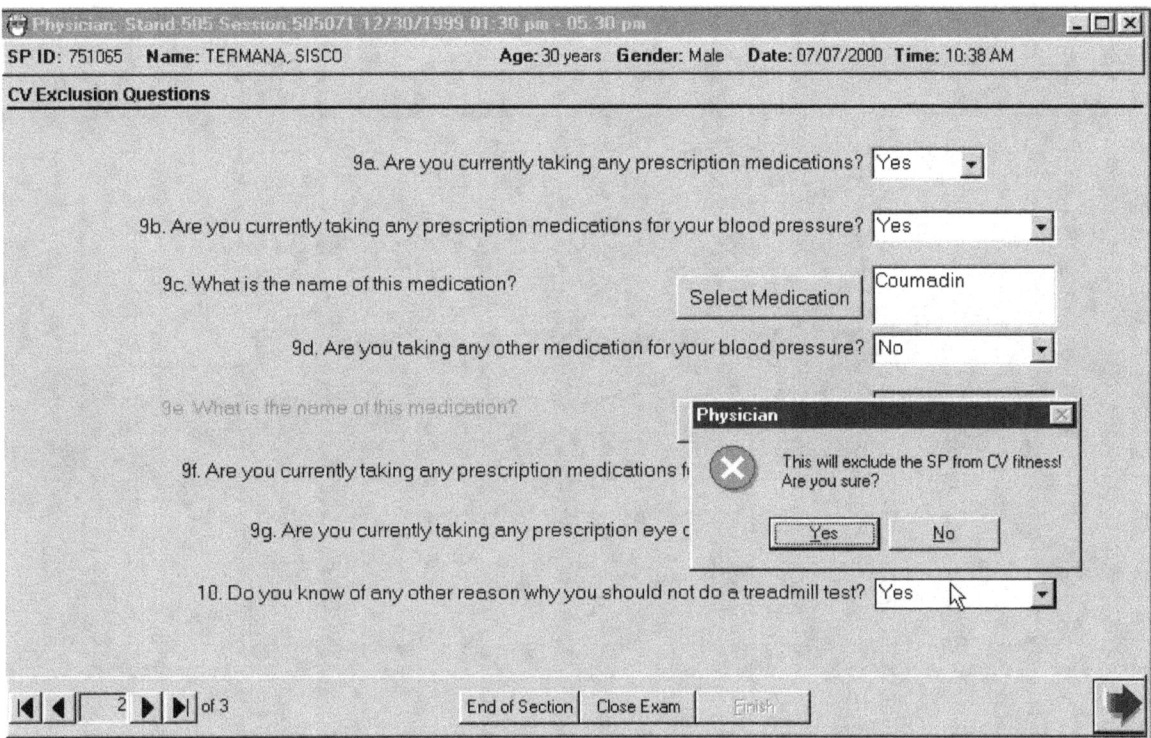

- Ask Question 10: "Is there any other reason why you should not do a treadmill test?"

- If the response to this question is "No," select the Next button to advance to the next screen.

- If the response is "Yes" or "Don't Know," the SP is excluded from the CV Fitness examination and the remaining questions are disabled.

- A message is displayed: "This will exclude the SP from CV Fitness! Are you sure?" If the response was correct, click "Yes" to the message.

- The CV exclusion status defaults to "Complete" and the CV Fitness component status defaults to "Not Done" with the comment "Safety Exclusion."

Exhibit 4-63. CV safety exclusion questions: Exclusion confirmation

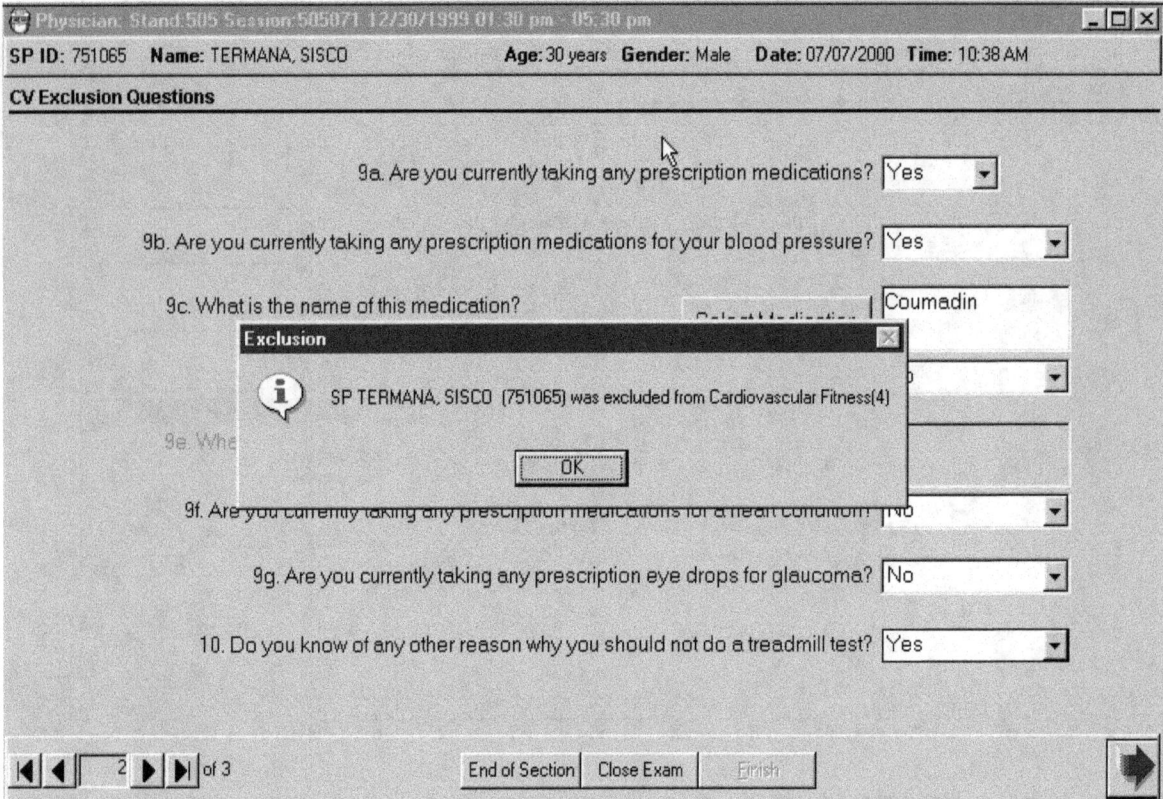

- When "Yes" is selected for the exclusion questions, a message is displayed to warn the examiner that this response will exclude the SP from CV Fitness. The message will ask if the examiner is sure. This message reads: "This response will exclude the SP from CV Fitness! Are you sure?" If the response was correct, the examiner clicks on "Yes." See above figures for examination.

- If the examiner clicks "Yes" to this message, the system will then exclude the SP from CV Fitness and will display a confirmation message: "SP <name, ID> was excluded form CV Fitness."

- Click OK to this message and proceed to the CV exclusion status.

4.7.13   CV Exclusion Status

Exhibit 4-64. CV Fitness exclusion completion status

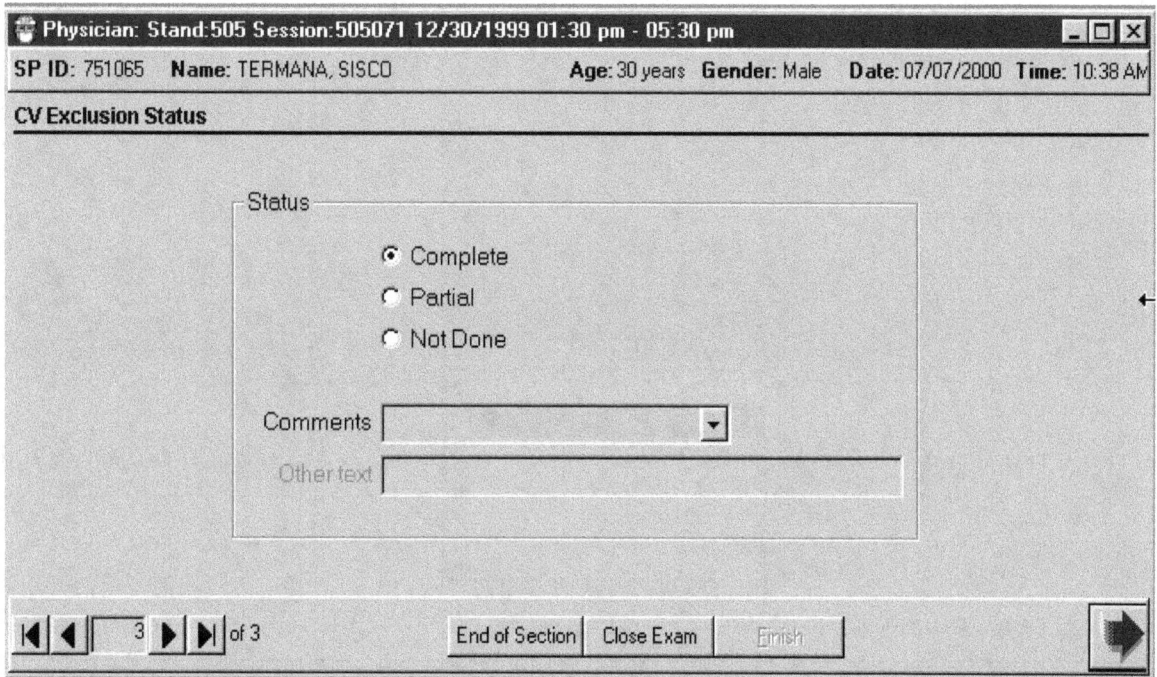

- If all CV exclusion questions are answered, the CV exclusion status defaults to "Complete."

- When the status is "Complete," no comment is required or allowed. The comment field is disabled.

Exhibit 4-65. CV exclusion status: Comments 1

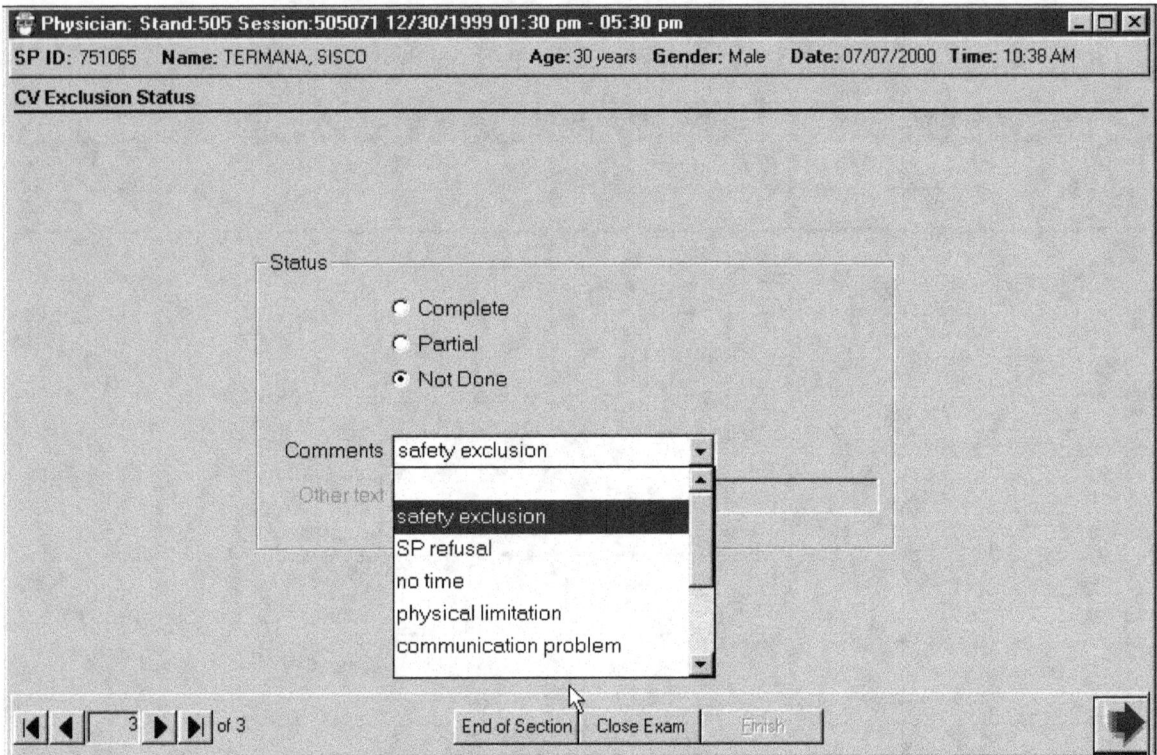

- If an SP is excluded from CV Fitness by a response from one of the CV exclusion questions, the CV exclusion status defaults to "Not Done" with the comment "Safety Exclusion" or "Physical Limitation" depending on the question.

- The CV Fitness component status will also be set to "Not Done" with the same comment.

- The "safety exclusion" comment is the default when the exclusion is initiated from this question.

Exhibit 4-66. CV exclusion status: Comments 2

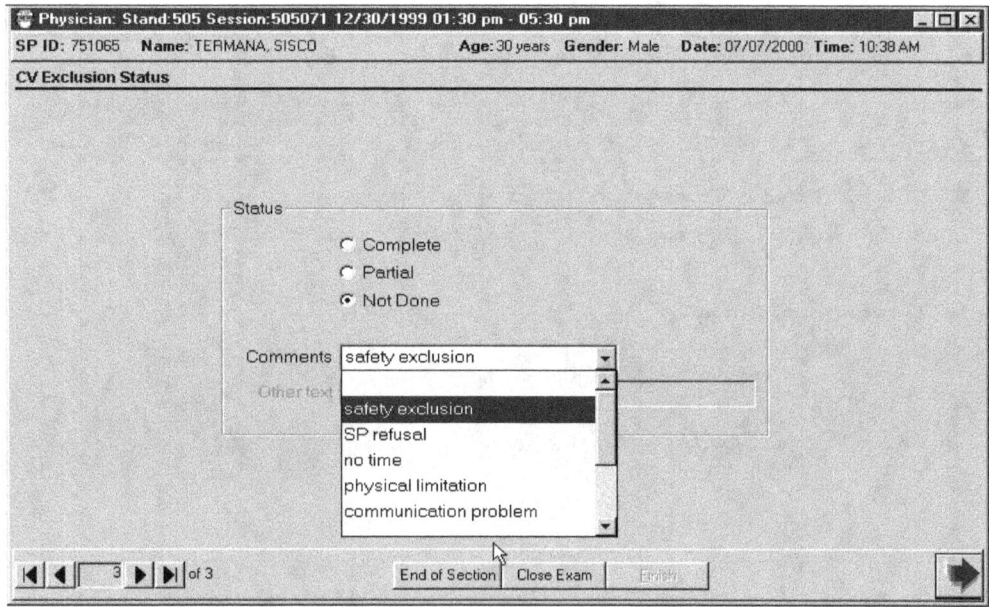

- If one or more data points are missing from the physician examination, ISIS defaults the status to "Partial." If no data points are collected, ISIS defaults the status to "Not Done."

- When the status is "Partial" or "Not Done" for other than the default safety exclusion, a comment must be entered in the Comment field. Guidelines for the comment selection option follow:

  Safety Exclusion: The SP is excluded from the exam due to a medical condition prohibiting collection of data. This would rarely be used for the physician component, but an example would be for blood pressure where there may be a shunt in each arm prohibiting taking the BP.

  SP Refusal: The SP refuses to complete the physician examination.

  No Time: There was not sufficient time in the MEC session to complete the examination. This would be unusual for the physician component. It could happen when the SP arrives late to the exam center, or when other SPs take longer than the usual time for the exam, or other unusual events on the MEC where the physician is involved at the expense of SP exams.

  Physical Limitation: This would be very rare, but could happen if the SP could not physically occupy the physician examination room.

  Communication Problem: This comment is selected when the physician and the SP are not able to communicate adequately to assure accurate data are collected. Examples could be language differences without an adequate interpreter, mental retardation to the point of lack of understanding, and no proxy.

4.7.14   STD and HIV Discussion of Tests and Obtaining Results

Exhibit 4-67. STD for SPs 14-17 years old

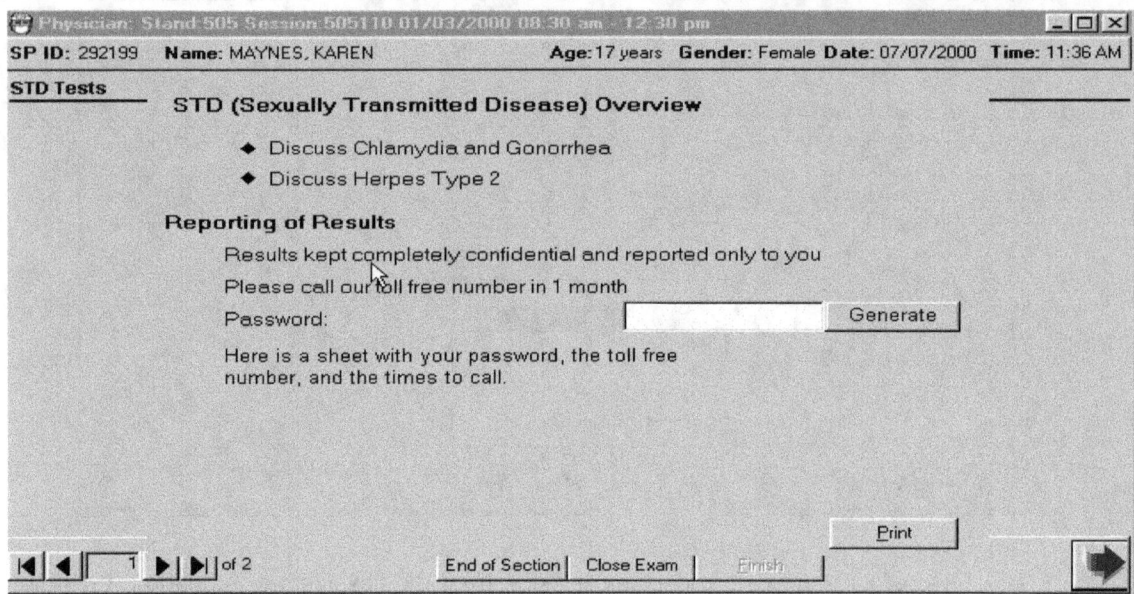

- If the SP is 14-17 years of age, the physician discusses the method for the SP to receive STD results.

- The physician asks the SP to give a password to use when calling to get their test results. If the SP cannot think of a password, the physician will give the SP a password by clicking on generate. The system will generate a password and display it in the password field.

- Other SP information on minors is given to the parents at the time of checkout from the MEC. Due to the sensitive and confidential nature of STD results, the information reports for 14- to 17-year-olds are printed in the physician's room. These test results are given only to the SP.

- Click on the "Print" button to print the information form for the SP. After discussing the mechanism for obtaining test results, put the STD and HIV information form in a sealed envelope.

- On the envelope, write the number on the SP's examination gown (the number corresponding to the number on the basket containing the SP's clothes). Put the envelope in your mailbox or give it directly to the assistant coordinator, who will put the envelope in the basket corresponding to the number on the envelope.

Exhibit 4-68. STD and HIV for SPs 18-39 years old

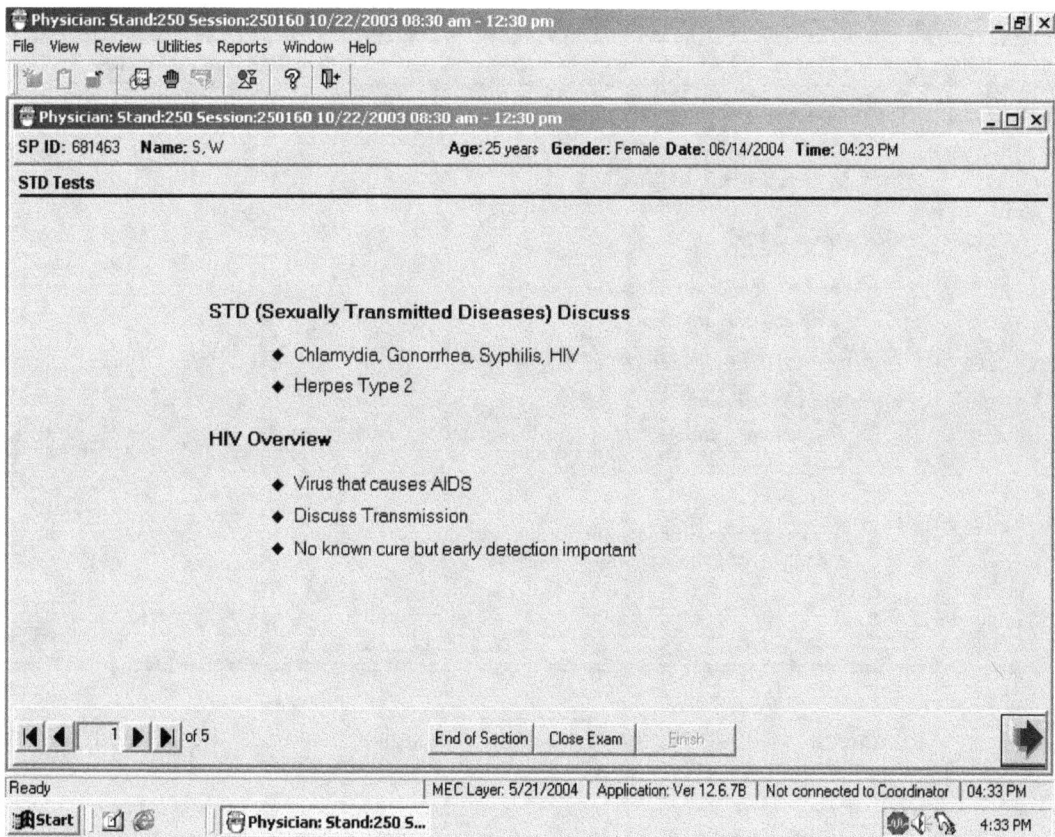

Exhibit 4-68. STD and HIV for SPs 18-39 years old

- If the SP is 18-39 years of age, the physician discusses the method for the SP to receive results for STD and HIV.

- The physician asks the SP to give a password to use when calling to get the test results.

- If the SP cannot think of a password, the physician give the SP a password by clicking on generate.

- The system generates a password and displays it in the password field.

- The SP is given a print out during MEC checkout with the information needed to call for test results. The information print out form is printed at the coordinator station and placed with the SP's information packet.

Exhibit 4-69. STD and HIV for SPs 40-49 years old

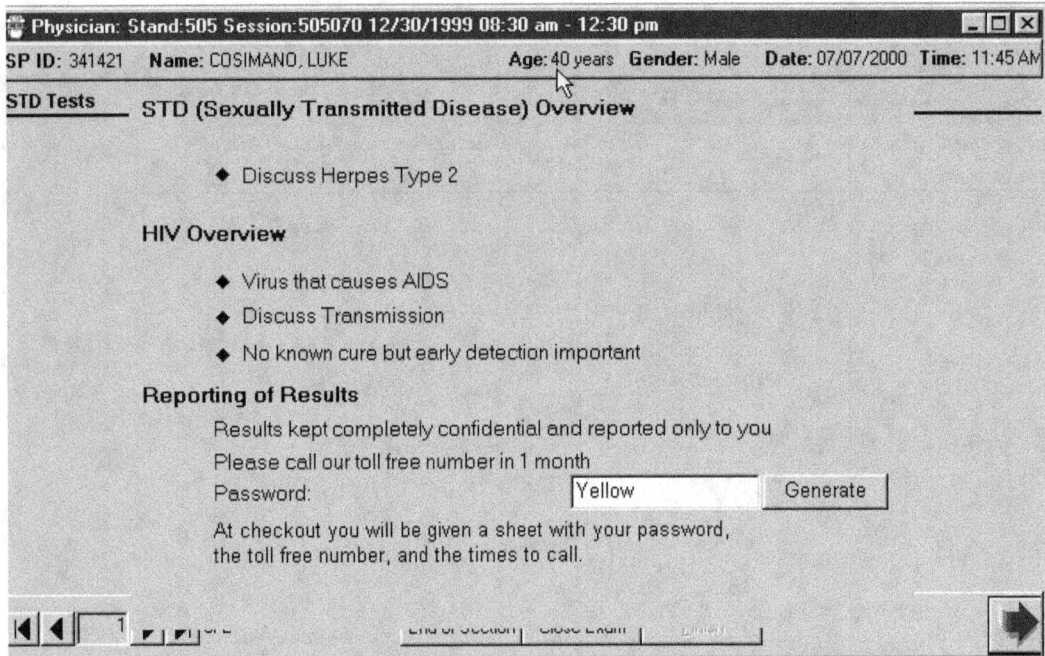

- If the SP is 40-49 years of age, the physician discusses the method for the SP to receive STD and HIV results.

- The physician asks the SP to give a password to use when calling to get test results.

- If the SP cannot think of a password, the physician will give the SP a password by clicking on generate.

- The system generates a password and displays it in the password field.

- The SP is given a print out at the time of MEC checkout with the information needed to call for test results. This information print out is printed at the coordinator station and placed with the SP's information packet.

Exhibit 4-70. Utilities menu for informed consent exclusions

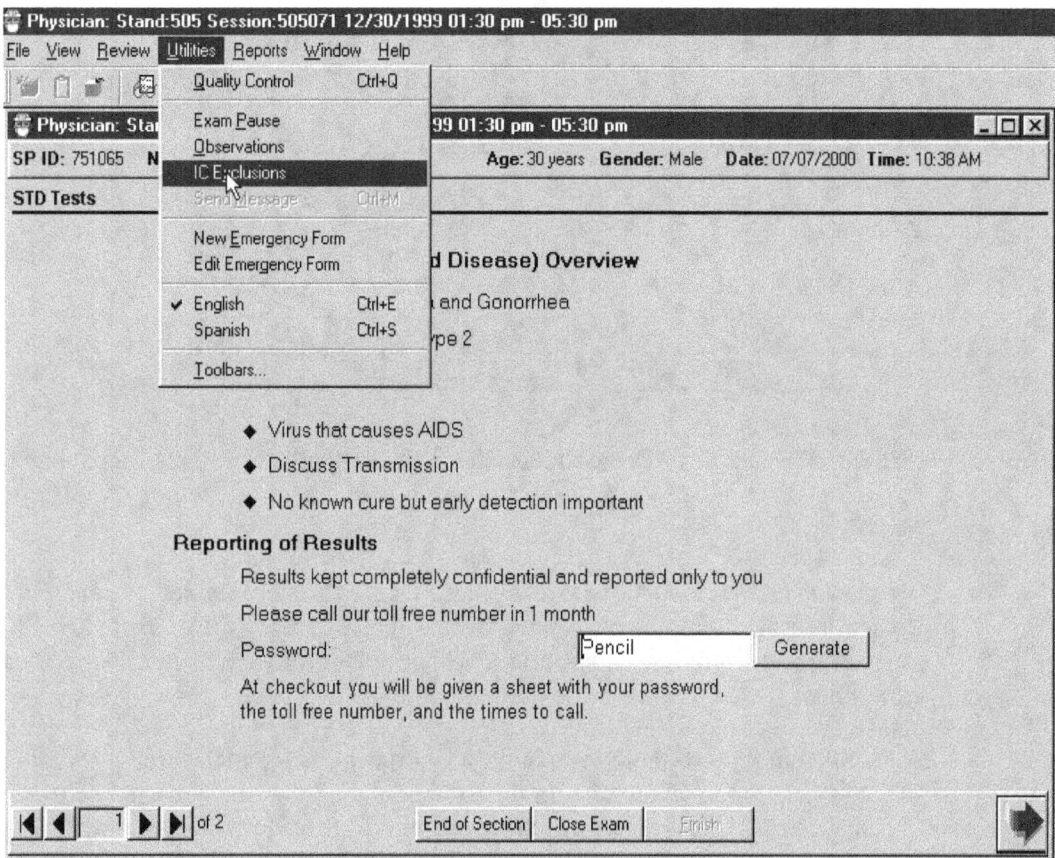

- SP's may refuse the STD and/or the HIV tests. They may do this at the Household Interview or in the phlebotomy room.

- They may also mention this to the physician and the SP can be excluded for STD and or HIV during the Physician's Examination.

- If the SP mentions that they want to refuse these tests, the physician advances to the "Utilities" menu from the toolbar and select "I/C Exclusions" (Informed Consent exclusions).

Exhibit 4-71. STD and HIV – Informed consent exclusion

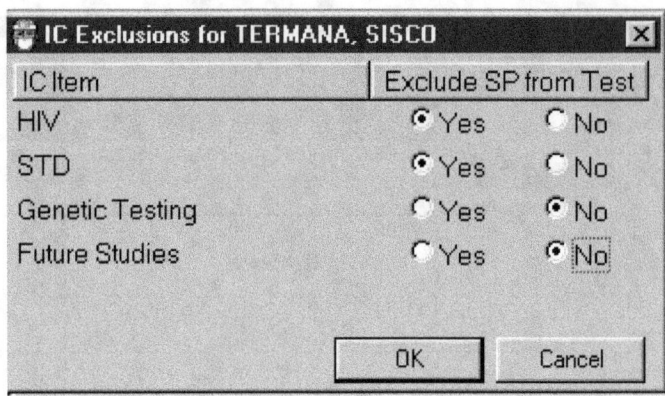

- Check HIV and/or STD to exclude the SP from these tests. This sends a message to the phlebotomy and laboratory examination component to exclude the SP from these tests.

- If the SP had previously agreed to these tests and later decided to refuse these test after discussion with the physician, the specimens can be still be excluded. Check one or both examinations as appropriate. This sends a message to the lab to discard the specimens.

- The SP could refuse these tests initially and later change their mind after talking with the physician or phlebotomist. In this situation, the informed consent exclusion should be unchecked. This will remove the exclusion for these tests in the laboratory.

Exhibit 4-72. SP refusal for STD and HIV testing

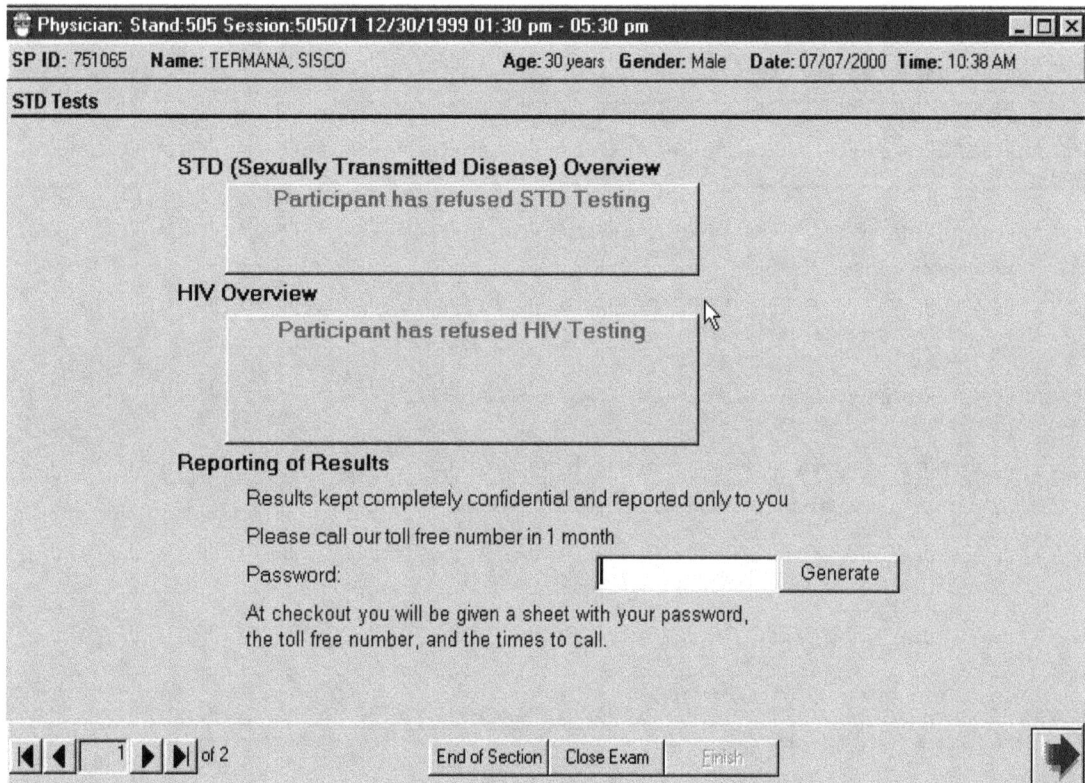

- If the SP refused to have STD and HIV testing either during the consent process or in the phlebotomy room, the screen in the physician's examination appears with a message over each section that was refused: "Participant has refused STD and HIV testing."

- If the SP refuses the testing it is not necessary to discuss the mechanism for getting results.

- It is not necessary to have the SP select a password.

- Select the Next button to go to the component status.

Exhibit 4-73. Password entry requirement for STD and HIV

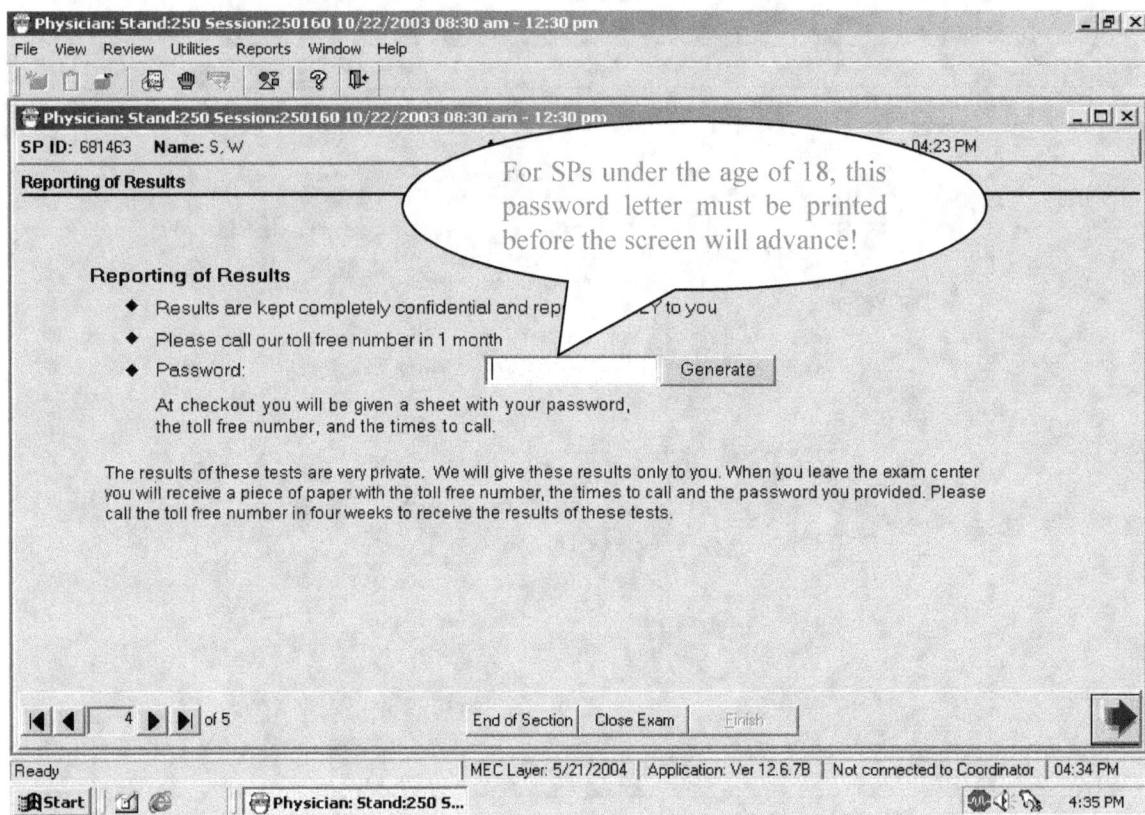

- If a password is not entered, a message is displayed: "Please enter the Password."

- Click OK to this message.

- Generate a password if one is needed.

- Select the Next button to go to the next screen.

Exhibit 4-74. STD and HIV test completion status

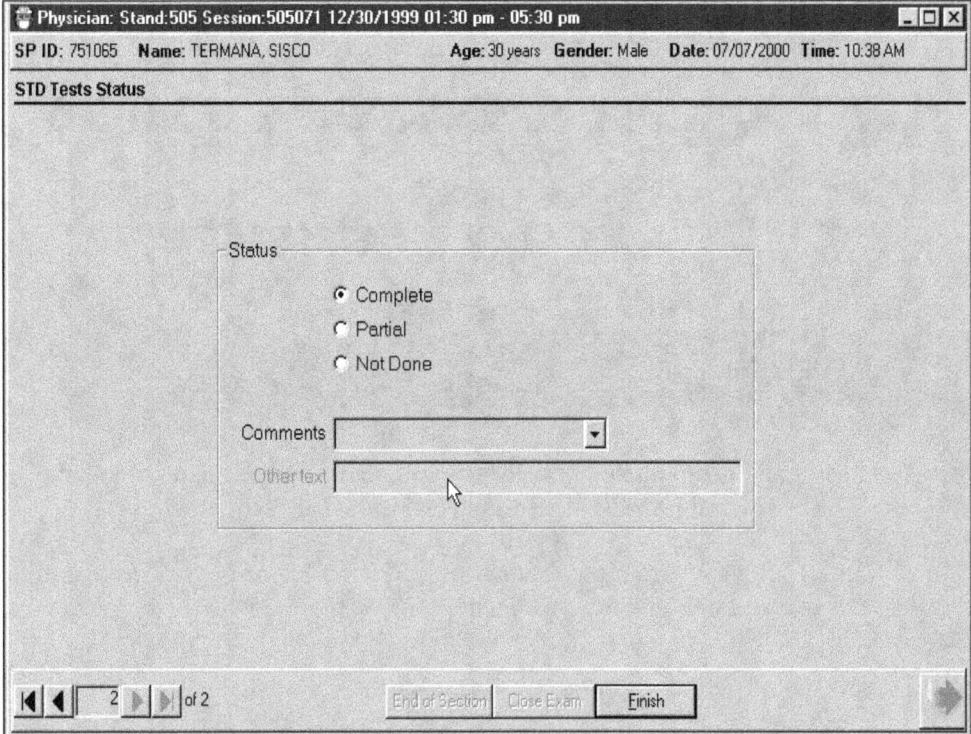

- The STD and HIV test completion status defaults to "Complete."

- Select "Finish" to close the examination.

4.7.15 Physician Look-up Table

Exhibit 4-75. Review menu for physician referral "look-up"

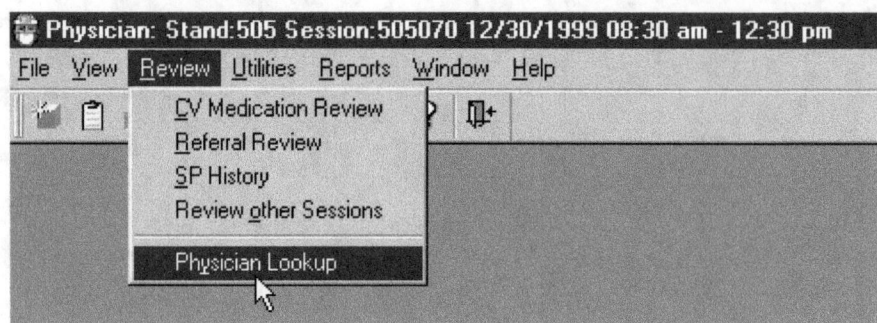

- Each stand is provided with a list of physician's and/or clinics who have agreed to see SP's on referral if the SP doesn't have a health care provider.

- Select "Review" from the toolbar to access the list of physicians and clinics. Choose "Physician Look-up" from the menu.

Exhibit 4-76. Physician/clinic "pick-up" box

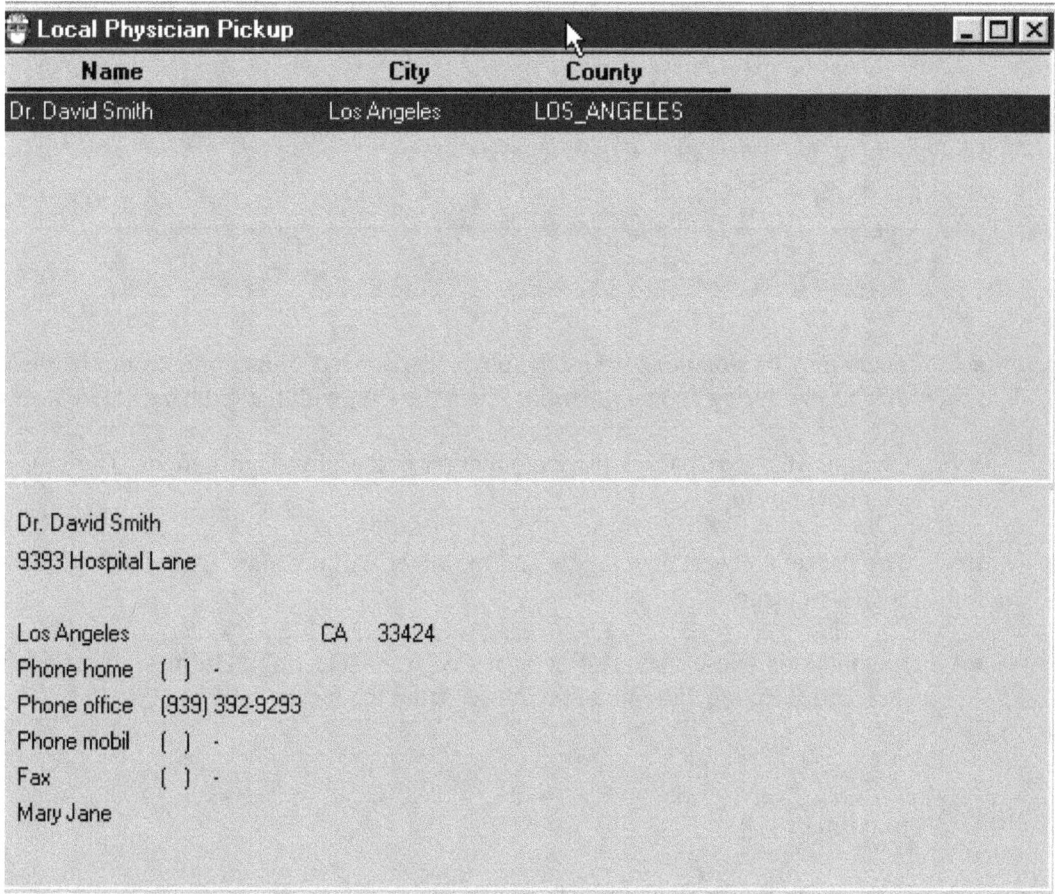

- The "Physician Pick-Up" box is displayed. Highlight the name of a physician or clinic.

- The complete address and phone numbers are listed in the lower part of the box.

4.7.16   Pausing an Examination

Exhibit 4-77. Pause an examination

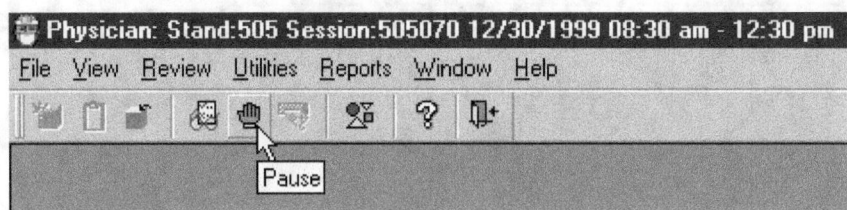

- There may be situations where the physician is needed in another room in the MEC. If this occurs during an examination, select the icon with the red hand (the Pause icon).

- Clicking this icon pauses the examination in the physician's room. The timer for the examination stops.

- The Pause icon acts as a toggle and the timer will not start again until the Pause icon is clicked again.

- Examination pause may also be accessed from selecting "Utilities" from the Toolbar and then selecting "Examination Pause" from the menu.

OMB Statement

Exhibit 4-78. Menu to select OMB statement

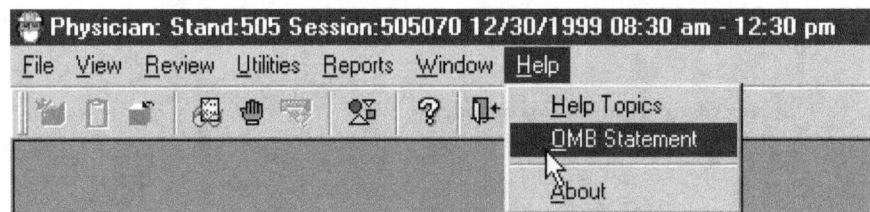

- The OMB statement is found under the Help menu on the toolbar. Choose Help, and then select OMB statement from the menu.

Exhibit 4-79. OMB statement

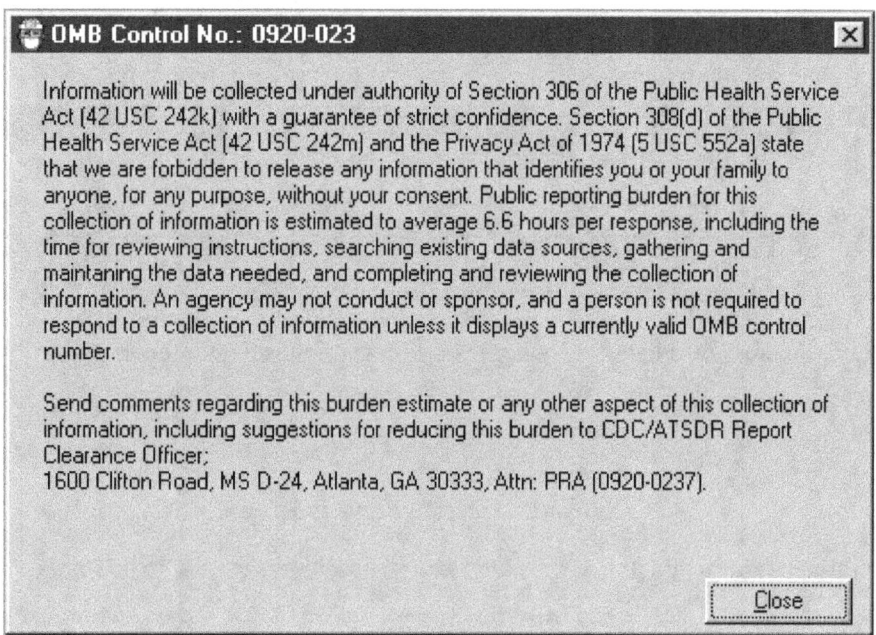

- The OMB statement is displayed. Click on "Close" to close this box.

4.7.17   Room Log

Exhibit 4-80. Menu for selecting room log

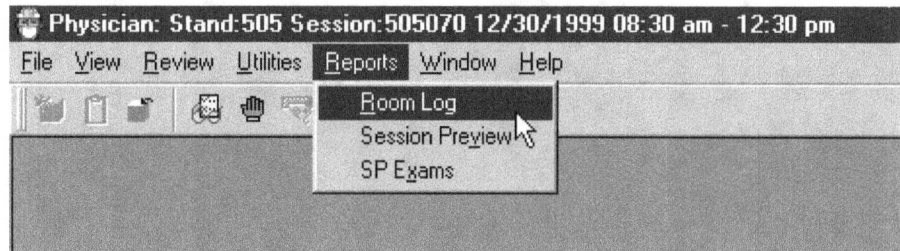

- The room log displays a list of the SP's who are eligible for this examination. All SP's are eligible for the Physician's Examination. The SP Examination Status report displays all SP's in the session along with the status and status comment.

- Choose "Reports" from the Toolbar and select "Room Log."

4.7.18   Session Preview

Exhibit 4-81. Session preview

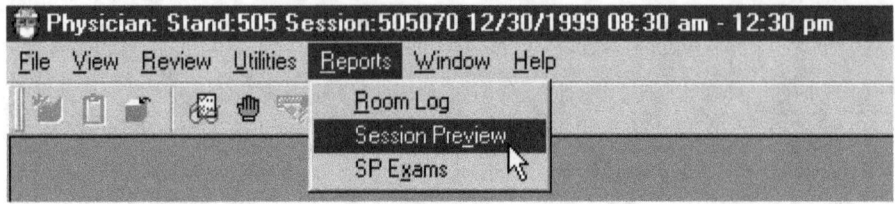

■   To preview a list of SP's in the current session, select "Reports" from the toolbar.

■   Select "Session Preview."

Exhibit 4-82. Session Preview Report

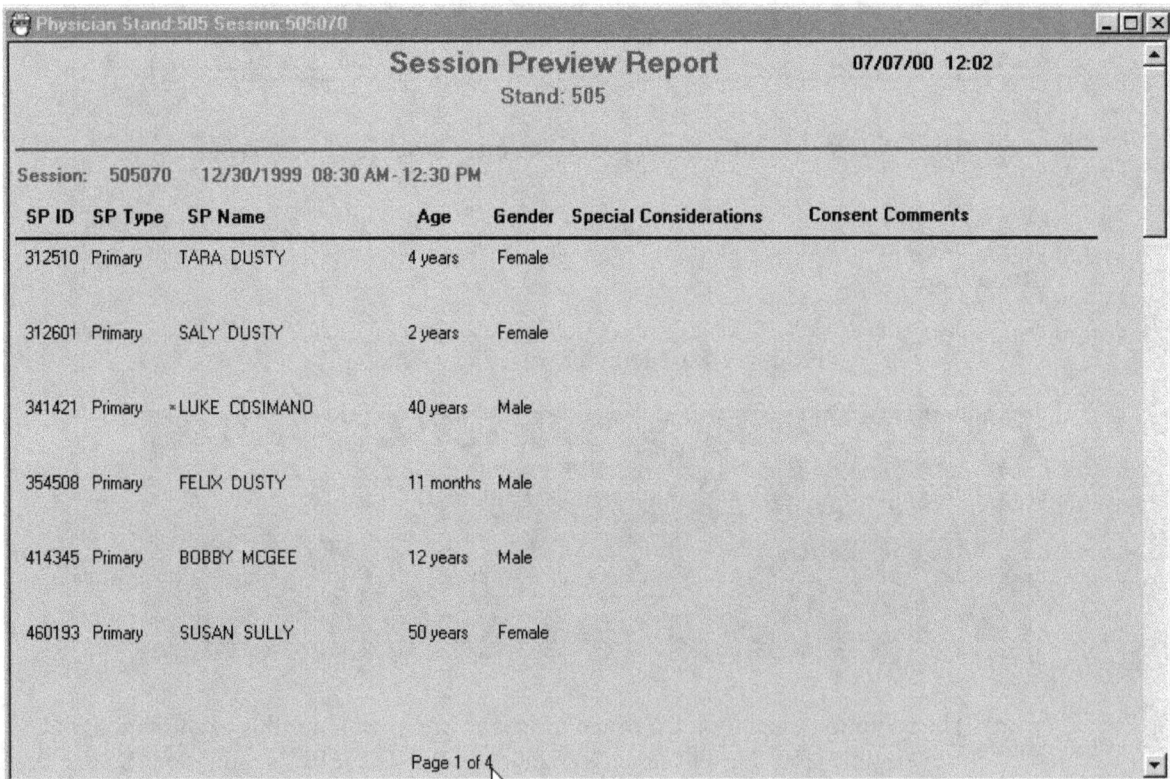

■   The "Session Preview Report" displays a list of SPs in the current session.

■   The ID, SP type, SP name, age, gender, special considerations, and consent comments are displayed.

■   This report provides information about special needs or consideration for each SP such as wheelchair bound, disabilities, and consent issues.

4.7.19   SP Examinations

Exhibit 4-83. SP examination

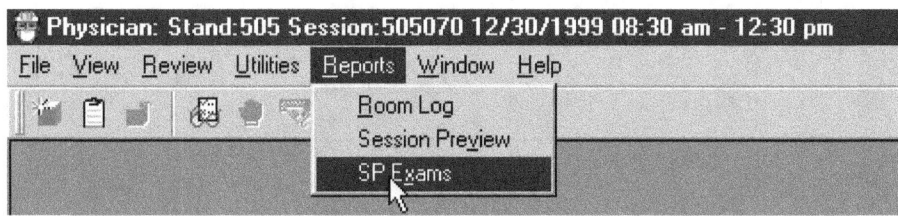

- To preview the status of the SP examinations in the current session, select "Reports" from the toolbar.

- Select "SP Examinations" from the menu.

Exhibit 4-84. SP Examination Status Report

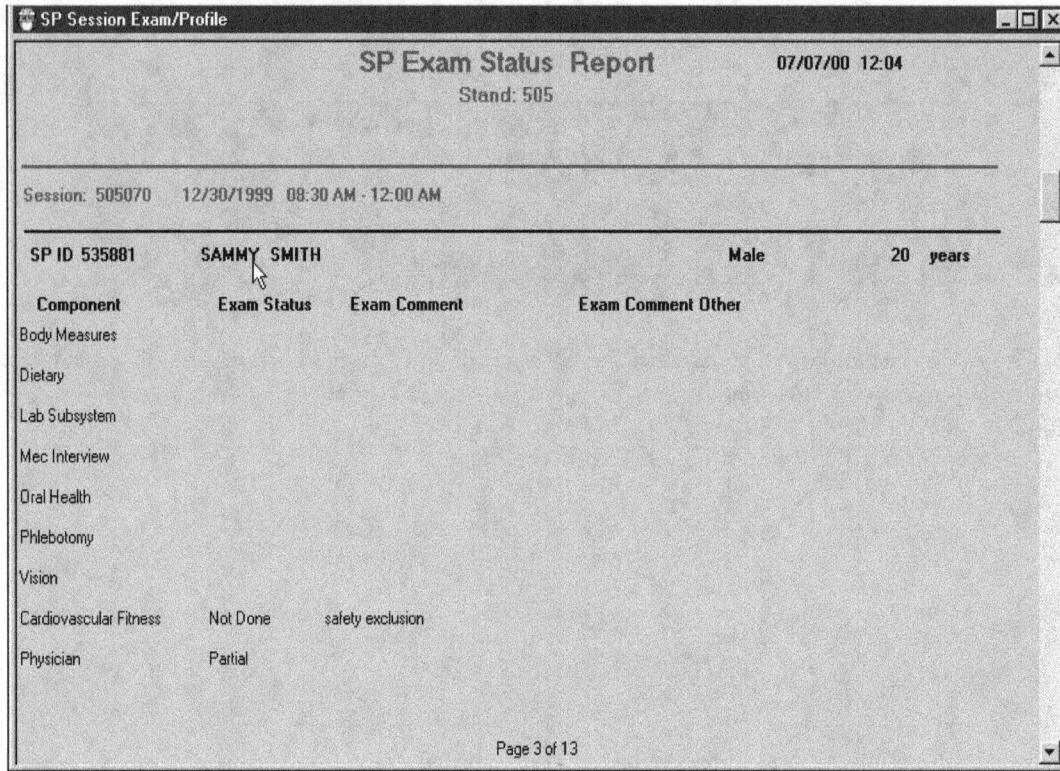

- The SP examination status report can be viewed for each SP in the session.

- The first column lists the components for which the SP is eligible.

- The second column displays the examination status: complete, partial, not done.

- The status remains blank until the SP has been to that component.

- If applicable, the status comment and "other" comment are also listed.

- Scroll up and down to view all SPs in the session. Page up and page down may also be used.

4.7.20   End of Section

Exhibit 4-85. End of section

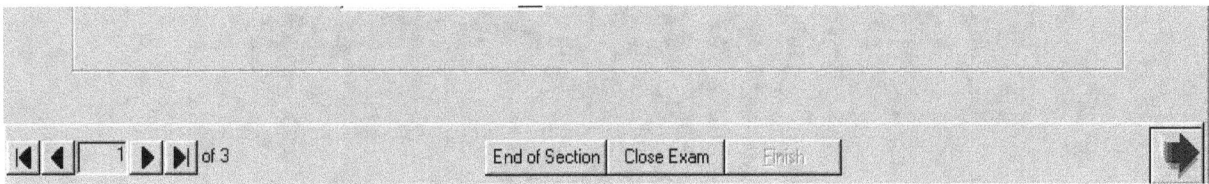

- The "End of Section" button is used to advance to the end of the current section without entering data in the required fields.

- The status defaults to "Not Done" and a comment is required. Select the appropriate comment for the situation.

- One potential situation if when there is not enough time at the end of a session to complete the entire examination, but the SP needs the STD and HIV information sheet to be able to obtain test results. The physician opens the examination, selects "End of Section" for the blood pressure and CV exclusion questions. The appropriate comment for both sections would be "No Time."

- The "End of Section button can be selected from each section.

- This allows the screens to advance through each section until the STD and HIV results screen appears.

4.7.21   Close Examination Button

Exhibit 4-86. Prematurely closing examination

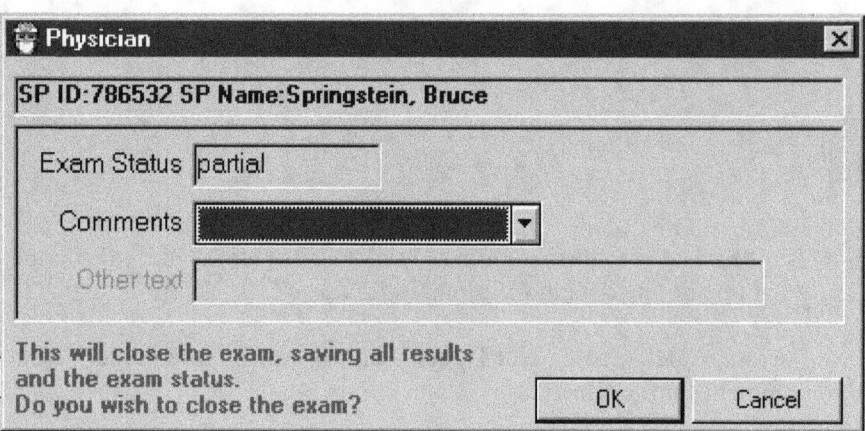

- The correct method of closing an examination is to select the "Finish" button after all the data have been entered.

- If there is a need to end the examination prematurely, the "Close" button can be selected at the bottom of the screen next to the "End of Section" button.

- When the "Close" button is selected, a pop-up box is displayed. The examination status defaults to "Not Done" or "Partial" depending on the stage of the examination when the "Close" button was pressed.

- Select the appropriate comment from the drop-down list.

5. REFERRALS

5.1 Medical Referrals

Although the primary purpose of the MEC examination is data collection, not diagnosis or treatment, the examination may produce findings that warrant further medical attention. There is an obligation to inform SPs of any abnormal results from the examinations and to refer SPs to appropriate providers for treatment. MEC physicians are responsible for referrals. Each examination component has a referral process built into the ISIS system. This automatic process alerts examining physicians to findings that may require a referral. SPs and their providers may already be aware of some findings, but others may have been revealed for the first time during the MEC exam. MEC physicians review the data provided and the categories set forth by the Physicians Advisory Group (PAG) to determine what type of referral, if any, is needed.

MEC physicians can arrange for a referral to a care provider for SPs who do not have a local provider. The local providers agree to accept referrals from the MEC examination prior to the arrival of the mobile examination team and prior to any examinations being carried out in the MEC. These advance arrangements are made through an advance arrangement team that includes a physician from the National Center for Health Statistics.

5.2 Referral Levels

There are three levels of referral for examination components. The levels are based on MEC component examination findings and represent an increasing severity and threat to the health of SPs. Level 1 is an urgent referral and Level 3 does not generate any referral. The Physician's Advisory Group (PAG) at the National Center for Health Statistics (NCHS) defined the action required for each referral level. The edit limits or ranges for referrals in each component were defined by the component specialists and consultants and subsequently reviewed and approved by the PAG. Based on the results of any component of the MEC examination, physicians place SPs in one of three referral categories.

5.2.1 Level 1 Referrals

These referrals are generated when there are major medical findings that warrant immediate attention by a health care provider, such as a dangerously high blood pressure, and emergencies. Level 1 referrals usually result in termination of the MEC examinations. SPs are transferred out of the MEC and into a hospital or other care facility. SPs who refuse treatment from this level of referral are asked to sign a release stating that they are aware of the examination findings, but they are refusing treatment against the advice of the MEC physician. SPs must sign the release form before leaving the MEC. The release is available in both English and Spanish.

5.2.2 Level 2 Referrals

The MEC physician generates these referrals when there are major medical findings that require attention by a health care provider in the next 2 weeks because they are expected to cause adverse effects within this time. Level 2 referrals allow SPs to continue MEC examinations; however, they are advised to see their primary care provider within 2 weeks following the examination. A high, but not dangerously high blood pressure is an example of a level 2 referral.

5.2.3 Level 3 Referrals

Level 3 referrals consist of no out of range medical findings or minor medical findings that an examinee already knows about, is under care for, or does not require prompt attention by a medical provider. Level 3 findings do not generate referrals. Examinees receive a report of the findings from many of the examination components before leaving the MEC. In addition, a detailed Report of Findings is sent from NCHS approximately 2 to 4 months after completion of the examination. The latter report contains the results of some findings that are not available before SPs leave the MEC.

Table 5-1. Table of referral levels

Level 1 Referral	(category 4)	Indicates major medical findings that warrant immediate attention by a health care provider.
Level 2 Referral	(category 3)	Indicates major medical findings that warrant attention by a health care provider within the next 2 weeks. These findings are expected to cause adverse effects within this time period and they have previously been undiagnosed, unattended, nonmanifested, or not communicated to the examinee by his/her personal health care provider.
Level 3 Referral	(categories 1 & 2)	Indicates no medical findings; minor medical findings that an examinee already knows about, and is under care for, or findings that do not require prompt attention by a medical provider.

5.3 Basis for Referral

Referrals may be based on data collected during MEC examination components (examination data related referrals) or based on subjective or objective observations made by any MEC examiner (observation referrals). These two types of referrals are described in detail in Sections 5.3.1 and 5.4 respectively.

5.3.1 Examination Data Related Referrals

Examination data related referrals are based on predefined criterion levels from the examination data. These criterion levels were defined by the physician advisory group and are built into the ISIS system such that when the limits are exceeded, the system automatically flags this information to the physician for the specific SP. The flag occurs when component data that are above or below the predefined limits are recorded. The examination components that send data related referrals to the physician system are the laboratory (pregnancy and complete blood count), lower extremity disease (LED), and blood pressure from the physician's examination.

5.3.1.1 Pregnancy Referrals

A positive test for pregnancy activates a system notification to the physician for all SPs. Urine pregnancy tests are done on all SPs between the ages of 12 through 59 years. In addition, pregnancy tests are done on SPs aged 8 through 11 years if they reported during the household interview that menarche had begun. The physician is the person who informs the SP of these results since some SPs may be unaware of their pregnancy at the time of the test. The physician discloses results of positive pregnancy tests to the SP, unless the SP is 18 or over and had already reported the pregnancy during the interview. SPs under 18 years of age always see the physician when a positive pregnancy test is reported. Negative pregnancy test results are provided to SPs only upon the SP's specific request. Physicians discuss the importance of prenatal health care in situations where SPs have not seen a health care provider when they have a positive pregnancy test. Referrals are facilitated if appropriate. SPs with no source of prenatal care are referred to a local public health clinic or primary care provider.

5.3.1.2 Age Specific Pregnancy Referral Requirements

SPs 18 years and over who have a positive pregnancy test are referred as described in Section 5.3.1.1 above. There are referral requirements based on child abuse laws for SPs under 18 years of age. While counseling the pregnant minor, physicians take a brief history to determine whether the pregnancy may have resulted from sexual abuse. MEC physicians received training on detecting and reporting child abuse from Dr. Judith Rubin, a pediatrician and researcher on the faculty at the University of Maryland Medical School. The index of suspicion for sexual abuse is based solely on what a minor discloses, rather than a full medical evaluation. Young women may refuse to provide information surrounding their pregnancy. If the information provided by a minor leads the physician to be concerned about possible, probable, or definite sexual abuse, *the parent/guardian is informed* and a report is filed with Child Protective Services (CPS). If the physician is unsure whether to report, the physician discusses the case with a social worker at Child Protective Services. When presenting the case, MEC physicians do not use the minor's name or any other identifier. If the social worker and physician agree that the referral to CPS should be made, the physician may provide the name and address of the minor. Physicians may follow up the verbal reporting with a written documentation of findings relevant to the reporting. These written reports are private, and are not collected in the NHANES database. The age specific requirements are described in Section 5.3.1.3 below.

5.3.1.3   Unmarried Minors Pregnancy Referrals

Federal law requires physicians to report child abuse. The finding of a positive pregnancy test in an unmarried minor (under age 18) requires physicians to conduct a brief evaluation to determine the level of counseling and referral necessary. The physician discloses a positive pregnancy test result directly to the minor.

If the minor is under 14 years of age, physicians discuss the circumstances of the pregnancy with the child, inform the parent, and report the case to Child Protective Services (CPS). Pregnancy in such a young age is probable child abuse. If the physician is informed that the child is already receiving prenatal care, the physician verifies this information directly with the provider. In cases where the child is already receiving prenatal care and has received a full medical evaluation, no report to CPS is indicated.

If the minor is 14 years and older, physicians disclose results directly to the minor and assesses (a) whether the minor is already receiving prenatal care or pregnancy counseling, (b) whether minor's parent/guardian is aware of the pregnancy, and (c) whether the pregnancy is a result of child sexual abuse. If a minor who is 14 years or older is already receiving prenatal health care, physicians confirm this with the local provider. No further referral or parental notification is necessary unless other examination findings meet the criteria for referral. If the minor is not receiving prenatal care, the physician discusses the importance of a medical evaluation and pregnancy counseling for the SP, and facilitates a referral. SPs with no source of care are referred to a local public health clinic or primary care provider. Because a parent/guardian should be informed of a minor's pregnancy if she is not receiving prenatal care, the physician will offer to help the minor tell her parent/guardian before leaving the MEC. If the minor strongly opposes the disclosure of the pregnancy test results to a parent or guardian, the physician respects the minor's confidentiality.

5.3.2   Blood Pressure Referrals – Adults

The MEC physician takes the BP on all SPs 8 years old and over. Table 5-1 provides the matrix of combinations of systolic and diastolic blood pressure results and the referrals that are generated when these BPs are present for adults. The left column specifies the minimum and maximum systolic pressure groupings. The first row specifies the minimum and maximum diastolic blood pressure (DBP) categories. The matrix cells specify the BP category severity for the SBP and the DBP combination. The category severity defines the MEC referral level.

Table 5-2.   Referral levels for adult blood pressure

(Systolic mm hg)	Diastolic (mm hg)					
	≤ 84	85 – 89	90 – 99	100 – 109	110 – 119	≥ 120
≤ 129	1	2	3	4	5	6
130 – 139	2	2	3	4	5	6
140 – 159	3	3	3	4	5	6
160 – 179	4	4	4	4	5	6
180 – 209	5	5	5	5	5	6
≥ 210	6	6	6	6	6	6

From the Sixth Report of the Joint National Committee on Detection, Evaluation, and Treatment of High Blood Pressure

Table 5-3   Blood pressure referral levels, category, and action required

Referral Level 1	(category 6)	Indicates major medical findings that warrant immediate attention by a health care provider.
Referral Level 2	(categories 4 & 5)	Indicates major medical findings that warrant attention by a health care provider within the next 2 weeks. These findings are expected to cause adverse effects within this time period and they have previously been undiagnosed, unattended, nonmanifested, or not communicated to the examinee by his/her personal health care provider.
Referral Level 3	(categories 1, 2, & 3)	Indicates no medical findings or minor medical findings that an examinee already knows about, and is under care for, or findings that do not require prompt attention by a medical provider.

Table 5-4.   Table of blood pressure referral comments

Statement for blood pressure in category 6	**Level 1 referral**	The participant's blood pressure is **severely high** based on the Sixth Report of the Joint National Committee on Detection, Evaluation, and Treatment of High Blood Pressure.
Statement for blood pressure in category 5	**Level 2 referral**	The participant's blood pressure is **very high** based on the Sixth Report of the Joint National Committee on Detection, Evaluation, and Treatment of High Blood Pressure.
Statement for blood pressure in category 4	**Level 2 referral**	The participant's blood pressure is **moderately high** based on the Sixth Report of the Joint National Committee on Detection, Evaluation, and Treatment of High Blood Pressure.
Statement for blood pressure in category 3	**Level 3 – no referral**	The participant's blood pressure is **mildly high** based on the Sixth Report of the Joint National Committee on Detection, Evaluation, and Treatment of High Blood Pressure.
Statement for blood pressure in category 2	**Level 3 – no referral**	The participant's blood pressure is **normal but at the high end of the normal range** based on the Sixth Report of the Joint National Committee on Detection, Evaluation, and Treatment of High Blood Pressure.
Statement for blood pressure in category 1	**Level 3 – no referral**	The participant's blood pressure is **normal** based on the Sixth Report of the Joint National Committee on Detection, Evaluation, and Treatment of High Blood Pressure.

Report of Findings Comments:

- Category 6 – Your blood pressure today is **<u>severely high</u>**.

- Category 5 – Your blood pressure today is **<u>very high</u>**.

- Category 4 – Your blood pressure today is **<u>moderately high</u>**.

- Category 3 – Your blood pressure today is **<u>mildly high</u>**.

- Category 2 – Your blood pressure today is **<u>normal but at the high end of the normal range</u>**.

- Category 1 – Your blood pressure today is <u>within the **normal range.**</u>

5.3.3 Blood Pressure Referrals – Children

Children's normal blood pressures vary by age, weight, and height. The table for children's blood pressures is found at Appendix A, Child Blood Pressure Values.

Referral Comments for Blood Pressure (Children)

Statement for blood pressure in category 4	**Level 1 referral**	The participant's blood pressure is **very high** based on the 1996 update of the Task Force Report on High Blood Pressure in Children and Adolescents.[*]
Statement for blood pressure in category 3	**Level 2 referral**	The participant's blood pressure is **high** based on the 1996 update of the Task Force Report on High Blood Pressure in Children and Adolescents.[*]
Statement for blood pressure in category 2	**Level 3 – no referral**	The participant's blood pressure is **normal but at the high end of normal** based on the 1996 update of the Task Force Report on High Blood Pressure in Children and Adolescents.[*]
Statement for blood pressure in category 1	**Level 3 – no referral**	The participant's blood pressure is **normal** based on the 1996 update of the Task Force Report on High Blood Pressure in Children and Adolescents.[*]

Report of Findings Comments:

- Category 4 – Your child's blood pressure today is <u>**very high**</u>.

- Category 3 – Your child's blood pressure today is <u>**high**</u>.

- Category 2 – Your child's blood pressure today is <u>**normal but at high end of normal range**</u>.

- Category 1 – Your child's blood pressure today is <u>**normal**</u>.

---

[*] National High Blood Pressure Education Program Working Group on Hypertension Control in Children and Adolescents. Update on the 1987 Task Force Report on High Blood Pressure in Children and Adolescents: A Working Group Report from the National High Blood Pressure Education Program. *Pediatrics*. 1996; 11:649-658.

5.3.4   **Lower Extremity Disease (LED) Referrals**

Referrals for Lower Extremity disease may occur for several reasons.

5.3.4.1   **Ankle Brachial Pressure Index (ABPI)**

Referral Levels for ABPI

Level 1	None
Level 2	≤ 0.5
Level 3	**$> 0.5 - \leq 0.9$**

Referral Comments for ABPI

Level 1		There is no Level 1 emergency referral for this component.
Level 2	≤ 0.5	This result indicates severe peripheral vascular disease. Participant should be evaluated within the next few weeks and followed on a regular basis.
Level 3	$> 0.5 - \leq 0.9$	This result indicates moderate peripheral vascular disease. Participant should be evaluated within the next few months and followed on a regular basis.

Report of Findings Comments for ABPI

Level 2 Referral	≤ 0.5	The blood pressure in your <left, right, both ankle(s) >, showed you have you have severely decreased blood flow to your <right foot, left foot, both feet>.
Level 3 Referral	$> 0.5 - \leq 0.9$	The blood pressure in your <left, right, both ankle(s) >, showed you have moderately decreased blood flow to your <right foot, left foot, both feet>.
No Referral	> 0.9	The blood pressure in your <left, right, both ankle(s) >, showed you have normal blood flow to your <right foot, left foot, both feet>.

5.3.4.2   Peripheral Neuropathy (PN)

Referral Levels for Peripheral Neuropathy

Level 1   There is no Level 1 emergency referral for this component.

Level 2   1 or more insensate sites (an "incorrect" or "unable to determine" response for 1 or more of the 3 sites on each foot)

Level 3   1 or less insensate sites; no referral required.

Referral Comments for Peripheral Neuropathy:

Level 1   There is no Level 1 emergency referral for this component

Level 2   This result indicates significant neuropathy, placing the sample person at increased risk of foot abnormalities and problems

Level 3   No referral required.

Report of Findings Comments for Peripheral Neuropathy:

Level 2 Referral	- 2 insensate sites on each foot	Based on testing your ability to feel things normally on the bottom of your feet, you have decreased sensation to your <right foot, left foot, both feet>.
No Referral	- ≤ 1 insensate site on each foot	Based on testing your ability to feel things normally on the bottom of your feet, you have normal sensation to your <right foot, left foot, both feet>.

5.3.4.3   Referrals for LED Observation Abnormalities

ABPI and monofilament testing is measured or tested by a health technician on all adults 40 years and older at household interview. Exclusions for these procedures are bilateral amputation, casts, ulcers, dressings, or other conditions that make BP readings at these sites impossible. The presence of these conditions on one limb does not exclude SPs.

5.3.4.4   Referral Levels for Observation of LED Abnormalities

There are no data related referrals for this observation. The health technician alerts the MEC physician if there is evidence of soft tissue pathology detected during visual inspection of the feet. These abnormalities would include, but are not limited to gangrene, cellulite, ulceration, ingrown toenail, and open wounds with purulent or other discharge. The MEC physician makes a determination whether a referral is necessary. The abnormality and subsequent referral can be made as an observation referral. There will be no report to the participant for this situation. The statement to the referral physician will be free text describing the MEC physician's clinical impression of the condition.

5.3.5   Laboratory Values

Urine and blood are collected for various laboratory tests on all SPs 1 year old and over. A complete and detailed description of these tests can be found in the laboratory procedure manual. Some laboratory findings are available prior to SPs leaving the mobile examination center. These findings are provided to the SPs, and when these findings are outside the predetermined criterion levels for referral, physicians decide whether a referral is needed. When a referral is indicated, the physician provides the information to the SP. Section 5.3.6.1 and Table 5-2 describe the laboratory findings and the parameters that generate referral advice to the physician.

5.3.5.1   Complete Blood Count (CBC)

The Beckman Coulter MAX® generates the CBC report. This machine directly measures the red blood count (RBC), white blood count (WBC), hemoglobin (Hg), and differential percentage. The mean corpuscular volume (MCV), red cell distribution (RDW), platelets (PLT), and mean platelet volume (MPV) are derived from histograms while other values are calculated. The reference ranges for normal values were calculated from the NHANES III data set, using 95 percent reference interval. All samples are run in duplicate.

The following values are transmitted to the physician for review:

- **Red Blood Count** – Elevated RBC may reflect primary polycythemia (polycythemia rubra vera) or secondary causes of polycythemia (stress erythrocytosis, diseases associated with low oxygen, certain renal disorders, etc.) Decreased RBC count may indicate anemia.

- **Hemoglobin** – Abnormal Hgb measurements usually reflect the same conditions as the RBC count and can define the type of anemia.

- **Hematocrit** – Abnormal hematocrit values usually reflect the same conditions as the RBC and can help define the type of anemia.

- **White Blood Count** – High values (leukocytosis) may indicate a primary condition such as leukemia or a secondary condition such as infection. Low values (leukopenia) may indicate the presence of autoimmune, neoplastic, drug-induced, congenital, or other conditions. See below.

- **Lymphocytes** – Elevated counts (lymphocytosis) may be primary (leukemias, lymphomas, monoclonal B cell lymphocytosis) or secondary (viral infection, acute physical stress, pertussis, and chronic disorders such as autoimmune disease and cancer). Depressed counts (lymphopenia) can reflect a variety of uncommon inherited disorders or the more frequent acquired conditions such as viral and certain bacterial infections, the effects of immunosupressive agents, and some chronic diseases.

- **Monocytes** – These cells, derived from the bone marrow are the precursors of tissue macrophages. Monocytosis is often seen in chronic infections (TB, brucellosis), acute protozoan and rickettsial diseases, and in neutropenia. Uncommon malignant disorders (monocytic leukemia, histiocytic lymphoma) and nonmalignant conditions (hemophagocytic syndromes) can also cause it.

- **Neutrophils** – Elevated neutrophils (granulocytosis) are seen in both primary (myelocytic leukemias, polycythemia rubra vera) and, more commonly, in secondary conditions (bacterial infections, chronic inflammation, corticosteroid use, cigarette smoking, etc.). Hereditary neutrophilia is rare. Decreased neutrophils (leukopenia) can also result from primary (myeloid malignancies, congenital disorders) and secondary (drug effect, viral infection, splenomegaly, autoimmune and hereditary disorders) conditions.

- **MCH** – The mean corpuscular hemoglobin, in picograms, is calculated from the ratio of Hgb to RBC. This measure of hemoglobin per RBC is used in conjunction with the MCV and the MCHC to further define anemias. For example, the MCH is elevated in macrocytic anemias and depressed in microcytic, hypochromic anemia.

- **MCHC** – The mean corpuscular hemoglobin concentration is derived from the ratio of the Hgb to the VPRC. It is also used to help define anemias, being elevated in macrocytic anemias and depressed in hypochromic anemias.

- **RDW** – The red cell distribution width is a measure of the homogeniety of the RBC population. It is analogous to anisocytosis seen on microscopic examination. Most macrocytic and microcytic anemias, especially with reticulocytosis, will cause an increased RDW. There is no known pathological cause of a decreased RDW.

- **Platelets** – A decreased platelet count (thrombocytopenia) can be caused by production abnormalities (radiation, drug-induced, cancer, folate or B12 deficiency, myelodysplasia syndromes, HIV, alcohol abuse, etc.), accelerated removal (ITP, SLE, drug antibodies, certain infections, etc.), and hypersplenism. Elevated counts (thrombocytosis) can be primary (myeloproliferative disorders such as CML and PRV, essential thrombocythemia) or secondary (acute trauma, chronic iron deficiency, inflammatory disease, cancer, splenectomy, etc.).

When the values from the Beckman Coulter® report are interpreted various interfering substances and conditions may affect these parameters:

- Abnormal BUN, glucose, or sodium levels could affect the MCV.

- Abnormal WBCs could affect lymphocytes, monocytes, and granulocytes.

- Abnormally small WBCs could affect white count, lymphocytes, monocytes, and granulocytes.

- Clumped platelets could affect white count, lymphocytes, monocytes, granulocytes, RBC, MCV, RDW, platelet count, and MPV.

- Cryofibrinogen and cryoglobulin crystals could affect white count, lymphocytes, monocytes, granulocytes, RBC, hemoglobin, platelet count, and MPV.

- An elevated WBC could affect RBC, hemoglobin, MCV, RDW, platelet count, and MPV parameters.

- Fragile WBCs could affect white count, lymphocytes, monocytes, granulocytes, platelet count, and MPV.

- Giant platelets could affect white count, lymphocytes, monocytes, granulocytes, RBC, MCV, RDW, platelet count, and MPV.

- Hemolyzed specimens could affect RBC, hemoglobin, platelet count, and MPV.

- Lipemic specimens could affect MCV.

- Severely icteric plasma causes increased hemoglobin. Evaluate CBC result carefully and report all parameters except the hemoglobin result.

- Nucleated RBC's could affect the white count, lymphocytes, monocytes, granulocytes, and hemoglobin values.

Table 5-5.   Reference ranges for complete blood count

Test	Units	Gender	1-5 years	6-18 years	19-65 years	66+ years
WBC	$(x10^3 \mu L)$	Male	4.3 – 14.1	3.7 – 11.9	3.9 – 12.1	3.9 – 12.3
Lymphocytes	%	Male	24.5 – 70.0	20.0 – 56.6	17.8 – 51.8	13.0 – 48.3
Monocytes	%	Male	0 – 12	0 – 12	0 – 12	0 – 13
Neutrophils	%	Male	21.4 – 70.5	33.2 – 74.7	39.7 – 77.3	44.7 – 81.9
Eosinophils	%	Male	0 – 10	0 – 11	0 – 8	0 – 8
Basophils	%	Male	0 – 2	0 – 2	0 – 2	0 – 2
RBC	$(x\,10^6 \mu L)$	Male	4.00 – 5.30	4.10 – 5.60	4.10 – 5.80	4.00 – 5.60
Hemoglobin	g/dL	Male	10.5 – 13.7	11.5 – 16.3	12.7 – 17.1	11.0 – 16.8
Hematocrit	%	Male	31.8 – 40.8	34.4 – 48.3	38.0 – 50.3	33.1 – 50.2
MCV	fL	Male	67.6 – 88.2	74.3 – 93.0	78.1 – 99.2	78.9 – 101.4
MCH	pg	Male	21.7 – 29.8	24.3 – 31.7	25.7 – 33.8	25.6 – 34.4
MCHC	μL	Male	31.5 – 35.0	31.9 – 35.1	32.0 – 35.3	31.8 – 35.1
RDW	%	Male	11.7 – 16.5	11.7 – 14.3	11.8 – 15.3	12.1 – 16.6
Platelets	$(x\,10^3 \mu L)$	Male	224 – 568	194 – 477	157 – 414	138 – 407
WBC	$(x10^3 \mu L)$	Female				
Lymphocytes	%	Female				
Monocytes	%	Female				
Neutrophils	%	Female				
Eosinophils	%	Female				
Basophils	%	Female				
RBC	$(x\,10^6 \mu L)$	Female				
Hemoglobin	g/dL	Female				
Hematocrit	%	Female				
MCV	fL	Female				
MCH	pg	Female				
MCHC	μL	Female				
RDW	%	Female				
Platelets	$(x\,10^3 \mu L)$	Female				

5.4　　Observation Referrals

　　Observation referrals are not related to specific examination data. An observation referral includes any observation by the technician or other examination staff about an SP's nonemergency condition that may require attention by the physician. An observation referral is sent through the ISIS process from any examination component technician and may be initiated during the examination, but is sent after the component examination is completed and the SP has left the component room. The technician initiating the referral enters a message in the observation referral box and sends it electronically to the physician. This referral sets a flag in the physician component and coordinator applications and SPs are not checked out of the MEC until the physician reviews and acts on this observation. Examples of observation referrals include referrals from a Dietary Interviewer when children or adult SPs are thought to be malnourished, or mental health referrals from a MEC interviewer. The physician will discuss the issue with the SP and refer as deemed medically necessary.

5.5　　Mental Health Observation Referrals

　　The MEC Interviewer asks the physician to see any SP who meets criteria for a potential Mental Health problem. The instructions to the MEC Interviewer are included in this section to inform the physician with regard to the reasons and circumstances that the MEC Interviewer may ask the physician to see an SP. In addition to the reasons stated in these instructions, the MEC Interviewer may ask the Physician to see an SP to evaluate a potential MH issue at other times.

Referral Protocol – Mental Health

5.5.1　　MEC Interviewer Process

　　Certain information volunteered or reported during the mental health interview should prompt a referral to the Mobile Examination Center (MEC) physician. These are listed below. MEC interviewers will complete a short referral form which will be given to the coordinator. The coordinator will be responsible for assuring that the examinee sees the MEC physicians prior to leaving the MEC. The physician is responsible for assessing the mental health problem and facilitating a referral.

5.5.2   MEC Interviewers

Adults 20-39 years of age should be referred to the MEC physician prior to leaving the examination center in the following circumstances:

- During CIDI interview, participant reported a time when he/she has thought a lot about committing suicide **and** that time period is still going on. (Questions E19 and E24a or E25o)

- During CIDI interview, participant reported a time when he/she attempted suicide **and** that time period is still going on. (Question E20 and E24a or E25o)

- Participant becomes visibly upset while answering questions about suicide (e.g. crying, unable to answer questions).

- Participant who makes homicidal threats.

Youths 8-19 years of age should be referred to the MEC physician prior to leaving the examination center in the following circumstances:

- During the CDISC interview, the youth reports he/she has thought seriously about killing him/herself during the **last four weeks** (21 – G).

- During CDISC interview, the youth reports he/she has tried to kill him/herself during the **last four weeks** (22 – G).

- Youth becomes visibly upset while answering questions about suicide (e.g. crying, unable to answer questions).

- Youth who makes homicidal threats.

- Youth 8-17 years of age who voluntarily discloses he/she has been sexually or physically abused in the recent past.

5.5.3   MEC Physician

The MEC physician should document the encounter with an SP referred by the MEC interviewer using an incident/emergency form.

5.5.4   Suicide

The MEC physician is not responsible for making psychiatric diagnoses; however, thoughts and plans for suicide should be considered seriously. The MEC physician should assess the need for a mental health referral for those who have either reported or voluntarily disclosed recent suicidal ideations or attempts.

Protocol for MEC physician receiving a referral from the mental health interview:

- Assess if the participant is currently suicidal. Simply ask the participant if he/she is depressed or thinking about suicide now. If so, then probe as to whether he/she has a plan and/or set a time for doing this. An person who is suicidal with plan to kill him/herself at a definite time is a *psychiatric emergency*.

Protocol for a participant who is in imminent danger:

- If the person is currently under psychiatric care, ask the him/her for permission to call their mental health care provider. The physician should negotiate a follow-up with the provider. If the participant does not have a provider, call the *<referral centers will be provided by advance team>*

Protocol for a participant who is not in imminent danger:

- If the participant is under the care of a psychiatrist or other mental health care provider, there may be no need to refer unless the participant provides some indication that his/her symptoms are worsening.

- If the participant has not seen a health profession for suicidal thoughts, then refer them to the following clinics or crisis hotline: *<referral centers will be provided by advance team>*

For minors under 18 years of age, the initial assessment should be done with the youth in private. If a referral is necessary, the participant's parent/guardian must be notified.

5.5.5   Homicidal Ideations/Threats

Threats to kill a person or person(s) should be considered seriously. The MEC physician should judge the mental stability of the participant. The physician should ask about specific plan for carrying out the threat and the time frame. A homicidal threat with a lethal weapon and plan must be reported to the 911 system.

5.5.6   Child Abuse

If a minor reports that he/she has been abused, the MEC physician should document the nature of the abuse. If warranted, the MEC physician should call *Child Protective Services at <number provided by the NHANES Advance Team>*. If the physician is unsure whether or not to refer, the physician should discuss the case with a trained Social Worker at Child Protective Services. When presenting the case, the MEC physician should not use the child's name or any other identifier. If the social worker and physician agree that the referral to CPS should be made, the physician may provide the name and address of the child.

5.6   Sessions Requiring Review

All MEC sessions with an SP requiring a physician's review for referral determination must be reviewed. The "Sessions Requiring Review" box is displayed every time the physician logs on to the application, and the physician must review these sessions. When the ISIS application first opens for the physician component, the "Sessions Requiring Review" screen opens by default. The purpose of this screen is to prompt the physician to complete reviews for SPs in all sessions. The physician can select which sessions to review.

Exhibit 5-1. Review all MEC sessions in the current stand

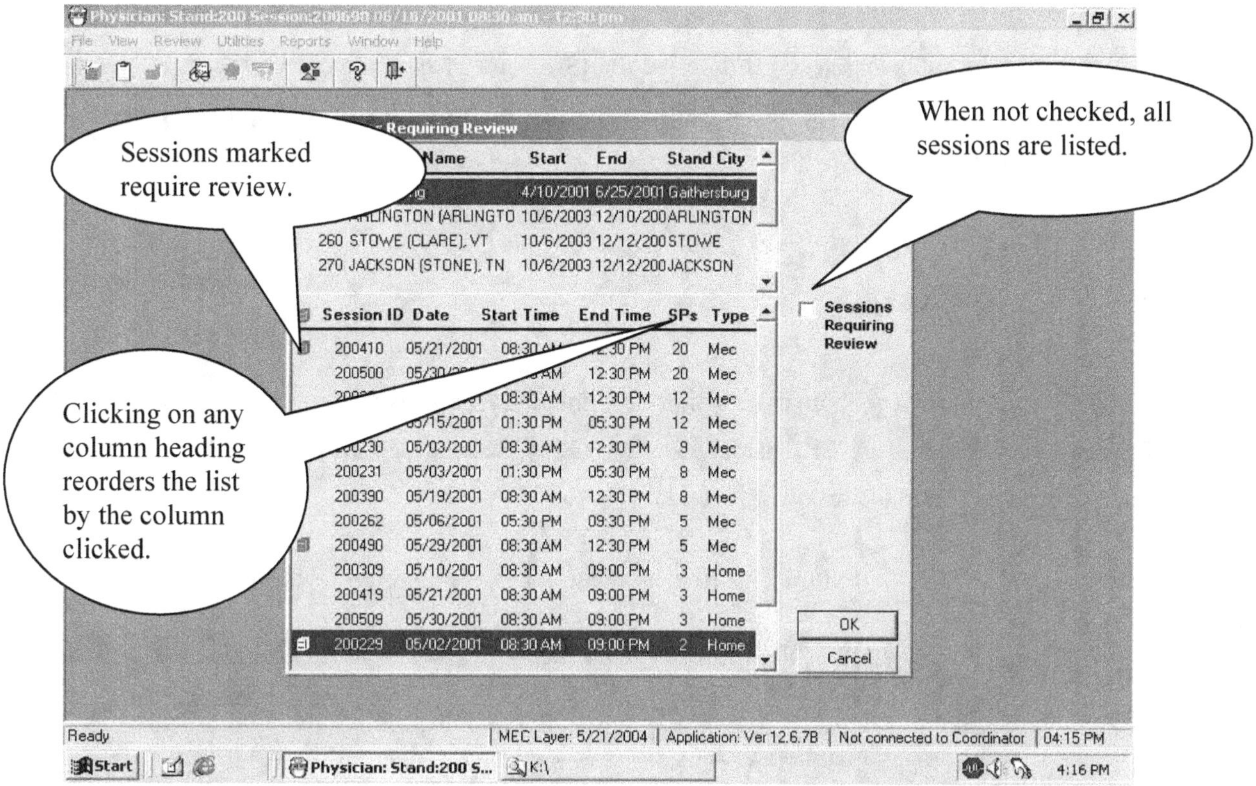

- When the Physician's application is opened, the "Sessions Requiring Review" pick list is displayed. If the physician does not want to review referrals at this time this screen may be closed by clicking on the "x" in the upper right hand corner or by clicking cancel in the lower right hand corner.

- The top part of the screen displays the current stand.

- The lower part of the screen displays the Sessions Review.

- To view all sessions in the current stand leave the box for "Sessions Requiring Review" unchecked. All sessions in the current stand will be displayed.

- To review a specific session, highlight and double click on that session and that session will be displayed.

- Click "Cancel" to exit without viewing any sessions.

- Close the screen when completed.

5.7   **Data Entry Screens for Referrals**

The following sections describe the ISIS screens and data entry process related to physician referrals. There are three types of screens related to referral: "Sessions Requiring Review," "Referral Review," and "Review in Box."

5.7.1   **Review Menu**

The review toolbar selection (Exhibit 5-2) has several review options: CV Medication Review, Referral Review, SP History, Review Other Sessions, and Physician Lookup. Each of these options is described in the following sections.

Exhibit 5-2. Review menu for selecting referral review

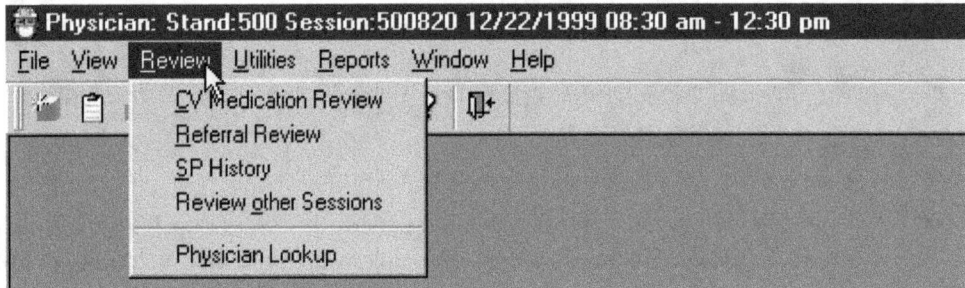

- ■   Use this drop down list to select the desired activity

- ■   Highlight the activity by pointing to it with the pointer

- ■   Click the activity to access the screens

5.7.2   Review Box

Exhibit 5-3. Referral review selection screen

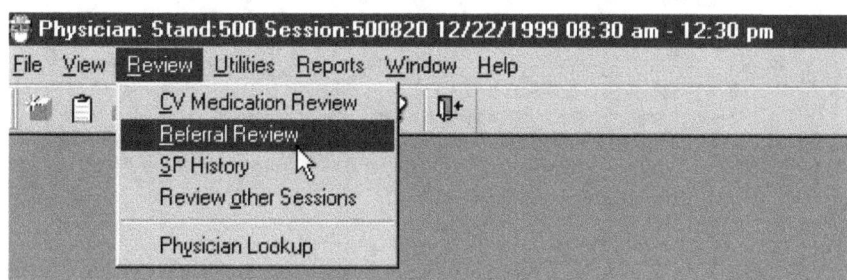

- The Referral Review Box option is the screen where all referrals can be viewed.

- To access the Review Box, first access the desired session (see Exhibit 5-1), then select "Review" (see Exhibit 5-2) from the toolbar, and last, select "Referral Review" from the drop-down list (see Exhibit 5-3).

- This will access the referrals for the current session.

5.7.3   Review Other Sessions

The "Sessions Requiring Review" is accessed from the "Review Other Sessions" drop-down list under the "Review" selection on the toolbar. The "Sessions Requiring Review" screens inform physicians which MEC sessions remain to be reviewed. The purpose of the review is to assure that all referrals are completed. This is especially important since some referrals may not be able to be completed while SPs are still available on the MEC. Physicians mark appropriate boxes about their referral decision for each SP.

Exhibit 5-4 shows the review selection, and drop down selection list for "Review Other Sessions" option that accesses the Sessions Requiring Review.

Exhibit 5-4. Review other sessions

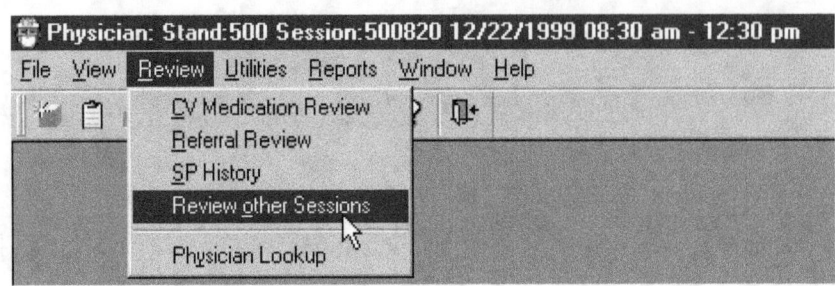

- When the "Review Other Sessions" option is clicked, the "Sessions Requiring Review" screen drop-down list is accessed. From this screen, physicians make choices about which sessions need to be reviewed.

5.7.4   Sessions Requiring Review

The top part of the "Sessions Requiring Review" screen displays the current stand location and number. The bottom part of the screen displays various sessions in the stand, depending on how they are selected by the physician.

Exhibit 5-5. MEC sessions requiring review

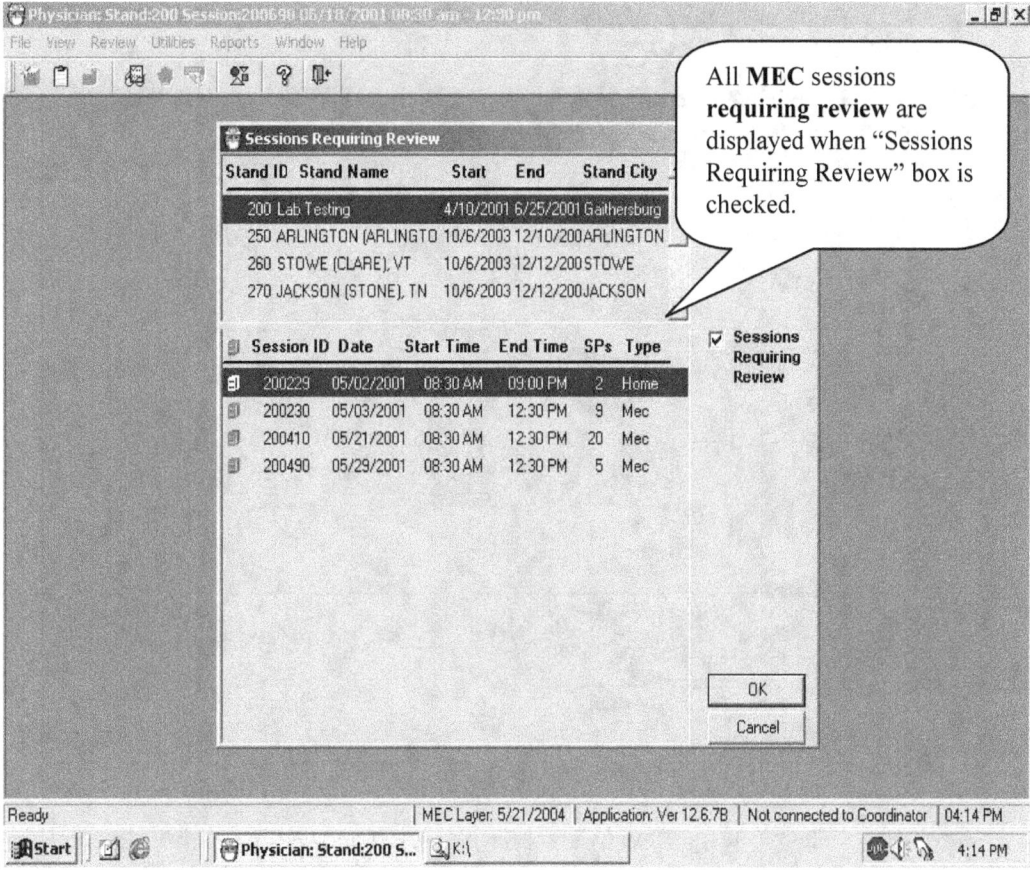

- When the "sessions requiring review" box is checked, all MEC sessions that require review are displayed.

- Referrals posted in the "Review Box" that the physician has not reviewed causes the application screen to display a <u>red marking beside the session indicating that the session requires review.</u>

- The <u>red mark remains</u> beside this session until the physician reviews all referrals in the session.

- When all referrals are completed or reviewed, the system removes the red flag.

5.7.5   Referral Review Screen

Exhibit 5-6. SPs referred for review for referral determination

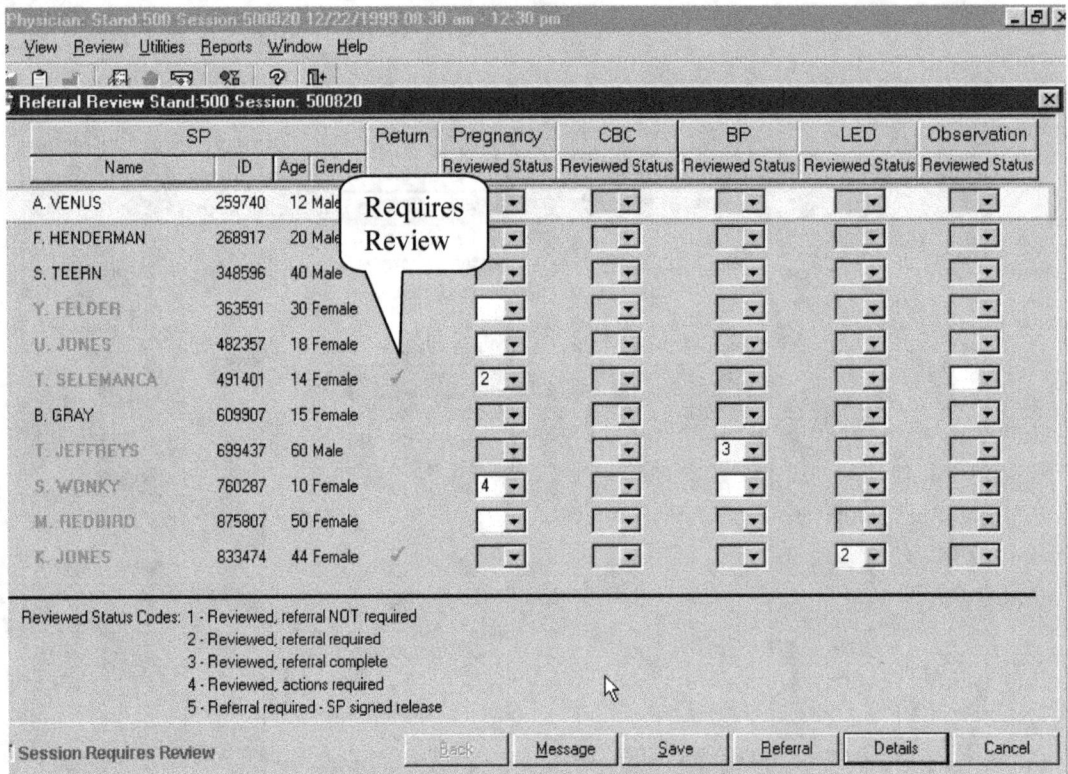

- The "Referral Review" box has the stand and session numbers on the top bar.

- Names of SPs requiring review are highlighted in red. The boxes for components requiring review are enabled. All other boxes are disabled or "grayed out."

- Note also that the SPs name is in red when a review is required.

5.7.6   Selecting SP for Detailed Referral Review

To complete the referral, the physician selects each SP in turn that has an indication that a review for referral determination is needed. The selection is made from the Referral Review screen.

Exhibit 5-7. SP selection from review in box

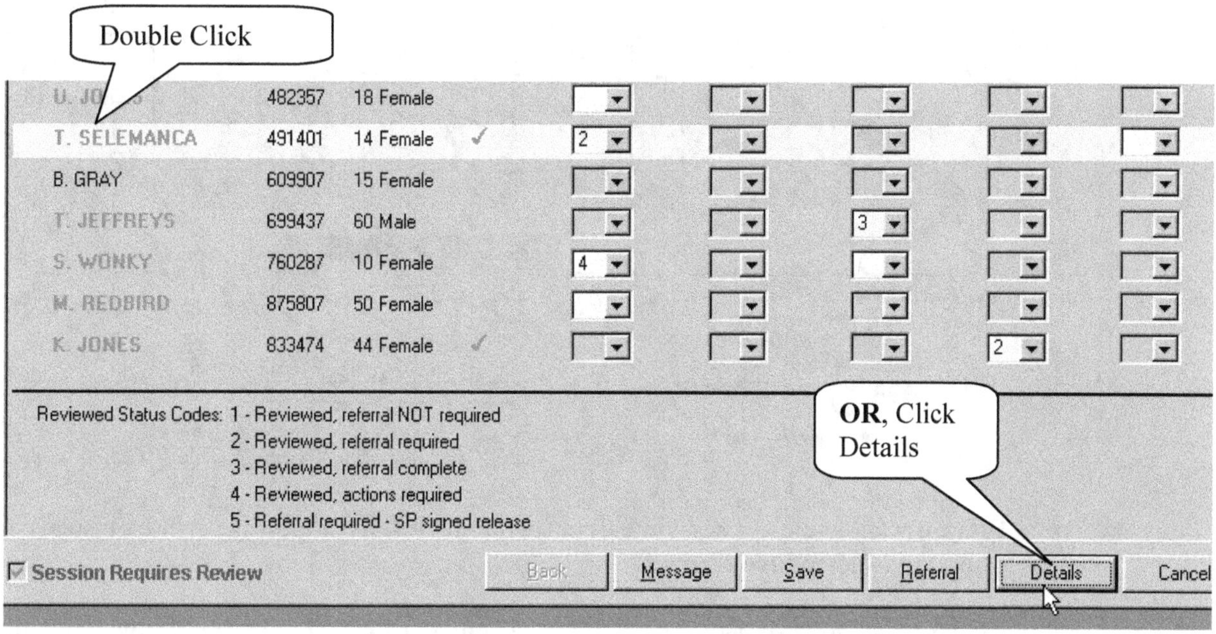

- To select the SP for review, move the cursor over the desired name.

- Highlight the name of the SP to be reviewed.

- Double click on the SP name, or, click the "detail" radio button.

Exhibit 5-8. Warning to save changes

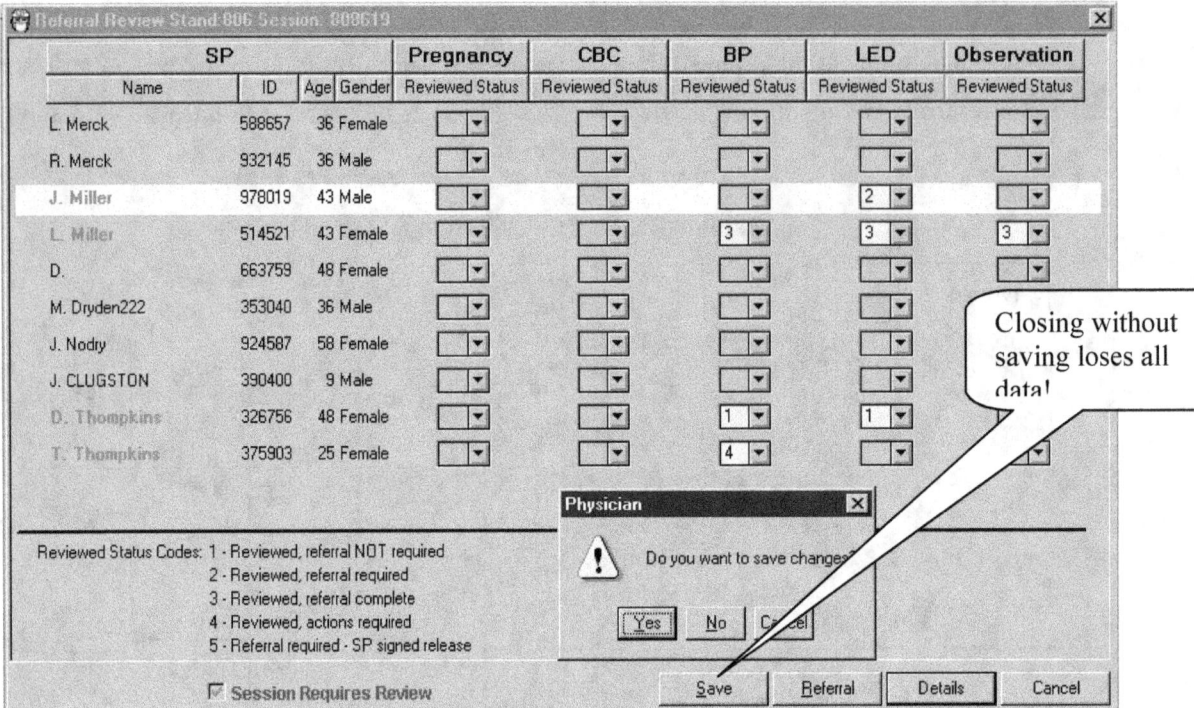

- If you want to close a session before saving the results, a message will be displayed: "Do you want to save changes?"

- Click "yes" to save and close this box. If all status codes are 1 and 3, the "Session Requires Review" box will be unchecked and the red flag will be removed from the session requiring review list.

Exhibit 5-9. Session requires review indicator

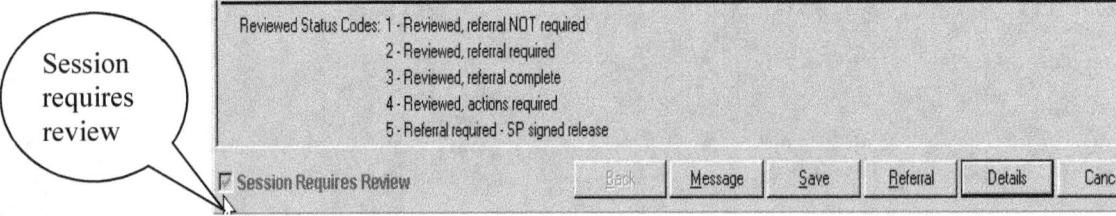

- A box at the bottom left of the screen is checked if the session requires review. The box is unchecked if no review is required.

- This box is especially useful if there is a long list of SPs. If the box is not checked, there is no need to scroll through the SP list.

Exhibit 5-10. Reviewed status codes legend

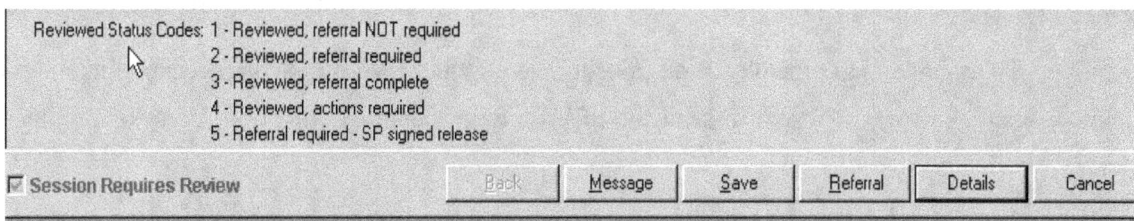

- The "Reviewed Status Codes" are listed at the bottom left of the screen.

- Code 1 – "Reviewed, referral not required": If findings were reviewed but the situation does not require a referral, select Code 1 from the drop-down menu.

- Code 2 – "Reviewed, referral required": If a referral is required but there is not enough time to do it or if the SP is in another exam, check Code 2. This keeps the referral session active. A referral Code 2 turns the Physician's Examination progress box on the coordinator's screen (for that SP) to green. This alerts the coordinator that the SP must return to see the physician before checking out of the MEC. (If the SP has not completed the Physician's Exam component, the box does not turn green. When the SP checks into the Physician's Exam the box turns green). The box remains green as long as there are referrals for that SP with a referral Code 2. After the code is changed from 2 to another code, the box turns blue.

- Code 3 – "Reviewed, referral complete": After the physician reviews the referral, sees the SP, and completes the referral letter, Code 3 is checked. If no other referrals are needed, the session will be considered complete.

- Code 4 – "Reviewed, action required": This is similar but not the same as Code 2. This code is marked when the SP has been reviewed and a referral generated, however, the physician wants to take further action but has not been able to complete the action at this time. This situation could occur when the physician needs to telephone a health care provider but has been unable to complete the process. This may be carried over to the next day, or the next session. When Code 4 is checked, the SP may be checked out of the MEC but this session continues to be flagged, requiring review until this and other referrals are coded as 1 or 3.

- Code 5 – "Referral required – SP signed release": When SPs refuse to accept a required referral, they sign a release form. The physician checks Code 5 which removes the red flag on the session if all other referrals are complete.

5.7.7   ISIS Message

To assure SPs see the physician prior to leaving the MEC, the physician can send a message to the coordinator to specify a time to send the SP to the physician examination room to complete the referral.

Exhibit 5-11. Message to coordinator

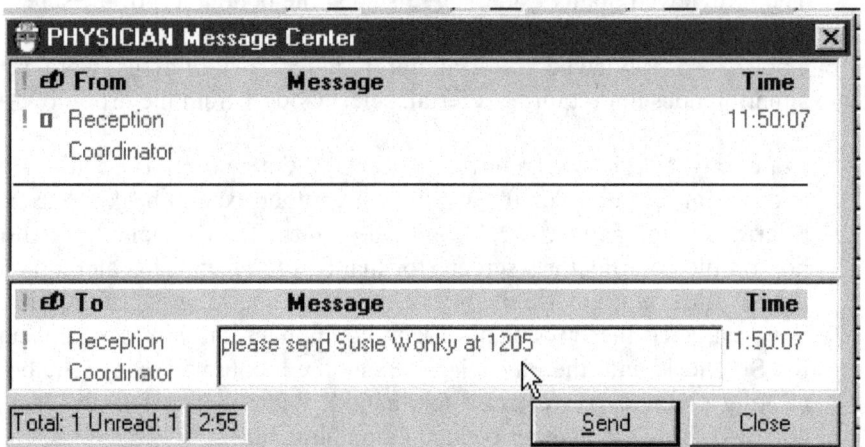

- Notify the coordinator when it is a good time to complete this referral.

- Click Message from the tool bar utilities, type a message, and send to the coordinator.

5.7.8   NHANES Release Form for SPs Refusing Referrals

Exhibit 5-12. NHANES Release Form

DEPARTMENT OF HEALTH & HUMAN SERVICES

Public Health Service
Centers for Disease Control and Prevention

National Center for Health Statistics
6525 Belcrest Road
Hyattsville, Maryland 20782

**NHANES
RELEASE FORM**

Date:

Stand:

This is to certify that against the advice of the staff doctor I:

(Check one)

☐   am leaving the Mobile Exam Center

☐   am removing _____
                        (name of sample person)
     from the Mobile Exam Center

☐   choose no further medical referral or immediate follow-up.

By so doing. I assume all responsibilities for my act.

Signed   _____

Relationship   _____

Witness   _____

- SPs who decline or refuse a medical referral, are asked to sign the NHANES Release Form (Exhibit 5-16). The date and stand number must be completed. The form is available in English and Spanish.

- This form is available for printing in the "Forms" directory.

- Ask the SP to place a check mark next to the correct ending for the reference sentence:

  "This is to certify that against the advice of the staff doctor, I:"

  ☐ am leaving the Mobile Exam Center

  ☐ am removing (name of sample person)

  ☐ choose no further medical referral or immediate follow-up."

- Ask the SP to sign this form.

- Obtain a witness signature for the form.

5.7.9 Review in Box for Pregnancy Details

The potential data for referral are selected from tabs for each SP that is referred: Pregnancy, CBC, BP, LED, and Observations.

Exhibit 5-13. Details for pregnancy referral

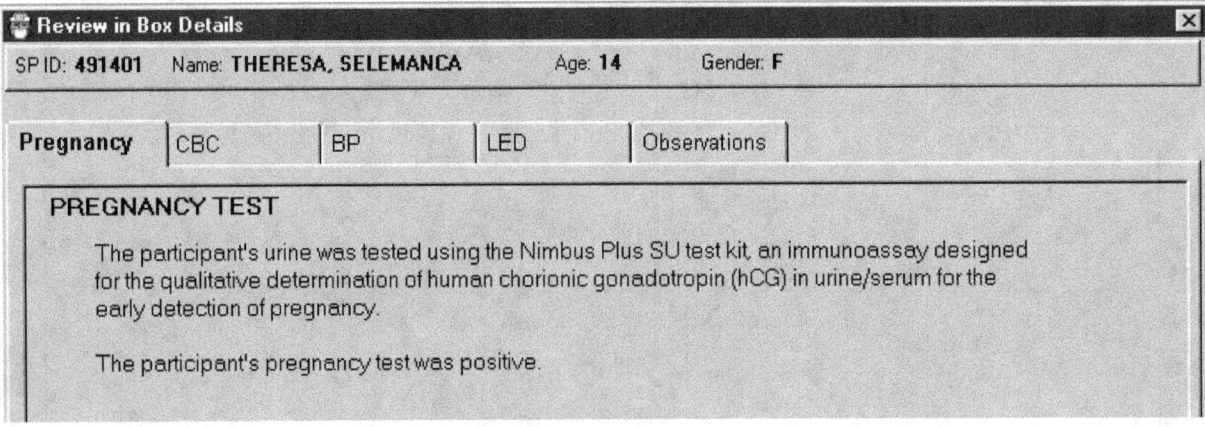

- If the Pregnancy tab is checked, the results of the pregnancy test in the lab are displayed. The results can only be one of the following for Pregnancy:

    - The pregnancy test is negative.

    - The pregnancy test is positive.

    - The pregnancy test is invalid.

- Complete the referral as appropriate.

5.7.10   Review in Box for CBC Details

Exhibit 5-14. Details of complete blood count referral (1)

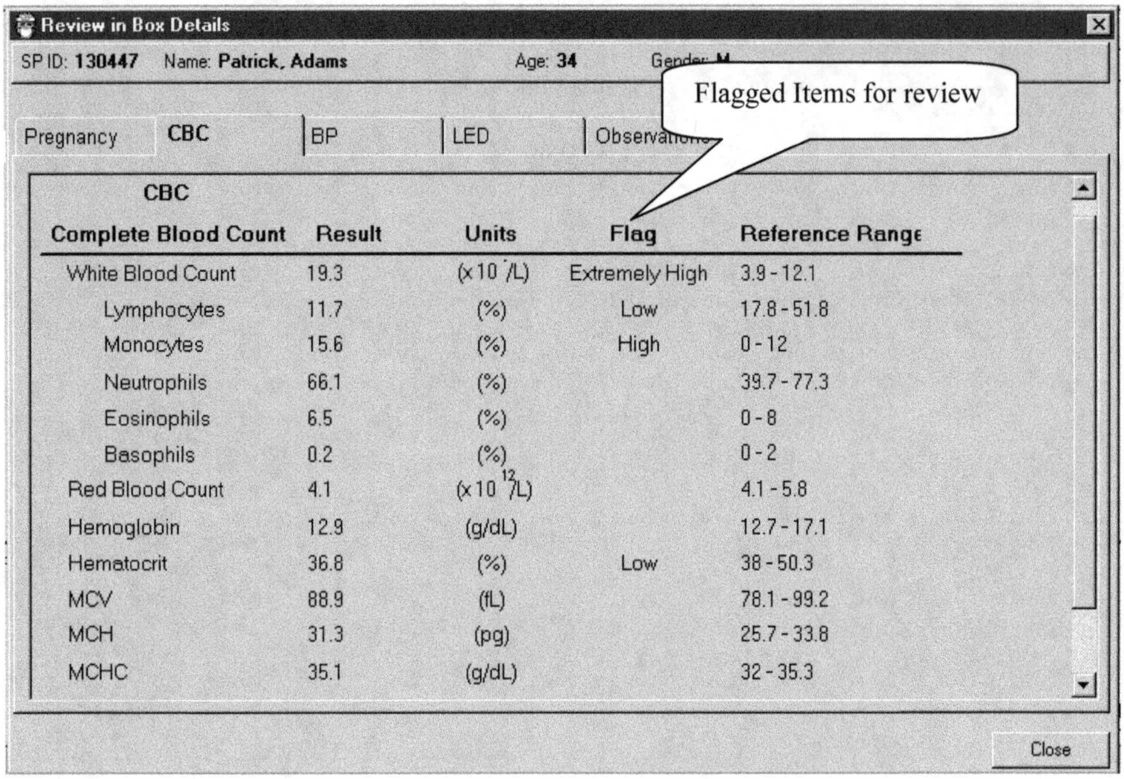

- Click on the CBC tab to review the results of the MEC laboratory CBC.

- The names of the tests are displayed in the left columns along with the units of measurement.

- The reference ranges are displayed in the far right column.

- The results and units of measurement are displayed in the next two columns.

- The flag items are displayed as "low, high, extremely high."

- Complete the referral as necessary.

Exhibit 5-15. Details of complete blood count referral (2)

Review in Box Details					☒
SP ID: **130447** Name: **Patrick, Adams**		Age: **34**	Gender: **M**		

Pregnancy | **CBC** | BP | LED | Observations

CBC

Complete Blood Count	Result	Units	Flag	Reference Range
Monocytes	15.6	(%)	High	0 - 12
Neutrophils	66.1	(%)		39.7 - 77.3
Eosinophils	6.5	(%)		0 - 8
Basophils	0.2	(%)		0 - 2
Red Blood Count	4.1	$(\times 10^{12}/L)$		4.1 - 5.8
Hemoglobin	12.9	(g/dL)		12.7 - 17.1
Hematocrit	36.8	(%)	Low	38 - 50.3
MCV	88.9	(fL)		78.1 - 99.2
MCH	31.3	(pg)		25.7 - 33.8
MCHC	35.1	(g/dL)		32 - 35.3
RDW	13.8	(%)		11.8 - 15.3
Platelets	456.0	$(\times 10^{9}/L)$	High	157 - 414

Clo

■   Scroll down the scroll bar to view the remaining CBC values.

Scroll down to assure review of all CBC values

5.7.11   Review in Box – Blood Pressure Details

Exhibit 5-16. Details of moderately high blood pressure referral

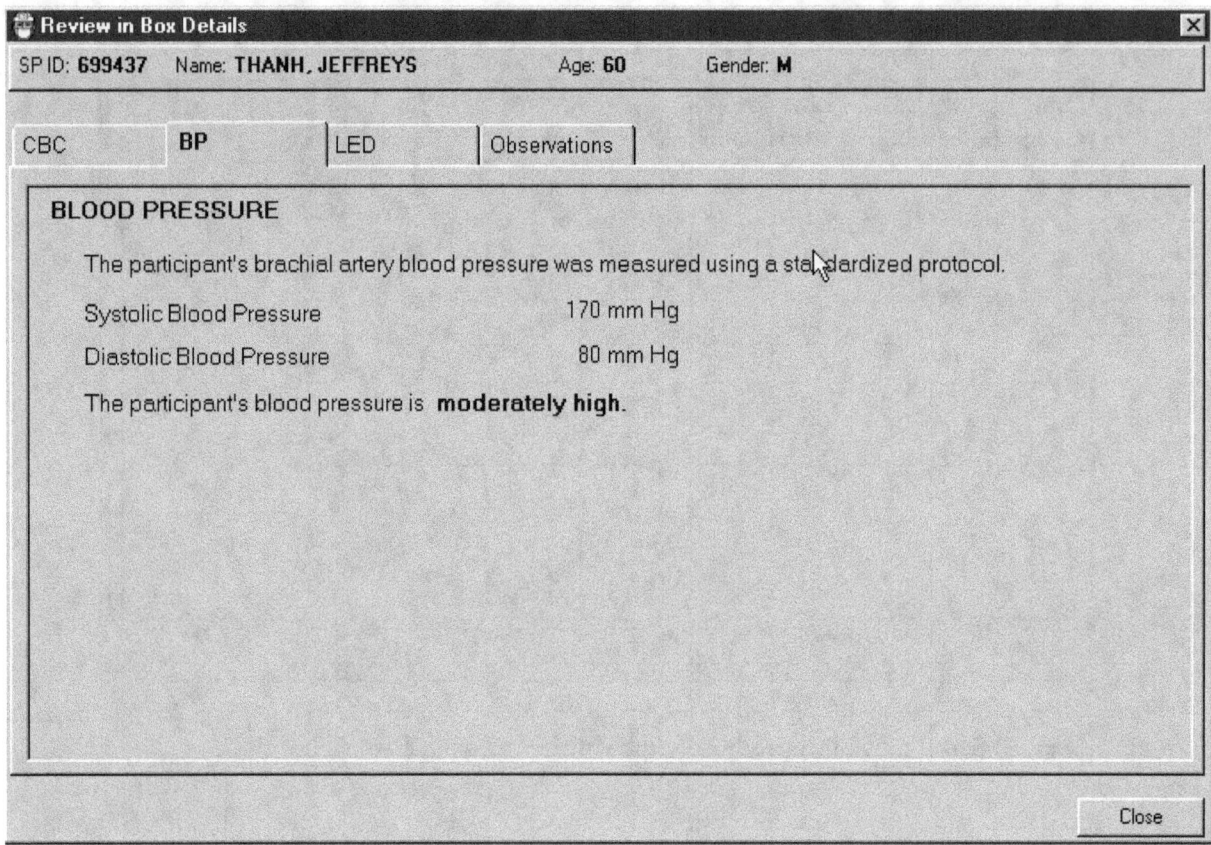

- Click on the blood pressure tab to view the BP results.

- Complete the referral if necessary and enter the appropriate code.

- The blood pressure in the above example is moderately high for the age group and is a Level 2 referral. These results are discussed with the SP and the physician gives a Level 2 referral letter to the SP. The SP may take this letter to their health care provider.

Exhibit 5-17. Details of very high blood pressure referral

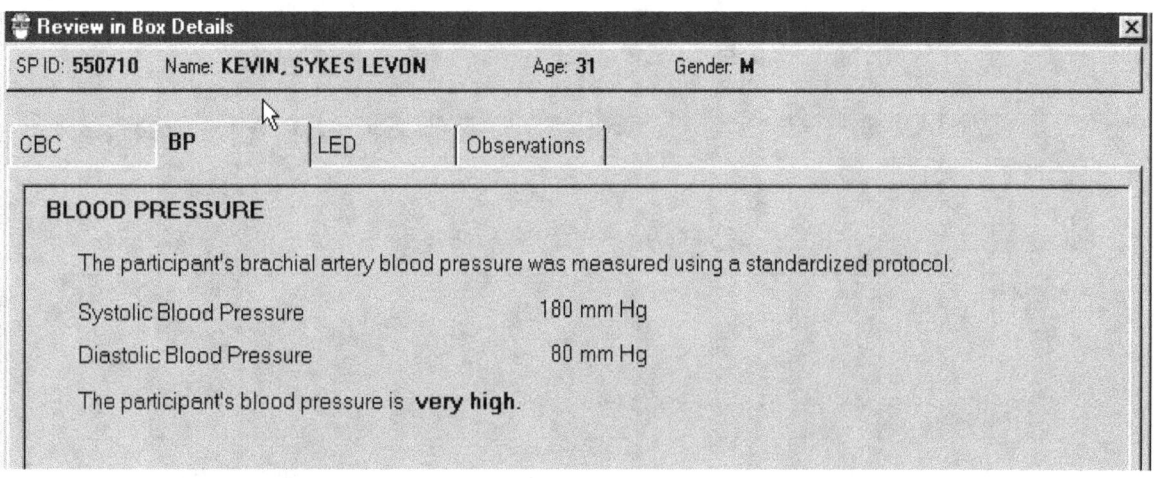

- The blood pressure in the above exhibit is very high for the SP in this age group. It is a Level 2 referral.

- Complete the referral as necessary.

- Click on the Close button to exit from this screen.

Exhibit 5-18. Details of severely high blood pressure referral

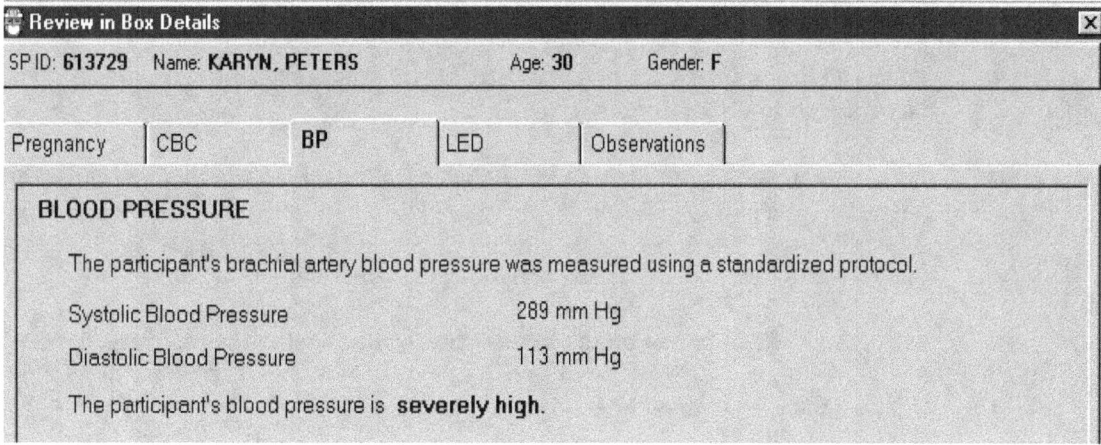

- The blood pressure in the above exhibit is severely high. This is a Level 1 referral. The physician should try to get an immediate referral to the SP's health care provider or to a local clinic.

- Complete the referral as necessary.

- Click on the Close button to exit this screen.

5.7.12   Review in Box- LED Details

Exhibit 5-19. Details of lower extremity disease referral

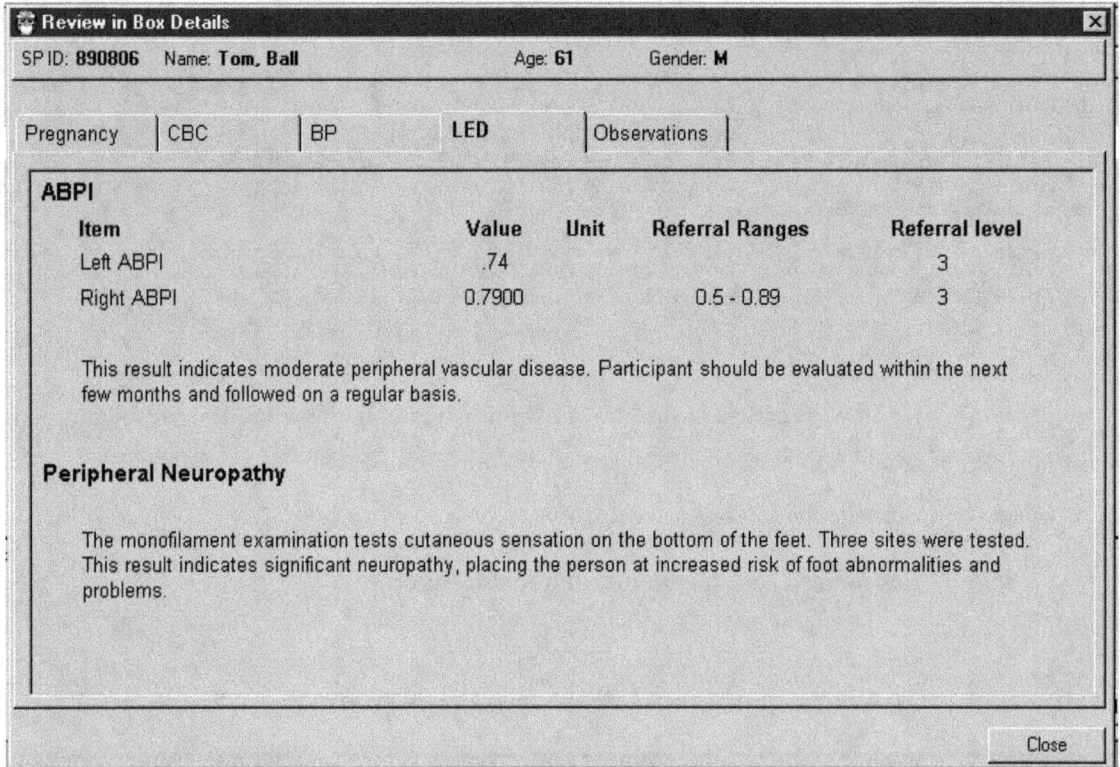

- This is an example of the Review in Box for the lower extremity disease (LED) exam. There are no Level 1 referrals for LED.

- The ankle brachial pressure index indicates a Level 3, which does not require a referral.

- The results for the monofilament test indicate significant neuropathy.

- Select the Referral button on the Review box screen to start the referral letter.

- Click on the Close button to exit this screen.

5.7.13   Review in Box – Observations Details

Exhibit 5-20. Details of Observations referral

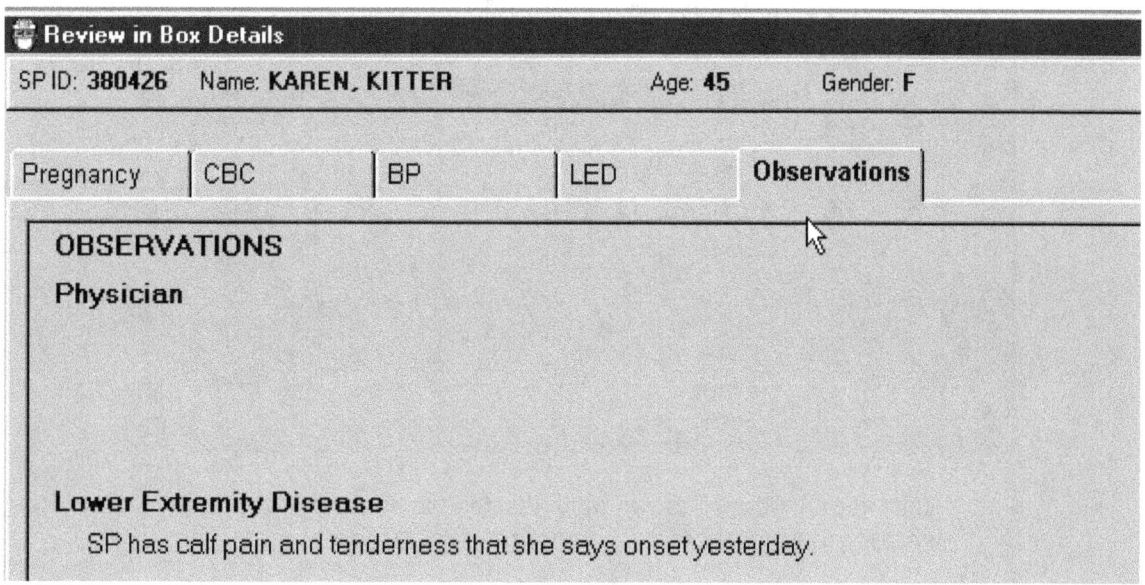

- This is an observation sent to the physician from the LED component. This SP is flagged in the physician's exam and in the coordinator system. The SP cannot check out of the MEC until the MEC physician has an opportunity to review this referral and make a decision on it.

- Click on the "Referral" button on the "Review in Box" screen to bring up the referral letter template.

- Click Close to exit this screen.

5.7.14   Observation Referrals

Observation referrals can be displayed by selecting "Observations" from the Utilities toolbar menu. This allows the physician to select any SP from the list of SPs referred for observation. The physician can also select the Observations tab from the Review in Box screen for the specific SP being reviewed.

Exhibit 5-21. Utilities menu for selecting Observations referrals

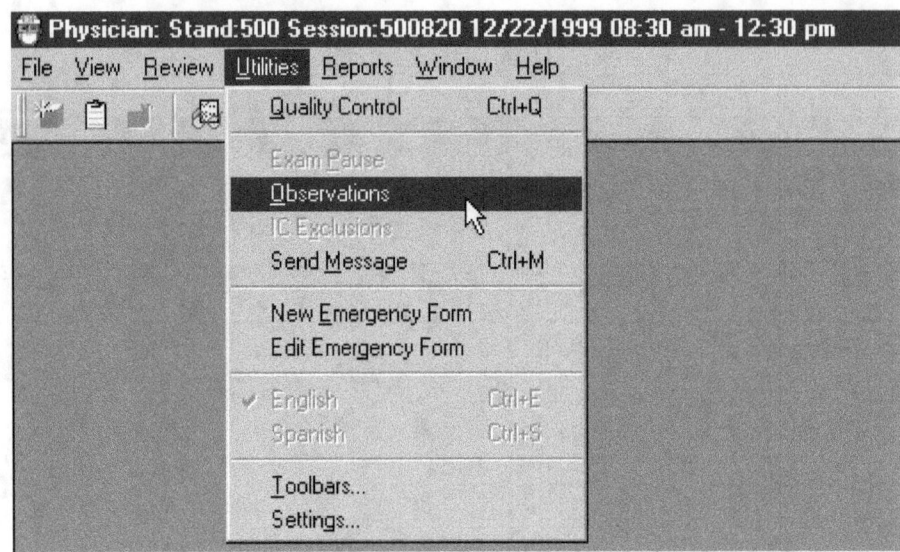

- Select the "Utilities" menu from the toolbar to access the Observations Referral window and then select Observations from the menu.

Exhibit 5-22. SP observation pick-list

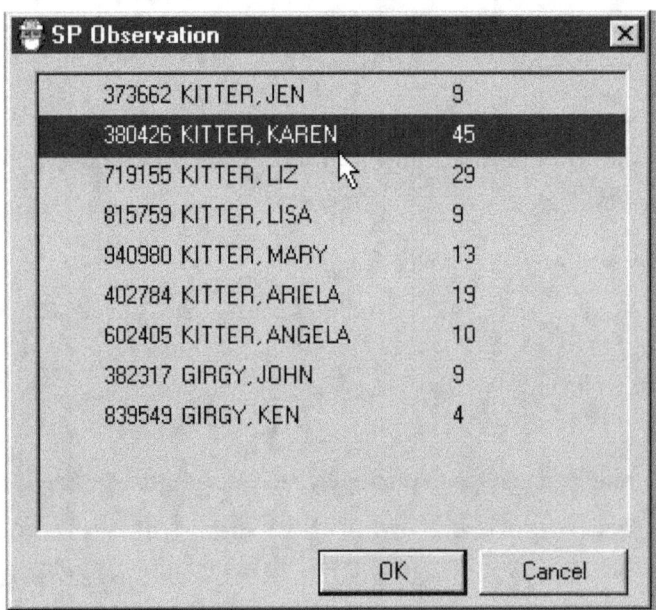

- The SP Observation pick list will appear with a list of all the names and ages of the SPs in the current session.

- Select the name of the SP for whom the observation referral is needed.

Exhibit 5-23. Observations referral box

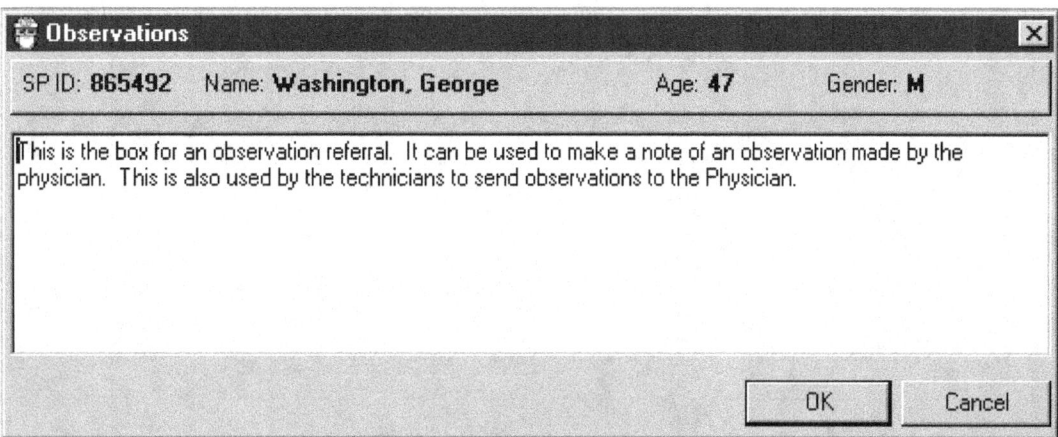

- This is the Observations referral box that will be displayed in the other components. The technician will open this box, write the information in the referral information box, and send it to the physician.

- This will be flagged in the Physician's Exam system and the SP will not be able to leave the MEC until the physician has reviewed this referral.

5.7.15   Referral Letter

Exhibit 5-24. Clinic pick-up referral letter

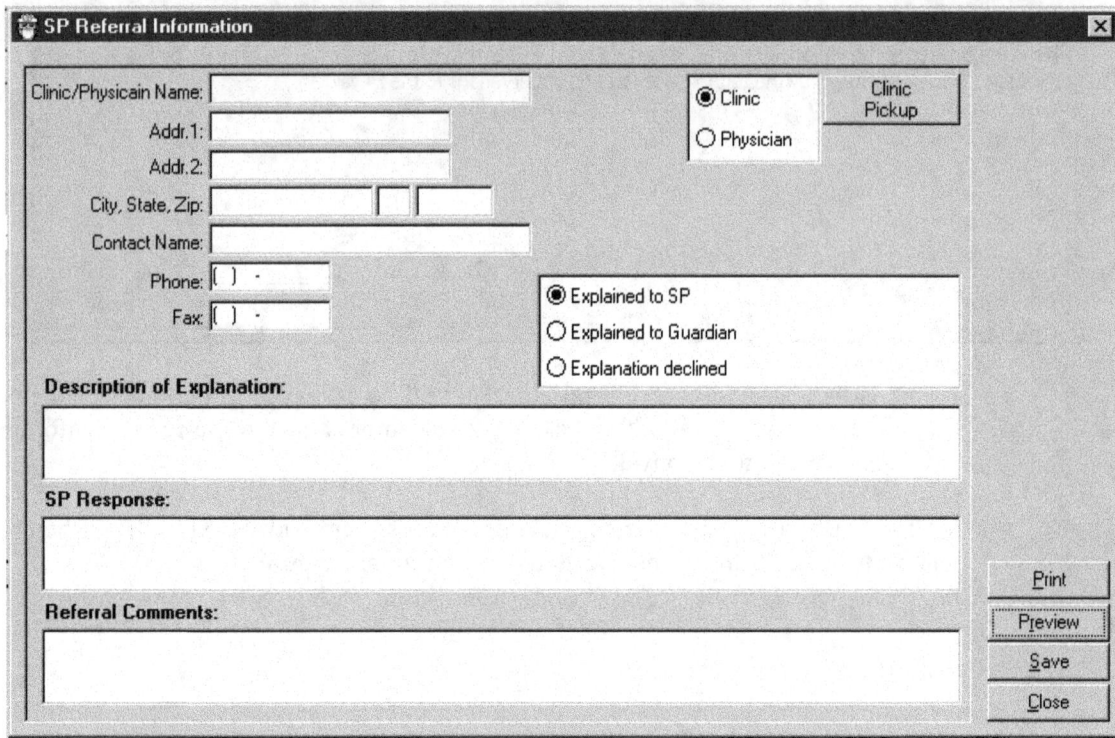

- When the "Referral" button is clicked, the above box is displayed. Click on "Clinic Pickup" to view a list of local clinics. Click on Physician to see a list of local providers.

- The address and phone number will appear in the appropriate boxes.

- Enter a description of your explanation of the referral to the SP, how the SP responds.

- The box at the bottom of the screen (Referral Comments) is for entering physician comments. These comments will appear on the second page of the referral letter.

5.7.16   Local Physician Pickup

Exhibit 5-25. Local physician and clinic pickup referral letter addresses

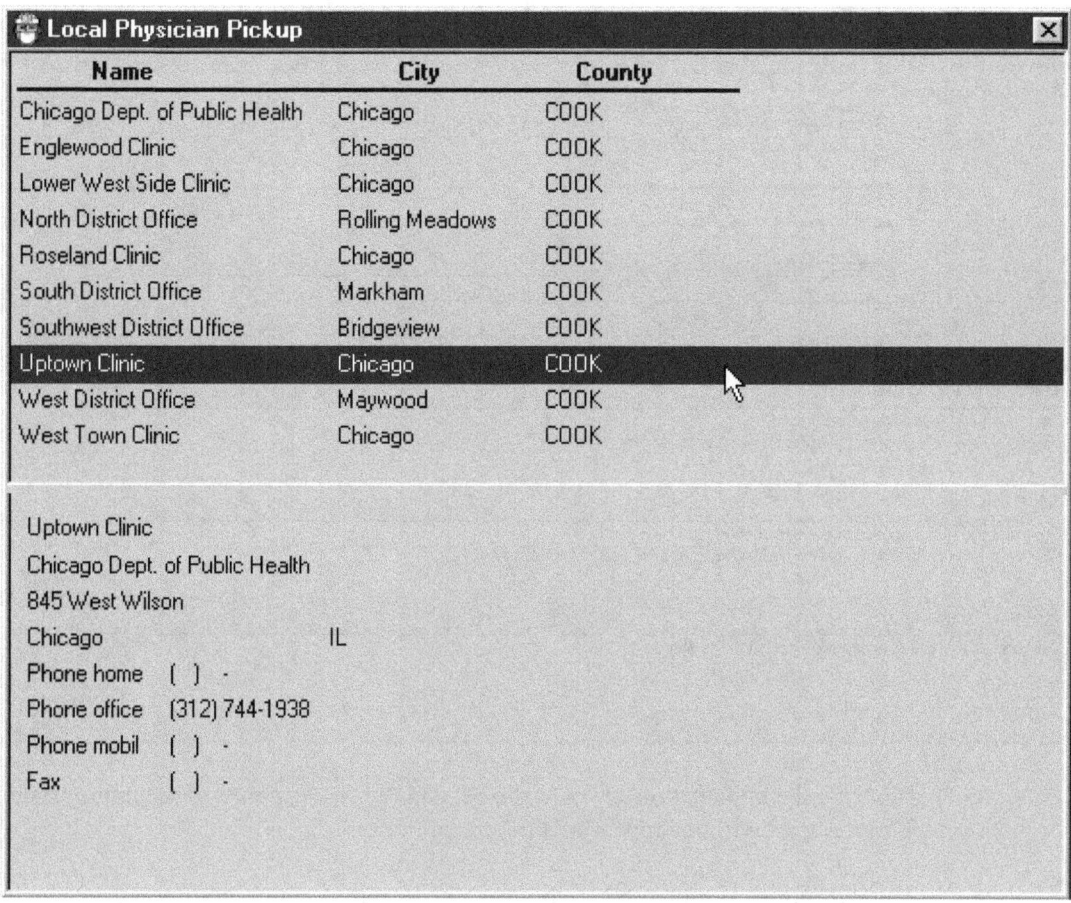

- Select the name of the clinic or health care provider.

5.7.17 Referral Address Information

Exhibit 5-26. Local physician and clinic pickup data entered for referral letter information

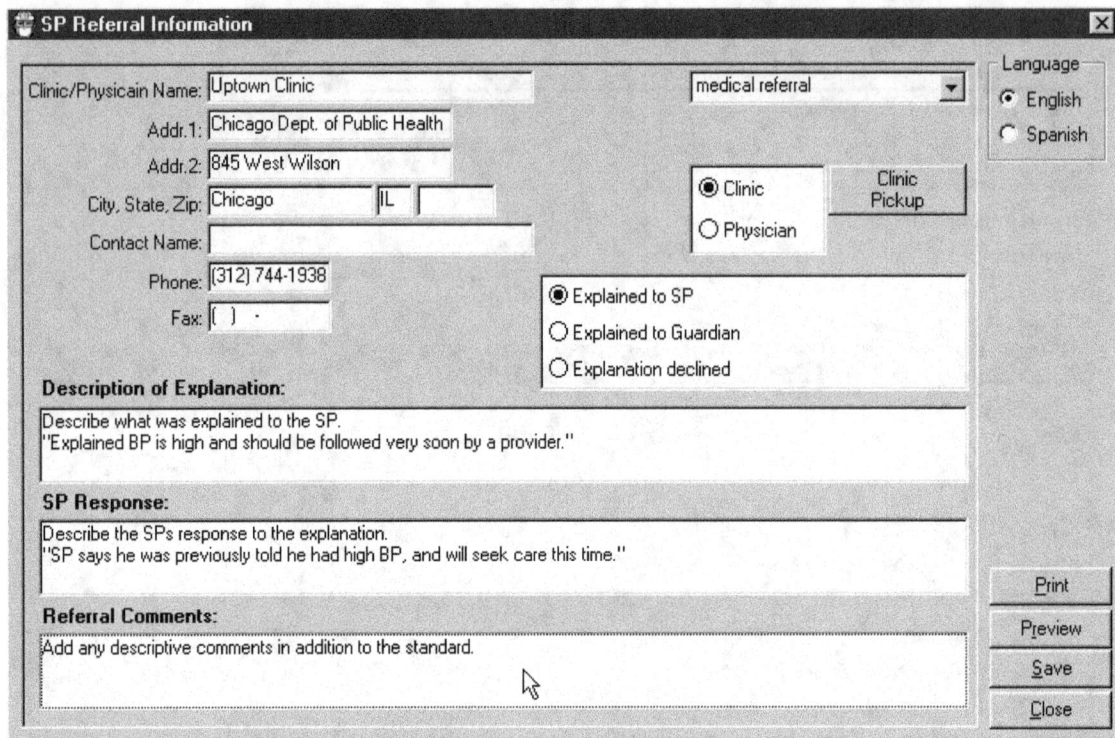

- Describe the explanation given to the SP and the SP response in the appropriate fields. These entries will not appear on the referral letter.

- The "Referral Comments" field may be used to enter comments to the referral physician.

5.7.18 Referral Letter Review

Exhibit 5-27. Preview referral letter

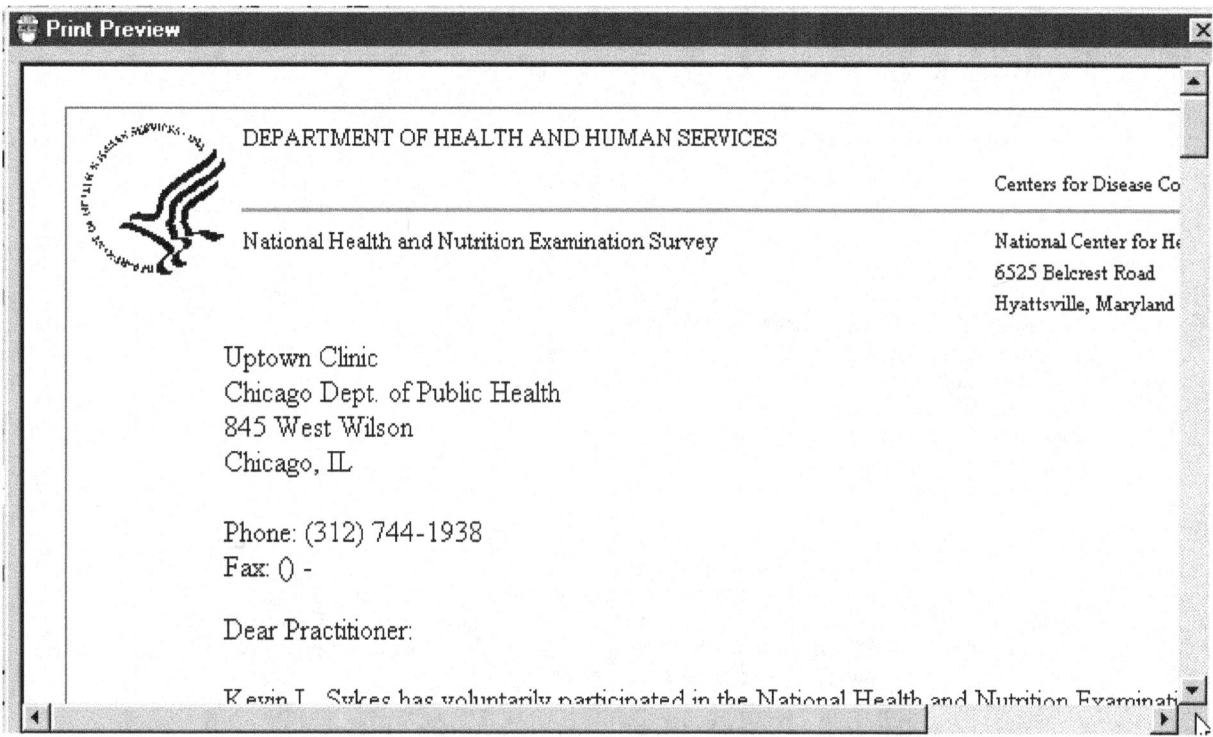

- Select "Preview" from the Session Review in Box screen.

- A preview of the referral letter will be displayed. Use the scroll bar to view all areas of the letter.

5.7.19   Referral Letter

Exhibit 5-28. Referral Letter Mock-up

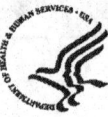

DEPARTMENT OF HEALTH & HUMAN SERVICES

Public Health Service
Centers for Disease Control and Prevention

National Center for Health Statistics
6525 Belcrest Road
Hyattsville, Maryland 20782

<Insert Clinics Name> or <SPs Physician>
<Insert Clinic Address>
<Insert Clinic City, ST, Zip>
<Insert Point of Contact>
<Insert Phone Number>

Dear Doctor:

<SP Name> has voluntarily participated in the fourth National Health and Nutrition
Examination Survey conducted at special facilities of the U.S. Public Health Service. The
objectives of the survey are to obtain information on the health and nutrition status of the U.S.
population. As a result of the testing that was done, it was noted that on **<Exam Date>**, a
finding was revealed that was outside the survey's medically acceptable range. This finding is
described on the attached Referral Comments page.

<Insert the following paragraph for SPs with Blood Pressure Level 1>
As indicated on the Referral Comments page the participant's blood pressure measurements
were severely high. The measurements were taken three times; and the values indicated are the
average of the last two measures. All survey participants with severely high blood pressure are
instructed to see their doctor or clinic the same day, or go to a hospital emergency room to
have their blood pressure rechecked.

This examination is intended to collect health measures for research. It is not a complete
physical exam. No attempt has been made to diagnose or treat medical conditions of the
participants. The findings disclosed to you are done so with the participant's permission.

Should you have any questions, you may contact me at the Mobile Exam Center. The phone
number is **<MEC Physician Phone>** until **<MEC Stand End Date>**. After that date you may
contact Dr. Kathryn Porter at the National Center for Health Statistics, Monday through Friday
9 AM to 6PM, EST. The toll free number is 1-800-452-6115.

Cordially,

<MEC Physician Name>, M.D.

- The data display for this referral letter includes all areas for referral in a single letter.

- See the next exhibit for the second page that will be attached to this referral.

Exhibit 5-28. Referral Letter Mock-up (continued)

Referral Comments for <SPs Name>

Blood Pressure

Systolic Blood Pressure: 118 mm Hg
Diastolic Blood Pressure: 73 mm Hg

Based on the Referral Level print the corresponding referral message from MEC_BP_Referral

Ankle Brachial Pressure Index

Left Ankle Brachial Pressure Index: 0.9
Right Ankle Pressure Index: 0.8

Based on the Referral Level print the corresponding referral message from MEC_ROF_Ranges

Toe Systolic Blood Pressure

Left Toe Systolic Pressure: 50 mmHg
Right Toe Systolic Pressure: 50 mmHg

Based on the Referral Level print the corresponding referral message from MEC_ROF_Ranges

Peripheral Neuropathy

Print Referral Statement from MEC_ROF_Ranges

CBC

Print all Lab Results – use same specs and format as Report of Findings

Exhibit 5-29. Example of referral comments

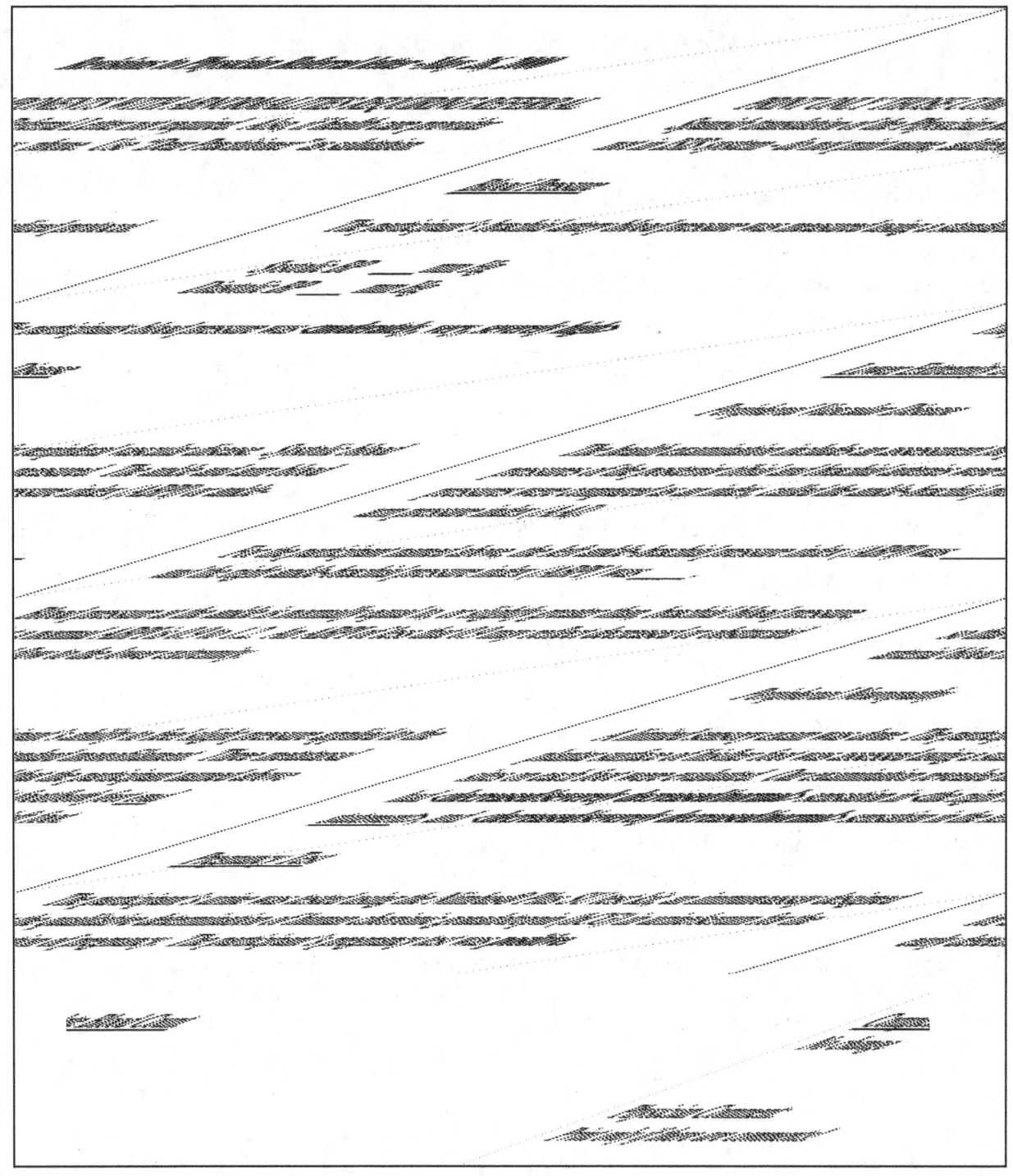

6. SAFETY ISSUES AND EMERGENCY PROCEDURES

6.1 Safety in the Mobile Exam Center (MEC)

The best approach to emergency situations in the MEC is to prevent problems from developing into emergencies whenever possible, and to be well prepared for those emergencies that cannot be avoided. It is the responsibility of all examination staff members to participate in maintaining safety in the MEC by staying alert for potentially unsafe conditions or unusual sample person (SP) behavior, and by being thoroughly familiar with the current NHANES procedures for emergencies.

Promotion of safety and prevention of accidents and emergencies in the MEC is of particular concern in NHANES in view of the proportion of elderly sample persons that will be participating in the survey. The number of elderly respondents will be significant as a result of an intentional oversampling and removal of the upper age limit on the examination.

6.1.1 Elderly Sample Persons

Care should be taken with all elderly sample persons to minimize confusion and ensure the safe completion of the examination. Elderly SPs should be escorted when moving between exam procedures and the coordinator's area, and should not be left alone for more than a few minutes, such as when changing clothes.

Instructions to elderly SPs should be provided in a clear, calm manner, and repeated as needed. It should not be assumed that the directions are understood until the SP offers an appropriate response. It may be necessary to guide SPs through each step required, such as providing a urine specimen or changing into a gown, to successfully complete a task. If the SP has difficulty understanding or performing tasks, try to offer one instruction or direction at a time and wait until the SP understands before proceeding.

Exam staff should be particularly alert to complaints or concerns from elderly SPs, as elderly SPs may not clearly communicate the extent of their discomfort or concern. Staff members will need to further investigate SP complaints and to refer all potential problems to the MEC physician.

6.1.2   Sample Persons in Wheelchairs

Some SPs may arrive for the examination in wheelchairs, and the exam staff will have to facilitate the SPs' entry into the MEC and their progress through the examination. The field office will alert the MEC manager and coordinator that an examinee is wheelchair bound so that the lift outside the LED examination room can be assembled.

SPs in wheelchairs will enter the MEC through the LED examination room, and then will be taken to the reception area where the coordinator will check them in and initiate the exam. The MEC trailers are large enough to allow passage of most wheelchairs. In the event a SP's wheelchair cannot move easily through the MEC, the SP may be transferred to the MEC wheelchair located in the handicapped bathroom. If the SP can bear sufficient weight on at least one leg or can otherwise support him or herself during the transfer, the physician and another exam staff member should assist him or her into the MEC wheelchair to facilitate movement throughout the MEC.

Sample persons who cannot bear most of their weight on one leg and need assistance in transferring to the MEC chair should not be lifted or moved out of their wheelchairs. Lifting or moving sample persons without their assistance could result in injury to a SP or staff member, and is unwarranted. SPs should remain in their wheelchairs and receive the exams that can be conducted in that position. When the transfer of a SP raises questions, the physician should make the decision to transfer or not transfer a SP.

6.1.3   Children in the MEC

Children in the MEC should be monitored at all times when not participating in an exam component. Young children should not be permitted to walk through the MEC unescorted, and should not interfere with the performance of any examinations.

When waiting for an exam, young or unruly children should remain in the reception area under the supervision of the MEC coordinator and assistant coordinator. Other staff members, when available, may be asked to assist the MEC coordinator and assistant coordinator during particularly busy sessions. Toys are available to entertain young children.

Staff members should be alert to the presence of children in the MEC, and always investigate the behavior of young children walking unattended through the exam center.

6.2 Safety Precautions

A number of precautions have been taken to promote safety in the exam center.

6.2.1 Mobile Exam Center Preparation

- Fire extinguishers have been placed throughout the MEC to allow rapid response to fire. Exit doors are present in every trailer.

- A drug kit, an automated external defibrillator, a portable oxygen tank, and portable blood pressure equipment is kept in one box in the physician's exam room in each caravan. All staff must be able to recognize and locate this equipment without delay.

- Pocket masks for CPR are in the following areas: The coordinator's station, vision room, CV fitness room, physician's exam room, MEC interview room #2, dietary interview room #1, LED room, the staff room, phlebotomy room, body composition room, anthropometry room, and dental exam room.

- The phone number "911" is to be used to activate EMS if applicable for the MEC location. The telephone number and address of the local fire and rescue squad will also be posted at the coordinator's station and in the staff room by the telephone.

- The address of the MEC will be posted in the coordinator's station and staff room so that the location can be reported correctly to EMS.

- The MEC is a "NO SMOKING" facility. Neither staff nor SPs may smoke in the exam center. Should a staff member or SP have the need to smoke, s/he should step outside the MEC.

6.2.2 Mobile Examination Staff Preparation

- All examination staff members are certified in cardiopulmonary resuscitation, Course Level C, and recertified biannually.

- A physician is required to be present when sample persons are in the MEC.

- All examination staff are required to be in the MEC while a session is in progress, and whenever SPs are in the MEC.

- All staff are required to be thoroughly familiar with the safety issues and emergency procedures.

- Mock emergency drills will be held periodically in the mobile exam center to simulate a medical emergency and permit practice of emergency procedures.

6.2.3   On-Site Preparations at Each Stand

- The field office or the advance arrangements team will contact and meet with local fire and rescue representatives to orient them to the location and structure of the MEC.

- The field office will provide advance notice to the MEC coordinator of any sample persons who will require assistance entering or moving through the exam center. The coordinator will inform the MEC manager so that appropriate preparations can be made.

- The physician will review the medication history from the household interview for each SP prior to the examination session in which the SP's appointment is scheduled. The SP medication information can be accessed by the physician in the ISIS Physician's Exam application.

6.3   Reporting SP Problems to the MEC Physician

Sample persons who report feeling ill or who appear to feel ill should be reported to the MEC physician at the earliest opportunity. At times sample persons may have nonspecific complaints such as viral illnesses, joint pain, or fatigue, that do not appear to warrant an emergency response. Exam staff members should offer to have the physician speak with a SP who has a particular complaint. If the SP is reluctant or refuses, and there is any question about the health or safety of the SP, staff members should consult the physician for recommendations on how to proceed through the exam.

6.4 Medical Management and Referrals

6.4.1 Medical Referrals

Although the primary purpose of the MEC examination is data collection, not diagnosis or treatment, the exam may produce findings that warrant further medical attention. There is an obligation to inform the SP of any abnormal results from the exams, and to refer the SP to the appropriate provider for treatment. The MEC physician is responsible for the referral process. Each exam component has a referral process built into the ISIS system, which will alert the physician to findings that may require a referral. Some of the exam findings may already be known to the SPs and their providers, but others may have been unknown up until the day of the MEC exam. Based on the results of any component of the MEC examination, the physician will place the examinee in one of three categories:

Level I   Major medical findings that warrant immediate attention by a health care provider e.g.; dangerously high blood pressure, emergencies.

Level II   Major medical findings that warrant attention by a health care provider in the next 2 weeks because they are expected to cause adverse effects within this time period.

Level III Minor medical findings that an examinee and his or her physician already know about. Medical findings that do not require prompt attention by a medical provider.

A Level I referral usually results in termination of the MEC exam, with a transfer of the SP out of the MEC and into a hospital or other care facility. If a SP refuses treatment, she or he must sign a release stating that she or he is aware of the exam findings and is refusing treatment against the advice of the MEC physician. The SP must sign the release form before leaving the MEC.

An SP with a Level II referral can continue the MEC examination, and will be advised to see his or her primary care provider within the 2 weeks following the exam. If the SP does not have a care provider, the MEC physician can arrange for the SP to see a local provider who has previously agreed to accept referrals from the MEC exam.

6.4.2 Medical Management

The following section describes some medical scenarios that may occur during the MEC examination and actions to be taken by the MEC physician. The section also provides guidance in determining the level of referral for an examinee.

6.4.2.1 Allergic Reactions

Examinees that experience allergic reactions will be treated according to the procedures adopted from Phil Lieberman, MD, Conn's Current Therapy, 1981, which states: "the therapy of anaphylaxis and anaphylactic reactions is subdivided into those procedures which are to be performed immediately and those which require a more detailed evaluation of the patient prior to transfer to the institution." Procedures that should be instituted immediately are:

1. The administration of epinephrine is the most important single therapeutic measure. Epinephrine should be administered at the first appearance of symptoms. Early administration can prevent more serious manifestations. The route of administration should be intramuscular or subcutaneous. Intravenous administration should be avoided if possible, being reserved only for those rare instances in which there is loss of consciousness and obvious severe cardiovascular collapse.

   The dose of intramuscular or subcutaneous epinephrine is 0.3 to 0.5ml of a 1:1000 concentration. Injections may be administered every 10 to 15 minutes until an effect is achieved or until tachycardia or other side effects supervene.

   The aforementioned subcutaneous and intramuscular dose is for adults. Children should receive a dose of 0.01 ml per kg of 1:1000 epinephrine to a maximum of 0.3 ml.

2. The airway should be checked immediately. Laryngeal edema and angioedema of the tissue surrounding the airway is the most rapid cause of death.

3. The SP should be placed in a recumbent position and his feet elevated.

4. Nasal oxygen should be started.

5. Vital signs should be obtained and monitored every 10 to 15 minutes for the duration of the attack.

After the procedures noted above have been done, a more extensive evaluation can be performed. The injection of epinephrine may be sufficient to prevent further symptoms. If, however, the SP continues to have difficulty, other measures are instituted as deemed appropriate according to the patient's evaluation.

6.4.2.2   First Aid for Choking

Infants, children, and adults who are choking as a result of a foreign body obstruction should be treated according to the guidelines recommended in basic life support courses.

For adults and children older than 1 year, the Heimlich maneuver is the treatment of choice. A series of six to ten rapid, upward abdominal thrusts can be performed until the foreign body is expelled. If the obstruction is not relieved using the Heimlich maneuver, the victim's airway should be opened using the tongue-jaw lift. If the object can be visualized, it can be removed with a finger sweep. If the object cannot be visualized, blind finger sweeps can be attempted on adults. Blind finger sweeps can cause further airway obstruction and should never be done on children.

For choking infants, place the infant face down on the rescuer's forearm in a 60-degree head-down position with the head and neck stabilized. A series of back blows and chest thrusts should be performed until the airway obstruction is relieved.

For further information on treatment of choking victims, both conscious and unconscious, consult the First Aid Handbook.

6.4.2.3   Seizures

Examinees who experience a seizure while in the MEC should receive immediate attention from the physician. The following steps should be taken to secure the safety of the examinee:

Step 1.   Position the examinee on the ground

Step 2.   Insert an oral airway if the jaw is relaxed (do not **force** any object into the mouth)

Step 3.   Remove glasses and loosen collar

Step 4.   Remove objects from vicinity of examinee to prevent injury

Step 5.   Monitor vital signs

The MEC physician must use his or her clinical judgement based on the examinee's past medical history, the type and duration of the seizure, the cause of the seizure, and current seizure medication to determine whether or not the person needs emergency medical care or can be sent home. The MEC physician is also responsible for maintaining an airway, giving any indicated medications, and directing care of a seizing examinee until an ambulance arrives or the seizure is over.

6.4.2.4   Hypoglycemia

Most conditions of hypoglycemia can be treated while the subject is conscious with the simple administration of juice and other first aid measures. If hypoglycemia is suspected in the case of an unconscious examinee, the following steps may be taken after emergency assistance is summoned:

Step 1. Recognition of hypoglycemia based on available history:

- Bizarre behavior and other clinical signs of possible glucose insufficiency should lead the physician to think of hypoglycemia. Hypoglycemia may develop in both diabetic and nondiabetic individuals.

Step 2. Basic life support:

- Immediate management includes positioning (supine), airway maintenance, oxygen administration, and monitoring of vital signs. The hypoglycemic examinee will not regain consciousness until the blood glucose level is elevated.

Step 3. Definitive management:

- An unconscious person with a prior history of diabetes mellitus is always presumed to be hypoglycemic unless other causes of unconsciousness are present. Definitive management of the unconscious diabetic usually entails the administration of a carbohydrate by the most effective route available. The most effective route is usually intravenous administration of 50 percent dextrose solution. The unconscious examinee must **never** be given anything by mouth, since this may add to the possibility of airway obstruction or pulmonary aspiration. In the absence of intravenous fluids, definitive management must await the arrival of local emergency assistance.

6.4.2.5   Use of Oxygen

When the oxygen tank is used in the MEC, the flow rate should be set between 3-6 liters/minute unless the person has Chronic Obstructive Pulmonary Disease (COPD), With the use of the nasal cannula a flow range of 3-6 liters/minute produces a forced inspiratory oxygen of 40 percent-50 percent.

If the sample person has COPD, the flow rate should be set at 2 liters per minute. At this rate, there is little to no danger of interfering with the hypoxic-breathing stimulus present in COPD.

6.5   Emergency Procedures

6.5.1   Medical Emergencies Overview

Before examinations begin at a stand, the MEC manager will have obtained information from the advance team about the types and availability of emergency medical services and oxygen suppliers in the area where the MEC is located. The MEC manager will also make the arrangements for the emergency medical service to tour the MEC prior to the start day of SP examinations. Emergency medical services can include those available at nearby hospitals, hospital ambulance services, and emergency services available from police and fire rescue squads as well as from other county or local rescue squads. The MEC manager will select the best services available from the standpoint of convenience to the MEC and availability of service and equipment. In some cases, it may be desirable to select two services. This information will be summarized on a fact sheet and posted by all the telephones in the MEC. The phone number "911" is to be used if applicable for the MEC location. However, the telephone numbers of the nearest police, fire, and rescue squads will also be posted. Execution of emergency procedures and the proper use of all emergency equipment will be the responsibility of the MEC physician. The primary response of the MEC physician should be to stabilize the examinee's condition and to expedite a safe transfer to the nearest emergency medical treatment facility.

The MEC examinations are designed to be safe for examinees. To ensure maximal safety the physician must be able to handle the initial management of an examinee in distress.

The response of the physician is limited by a number of factors. There are no nurses, respiratory therapists, physician's assistants, or other specialized staff that are necessary for a high level emergency response. The MEC is not a diagnostic or treatment center, and the liability insurance obtained for Westat physicians does not cover any type of treatment procedure (except emergency stabilization). Within these restrictions, the appropriate response of the physician should be, as previously stated, to stabilize the examinee in distress and facilitate a safe and expedited transfer to the nearest medical facility.

The physician is responsible for directing the care of a patient in the event of an emergency. Staff members are responsible for the tasks assigned to them under the direction of the MEC manager and the physician.

The best overall approach to medical emergencies is prevention. The physician may be called upon to decide if some procedures should not be administered to certain examinees to avoid potential medical problems if the examinee does not fit easily into the preexisting medical exclusion categories for that procedure. The examining physician can at his/her discretion proscribe certain procedures such as cardiovascular fitness and other tests if he/she believes the test may endanger an examinee's health. The specific reasons for excluding the examinee should be recorded in the system in the comment drop-down list.

A first aid manual entitled *The American Medical Association's Handbook of First Aid and Emergency Care 1990*, will be available as a reference review guide. Standard first aid approaches are to be followed for common problems such as faints, minor seizures, falls, and other minor injuries. The MEC physician will determine the level of treatment and referral based on the circumstances of each case. Caution should be exercised and there should be no hesitation to send an examinee to an emergency room when circumstances warrant.

The physician is to be notified immediately of any situation involving an examinee whose safety is of concern. Any questionable situation should be considered an emergency and evaluated by the physician. In addition to the equipment and supplies that are transported to the site at the time of the emergency, a list of the medications (prescription and nonprescription) that the examinee is currently taking will be available. The medication list may provide pertinent medical history information to the physician so that a more accurate assessment of the examinee can be made and the appropriate emergency treatment given. The medication list is the one obtained by the interviewer in the household questionnaire, and is available in the Physician's Exam ISIS application.

When ambulance personnel trained in emergency medical care arrive to transport an examinee in distress (Level I referral) the physician should make an assessment of whether he or she should accompany the examinee to the emergency room. The decision should be based on maximizing safety for the examinee. If the physician determines that he/she should accompany the examinee to the hospital, the MEC must be closed. The field office will contact the examinee's family as soon as possible to inform them of the incident and the medical facility to which the examinee was taken. The physician may also contact the examinee's designated primary health care providers as soon as possible to inform them of the occurrence and name of the medical facility to which the examinee was taken.

6.5.1.2 Emergency Supplies and Equipment

A limited number of emergency supplies will be located in the physician's room. The supplies on hand will be an oxygen tank, nasal cannulas, a portable blood pressure kit, a stethoscope, an automated external defibrillator, a drug kit, and an ambu bag and pocket CPR mask. The drug kit contains the following items:

Albuterol (17g)	Metered dose canister	90 mcg/puff	Inhaled
Ammonia	Ammonia Aspirol	0.3 ml	Inhaled
Epinephrin-adult	EpiPen	0.3mg 1:1000	IM injection
Epinephrin-peds	EpiPen Jr.	0.15mg 1:2000	IM injection
Glucose – tube	Insta-Glucose 31 gm	1-2 tbsp	Oral
Nitroglycerin (25 tabs)	Nitrostat	0.4mg 1/150gr	Sublingual

Please note the drug kit does not contain antiarrythmic medications or narcotics. Only the physician should administer emergency procedures and use the contents of the emergency supplies other than the stethoscope and blood pressure cuff.

6.5.1.3   MEC Standard Medical Emergency Protocol

Due to the limited space in the MEC trailers, congregations of more than three or four people in one room are almost impossible. Subsequently, staff response to an emergency has been designed to limit the number of people needed to be together at one time. For example, a true cardiac or respiratory arrest requires only three people to be close to the patient for an extended period of time; two staff members to perform CPR and one physician. Two staff members will act as a runner and a recorder, but will be required to do so without hindering the performance of CPR or the physician's access to the patient. Once an ambulance arrives, the path to the victim must be clear to allow transfer to EMS staff. If possible, the closest emergency exit door should be opened for EMS personnel to transfer the patient to an ambulance. Other types of emergencies, such as a fall or a seizure, will require the presence of the physician and only one or two staff as requested by the physician and the MEC manager. There should be no spectators in the vicinity that may inhibit care of a patient.

6.5.1.4   Staff Roles in an Emergency

First Responder

The first responder is the person who either discovers the victim or is with the victim at the time of the event. Do not leave the victim alone at any time. Call for another staff member to alert the coordinator and the physician of the situation immediately and initiate CPR if needed. The first person who responds to your call will be the runner for the event. If another staff member is immediately available, call for that person to assist you with CPR. If no one is available, continue one-person CPR until someone arrives to assist you. Once the physician arrives, explain briefly what happened and s/he will direct care of the patient while you and your partner continue CPR. The physician will also ensure that there is a designated recorder for the event. If the physician is the first person on the scene, she or he should call for help to alert the coordinator and MEC manager immediately and then initiate CPR if needed. The physician should continue one-person CPR until two other staff members arrive to take over CPR while the physician directs care of the patient. The MEC manager will confirm that all roles in the emergency response have been filled, and that all unneeded staff are clear of the area. If the coordinator has taken on a role in the emergency, the MEC manager will assign another staff member to take over for the coordinator. The coordinator will then return to the reception area to manage the SPs in the MEC. If the MEC manager is not in the MEC at the time of the event, the chief health technologist should be notified to follow the MEC manager's emergency protocol responsibilities.

Coordinator

The coordinator's responsibilities in the event of an emergency are as follows:

1. Activate the Emergency Medical Services (EMS) system by calling 911 or other emergency number posted at the coordinator station. Request an ambulance for a medical emergency and give the location of the MEC, which will be posted at the coordinator's station.

2. Notify the MEC manager of the emergency and provide any information you have regarding the need for staff assignments. If the MEC manager is not in the MEC at the time of the event, notify the chief health technologist who will then follow the MEC manager's emergency protocol responsibilities.

3. Retrieve any SPs left unattended in exam rooms while staff members are assisting with the emergency. Staff should remain in the exam rooms with the SPs if they are not called upon to assist in the emergency. All other SPs should remain in the reception area with the coordinator. If the event occurs in the reception area, SPs in the reception area should be escorted to other exam rooms.

4. Remain in the reception area with the SPs or designate another staff member to do so. Maintain calm and assure SPs the situation is under control.

MEC Manager

The MEC manager's responsibilities in the event of an emergency are as follows:

1. Check that the following staff are on the scene: 1 runner, 1 recorder, 2 people performing CPR, and the physician.

2. Check that all other staff members are clear of the area.

3. Post the assistant coordinator or other available staff member outside the MEC to direct EMS to the site of the emergency.

4. If possible, open the emergency exit closest to the site of the emergency to facilitate transfer of the patient to EMS.

5.   Contact the field office immediately after the SP has left the MEC to inform the field Office manager of the emergency. The field office will notify the SP's family of the event if the SP came alone to the MEC.

If the MEC manager is not available at the time of the emergency, the chief health technologist will follow the protocol for the MEC manager's responsibilities.

Assistant Coordinator

The assistant coordinator will be stationed outside the entrance to the MEC and will direct EMS into the MEC and to the site of the emergency. If an emergency exit door has been opened, the assistant coordinator will direct EMS to the emergency exit door to facilitate transfer of the victim. If the assistant coordinator is not available, another staff member can be designated to guide the EMS team.

MEC Physician

The MEC physician is responsible for directing care of the SP until EMS arrives. Once the emergency equipment is on the scene, the physician should ensure that a staff member is recording events on the MEC Incident/Emergency Report form. The physician should not perform tasks such as CPR unless the physician is the first person on the scene. If the physician is the first responder, she or he should begin CPR until two other staff members arrive. The physician is also responsible for the operation of the automated external defibrillator and the administration of medications. The physician will follow the ACLS algorithm and emergency protocols as outlined in the physician manual. When ambulance personnel trained in emergency medical care arrive to transport a SP in distress (Level I referral) the physician should make an assessment of whether she or he should accompany the SP to the emergency room. The decision whether or not to provide an escort to the hospital should be based on maximizing safety for the SP. If the physician determines that she or he should accompany the SP to the hospital, the MEC must be closed. If possible, the physician should obtain consent from the SP or the SP's family to contact the SP's designated primary health care provider as soon as possible to report the occurrence and give the name of the medical facility to which the SP was taken.

Recorder

Any staff member could be called upon to act as recorder for the event. The recorder will be responsible for documenting the time of the emergency and the sequence of events that follow the initiation of emergency care on the MEC Incident/Emergency Report form (Exhibit 6-3). The order of the events and time sequence are the critical elements in documentation. MEC Incident/Emergency Report forms will be kept in the physician's emergency kit and are available on ISIS by clicking on the ambulance icon in the Toolbox. Instructions for completing this form are found in Exhibit 6-4 of this manual.

Runner

Generally, the first person to respond to the call for help will be the runner for the event. The runner's first responsibility is to notify the physician, the coordinator, and the MEC manager of the event. Once the appropriate people have been notified, the runner is responsible for retrieving supplies and equipment, and making phone calls as directed by staff at the scene.

Other staff members should remain clear of the site and assist in keeping order in the MEC unless asked to help. No SPs should be left alone in the MEC. If a staff member has a role in the emergency and is in the process of examining a SP, the SP will be returned to the reception area while the staff member is in the emergency. All other staff will remain in the exam rooms with SPs until the crisis has passed. The coordinator is responsible for managing SPs in the reception area. The MEC manager is responsible for managing the MEC staff. In the absence of the MEC manager, the chief technologist will manage the MEC staff response during the emergency.

6.5.1.5 The Physician's Role and AED Operation

As explained previously, the MEC is not a diagnostic or treatment center, and the liability insurance obtained for Westat physicians does not cover any type of treatment procedure (except emergency stabilization). The primary response of the MEC physician should be to stabilize the examinee's condition and to expedite a safe transfer to the nearest emergency medical treatment facility. MEC physicians are required to be BLS certified. The physician is the only person responsible for the operation of the automated external defibrillator (AED), and the administration of oxygen and medications (Exhibit 6-1)*. The AED can be placed on a patient for the purpose of monitoring a heart rhythm, but only one lead will be displayed. The physician is not expected to make a diagnosis based on the AED monitor. The AED should be used only for monitoring a heart rate, or when ventricular tachycardia or ventricular fibrillation is suspected or imminent. Any patient who is unconscious is a candidate for application of the AED. The AED will advise a shock only in the event of ventricular tachycardia or fibrillation. The AED does not have cardioversion capability, nor will the physician be able to deliver a shock if the AED does not advise a shock. As there are no antiarrythmic medications in the emergency drug kit, the response to a cardiac emergency is basic life support with defibrillation if indicated.

6.5.1.6   Documentation

After the SP has left the MEC, the physician should make sure that the incident and outcome are documented in the automated system in the physician's ISIS application. The physician will also complete a full report on a separate form, the MEC Incident/Emergency Report form, described below. The recorder will also use this form to record events on the scene. The recorder's notes of the event will be especially important in the completion of the physician's report, and should be kept with the physician's documentation of the incident. The MEC manager should review the final report prepared by the physician and add any information not included in the physician's report. The MEC manager's addendum should include only information about the event that is not in the physician's report. Any discrepancies in reports should be brought to the attention of the Director of MEC Operations before being made final. Notification and documentation of the emergency incident should be directed to Catherine Novak, Director of MEC Operations, as soon as possible.

6.5.1.7   MEC Incident/Emergency Report Form

A hard copy form entitled "MEC Incident/Emergency Report" will be utilized for recording the sequence of events or actions that are taken during the emergency response. An example of the form is shown in Exhibit 6-3. Guidelines for completion of the form are in Exhibit 6-4. During the emergency,

---

* All exhibits are located at the end of this chapter.

the recorder will use the form to record vitals, treatments, and some patient outcomes. The physician will then use the recorder's notes to complete a final official MEC Incident/Emergency Report Form. The MEC manager will then review the final form with the physician and make any necessary additions.

The NHANES Emergency Protocol Checklist (Exhibit 6-2), and the MEC Incident/Emergency Report Form Documentation Guidelines (Exhibit 6-4) are located in the emergency kit in the physician's exam room. The NHANES Emergency Protocol Checklist is also located in the major hallways of the MEC.

6.6   Psychiatric/Behavioral Problem Procedures

There are situations that may arise regarding SP behavior that will require special handling. They include:

- Previous psychological injuries, deterioration and/or deprivation - Due to changes in mental status, the SP may seem confused or may actually have dementia.

- Inebriation due to intoxication with alcohol and/or drugs - The SP will be less able to grasp ideas, reason, problem-solve, calculate, and attend to the tasks at hand. Therefore, the potential for injury, trauma, and violence is present.

- Belligerence - This will include SPs with noncompliant or abusive behavior.

- Suicidal/Homicidal Ideation – If a SP expresses intent to harm him/herself or someone else, the SP should be referred to the physician. The physician will evaluate the SP and determine the need for a referral to a psychiatric facility.

If the SP is so demented, confused, intoxicated, or belligerent that it is impossible to continue the examination, the MEC manager should calmly terminate the MEC examination and have the examinee leave the center without delay. For those examinees who require assistance going home, have a family member escort them home or call a cab.

Suicidal and homicidal ideation are considered psychiatric emergencies and are generally handled by referral. Guidelines for handling SPs who express suicidal or homicidal intent are included in the physician's manual.

For any psychiatric emergency, an incident form should be completed, and the incident reported by telephone to the Director of MEC Operations as soon as possible.

6.7   Natural Disaster Procedures

In the event of an unforeseeable occurrence (i.e., hurricane, tornado, fire, etc.), certain procedures should be followed depending on whether the event happens prior to or during an examination session.

6.7.1   Disaster Prior to an Examination Session

- Predicted Event - The stand coordinator should contact the home office for instructions regarding whether to cancel the session. If the session is cancelled, the stand coordinator will then notify the MEC manager, who in turn will notify the MEC staff.

- If residents of mobile homes and trailers have been notified to evacuate, the stand coordinator should make the decision to cancel the session. S/he should then call the home office to report the occurrence and cancellation of the session and notify the MEC manager. The MEC manager should notify the MEC staff.

- The stand coordinator and MEC manager may place the staff on stand-by procedures, with instructions to be ready to work but accessible by phone at home awaiting orders from the MEC manager regarding status of operations.

6.7.2   Disaster During an Examination Session

If an examination session is underway and SPs are in the MEC when the MEC manager or coordinator is notified by the field office of a pending natural event, the following procedures should be followed:

- The MEC manager and the physician should make a joint decision regarding closing the MEC and/or canceling the session. The first priority should be the safety of the SPs and staff.

- The MEC staff and SPs should evacuate the MEC as soon as possible and go directly to a safe haven, such as a building close by or the staff hotel. The staff and SPs should remain at this site until the impending event is over and it is safe to proceed outside.

- After the event, the MEC manager and the physician should decide whether or not to continue the exam session if the SPs are willing to stay for the rest of the session.

- If either the decision is made to cancel the session or the SPs decline to remain, the appointments for those SP's will need to be rescheduled by the field office.

- It is essential for the MEC manager to notify the stand coordinator of the outcome of events. The stand coordinator should then notify the home office immediately.

- Examiners who were conducting an exam or interview at the time evacuation of the MEC was ordered should interrupt the exam in the ISIS system. The reason for interruption of the exam must be accurately documented in ISIS and in room logs as soon as possible after the MEC is reopened.

- The MEC coordinator should be sure to document the reason for exam components omitted because of the closure of the MEC.

Exhibit 6-1. AED Algorithm

Automated External Defibrillation (AED) Treatment Algorithm
Emergency cardiac care pending arrival of EMS personnel

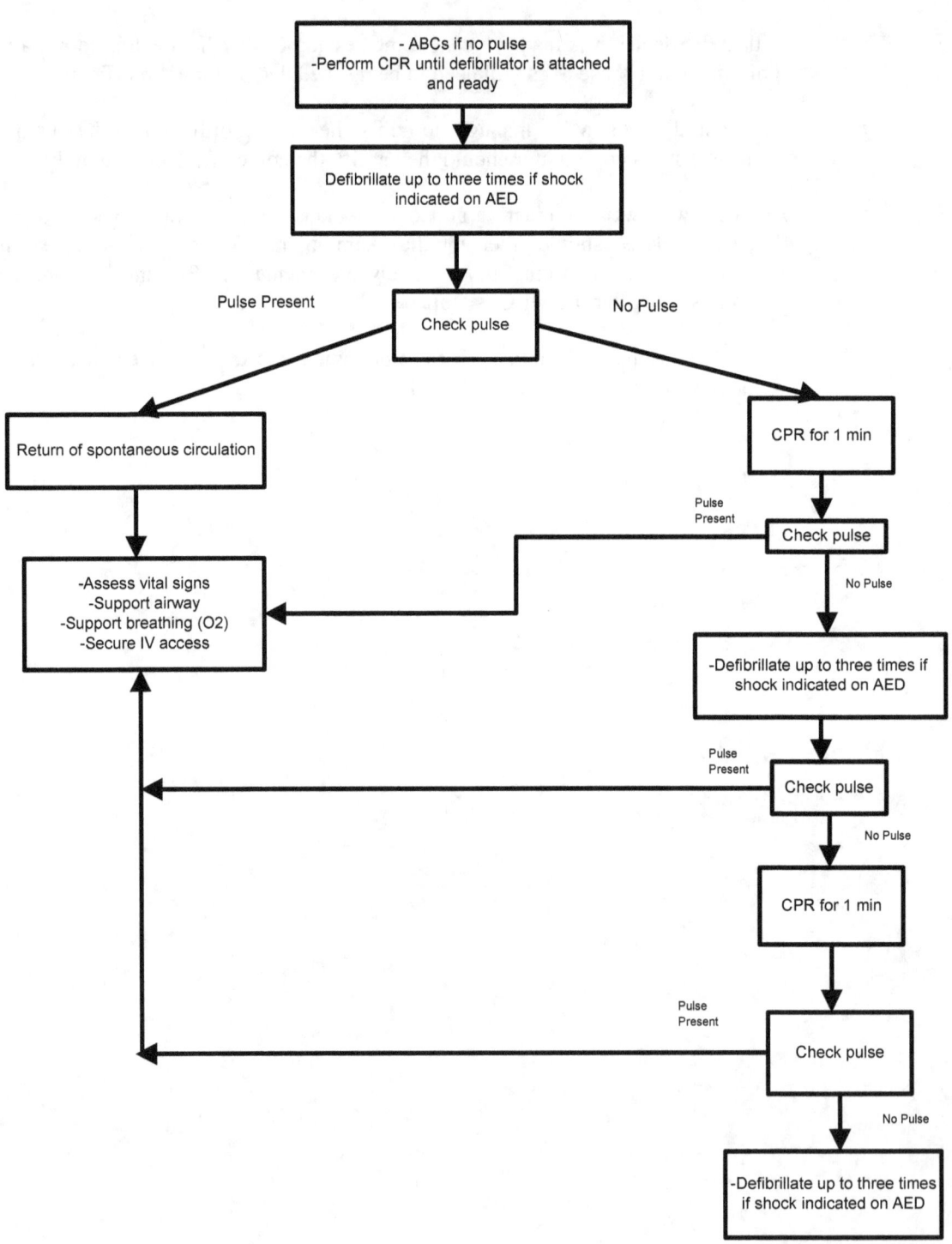

Exhibit 6-2. NHANES Emergency Protocol Checklist

NHANES Emergency Protocol Checklist

Call for help and initiate CPR if needed

Send runner to notify physician and coordinator of the emergency

MEC Coordinator:
Activate EMS by calling 911 or other emergency number
Retrieve unattended SPs and return them to the reception area
Remain with SPs in reception area, and provide reassurance

Physician:
Direct staff care of victim
Operate automated external defibrillator
Give medications
Determine if victim needs a physician escort to the hospital

MEC manager:
Ensure adequate staff for emergency response
Open the emergency exit door closest to the scene
Post assistant coordinator or other staff member outside the MEC to
greet ambulance personnel
Notify the field office of the event once the SP has left the MEC

Runner:
Notify staff, obtain equipment and supplies as directed

Recorder:
Record events on the MEC Emergency/Incident Report Form

Assistant coordinator:
Direct ambulance personnel to emergency site

Staff not requested to be involved in the emergency must stay away from the scene, remain in the exam rooms with SPs, and assist in maintaining order in the MEC.

Exhibit 6-3. MEC Incident/Emergency Report form

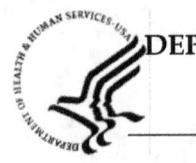 **DEPARTMENT OF HEALTH & HUMAN SERVICES**

Public Health Service
Centers for Disease Control and Prevention

National Center for Health Statistics
6525 Belcrest Road

MEC INCIDENT/EMERGENCY REPORT

Incident/Emergency	**Person Type**
◯ Incident ◯ Emergency	◯ SP ◯ Tech ◯ Other

General Information

Physician Name:	Recorder Name:
Emergency Date:	Runner Name(s):
Start Time: End Time:	Who Called 911:
Location:	Who Found:
Description:	

Personal Information

Person ID:		Age:	Gender:
Last Name:	First Name:		Middle Name

DEPARTMENT OF HEALTH & HUMAN SERVICES

Exhibit 6-3. MEC Incident/Emergency Report form (continued)

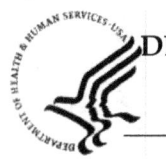

DEPARTMENT OF HEALTH & HUMAN SERVICES

Public Health Service
Centers for Disease Control and Prevention

National Center for Health Statistics
6525 Belcrest Road

Vitals

Time	Heart Rate	Systolic BP	Diastolic BP	Respiratory Rate	Comments

Treatment

Time	Medication/Equipment	Comment

Page 2 of 5

Exhibit 6-3. MEC Incident/Emergency Report form (continued)

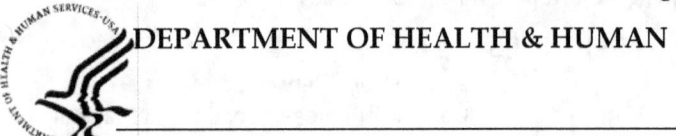

DEPARTMENT OF HEALTH & HUMAN SERVICES

Public Health Service
Centers for Disease Control and Prevention

National Center for Health Statistics
6525 Belcrest Road

Symptoms

Observation

Assessment

Plan

Exhibit 6-3. MEC Incident/Emergency Report form (continued)

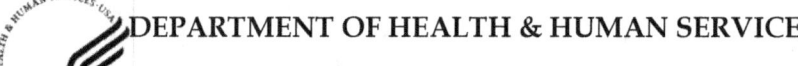

DEPARTMENT OF HEALTH & HUMAN SERVICES

Public Health Service
Centers for Disease Control and Prevention

National Center for Health Statistics
6525 Belcrest Road

Urgent Care

☐ Transported to Hospital	Hospital Name:
Ambulance Arrival Time:	Ambulance Departure Time:
Emergency Service Name:	
☐ Physician Accompanied SP to Hospital	

Notification

☐ Family Member Notified	Name:	Date/time:
	Relation:	
☐ Family Physician Notified	Family Phys Named:	Date/time:

Signature:_____   Date:_____

Exhibit 6-3. MEC Incident/Emergency Report form (continued)

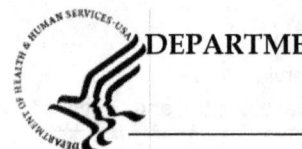

DEPARTMENT OF HEALTH & HUMAN SERVICES

Public Health Service
Centers for Disease Control and Prevention

National Center for Health Statistics
6525 Belcrest Road

Vitals

Time	Heart Rate	Systolic BP	Diastolic BP	Respiratory Rate	Comments

DEPARTMENT OF HEALTH & HUMAN SERVICES

Exhibit 6-4. MEC Incident/Emergency Form Documentation Guidelines

The Vitals and Treatment sections on page 2 should be completed first during the emergency. If the spaces on page 2 are insufficient, the last page should be used for recording vital signs. The 'comments' section of the last page can be used to record treatments. The remaining sections should be completed as soon as the emergency is over. The recorder should collect most of the information requested on page 1 before turning the notes over to the physician for compilation of the final report. The following information is to be documented:

Page 1:

- Check either Incident or Emergency, depending on the event. The difference is to be determined by the physician and the MEC manager;

- Check whether the person was a SP, a tech, or other (such as a guest or someone who has accompanied a SP to the exam);

- Names of the physician, runner, recorder, person who called 911, and person who found the victim;

- Date of the emergency response;

- Time that the emergency response started, beginning from the time the victim was found;

- Time that the emergency response ended, i.e.; time the ambulance arrived or time the victim left the MEC;

- Location of the emergency in the MEC;

- Description of the victim upon discovery; and

- If the victim is a SP, escort, or guest, the sample number, age, gender, and first and last names should be recorded. If the victim is a staff member, the first and last names are sufficient.

Page 2:

- Vitals and Treatment sections to be recorded at the time of the event by the recorder.

Page 3:

- The sections Symptoms, Observation, Assessment, and Plan are to be completed by the physician after the event.

Exhibit 6-4. MEC Incident/Emergency Form Documentation Guidelines (continued)

Page 4:

- The section Urgent Care is to be completed by the physician if the SP is transported to a hospital;

- The section Notification will be completed by the MEC manager after notifying the field office of the emergency; and

- If the physician has obtained consent from the SP or the SP's family to contact the SP's care provider, the physician must record the name of the physician and the date and time the physician was notified of the SP's status.

7. DOCUMENTATION OF INCIDENTS AND EMERGENCIES

7.1 Incident Forms

If an incident occurs in the MEC, the physician is called to assess the SP. The physician completes an incident form as soon as possible after the incident has occurred. Blank incident/emergency forms are kept in the emergency kit in the Physician Exam Room. Blank incident/emergency forms may also be printed directly from the ISIS system using the following steps:

- At the Desktop, open Microsoft Word.

- Select File.

- Select Open.

- Go to the Network Drive.

- Select MEC STAFF 'H.'

- Select 'Blank Forms.'

- Select 'Incident/Emergency Forms.'

- A blank form will be opened in 'Read-only' mode.

- Select 'Print' and press OK to print a hard copy of the blank form.

The blank form can be used to temporarily record the details of the incident if it is not convenient to enter the information directly into the system.

At a convenient time, the information is entered directly into the system.

See Exhibit 7-1 for details of data entry.

Exhibit 7-1. Utilities menu for Incident/Emergency Form

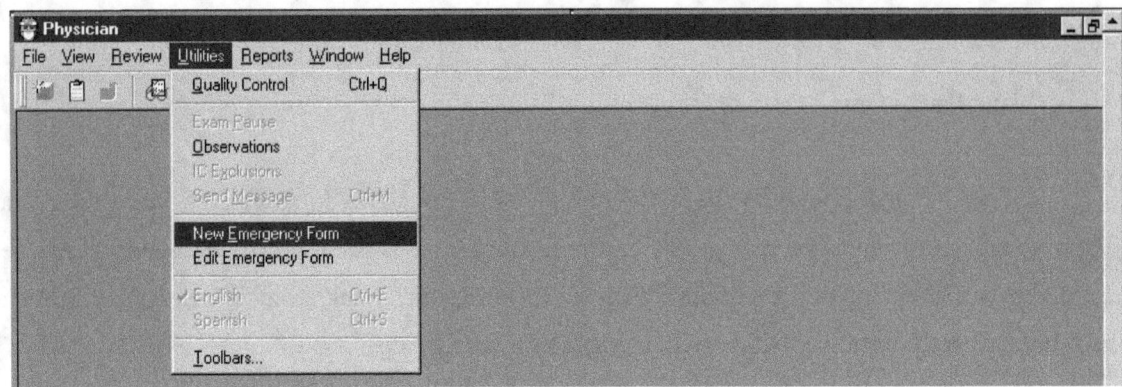

At the 'Utilities Menu', select 'New Emergency Form' and press 'Enter.'

Exhibit 7-2. Incident Form – blank

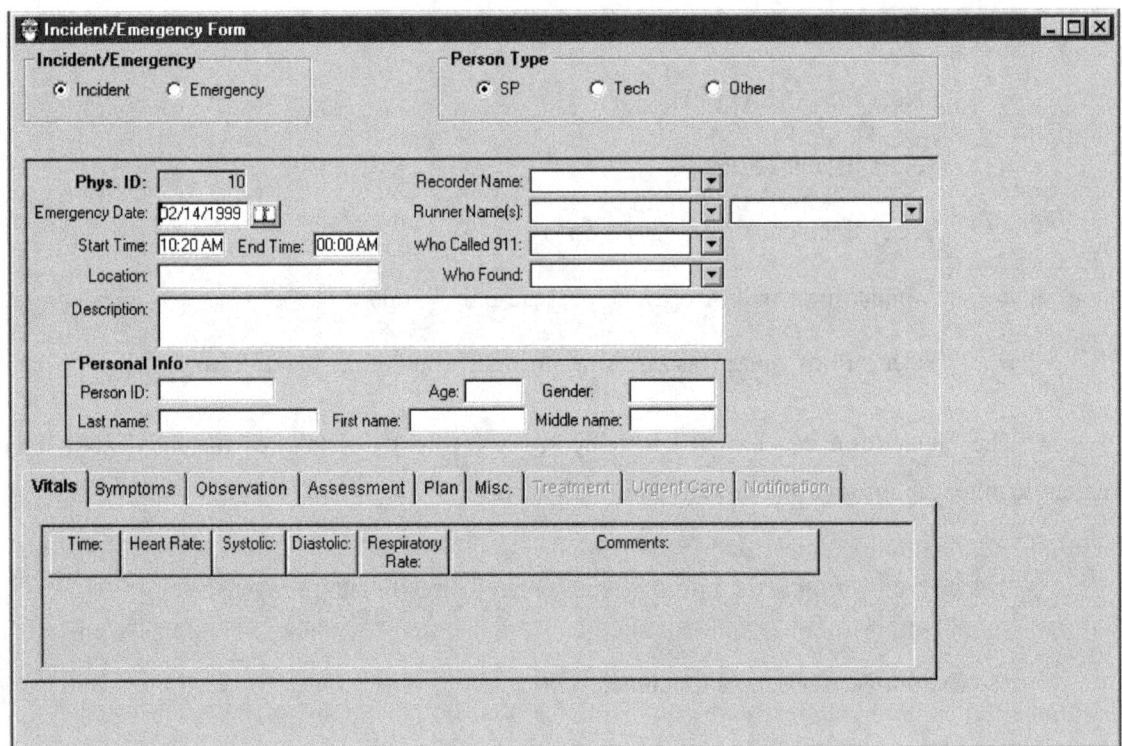

- Select 'Incident' or 'Emergency' as appropriate.

- Select the 'Person Type.' The choices are 'SP,' 'Staff,' or 'Other.' 'Other' may include visitors or guests.

- The 'Date' is automatically entered as the current date. If the incident occurred on an earlier date, the date entered should be the date the incident occurred. The date is a required field.

- The 'Start Time' is automatically entered as the time the form was opened. If the incident occurred at an earlier time, the time entered should be the time the incident started. The start time is a required field.

- NOTE: 'AM' is changed to 'PM' by pressing 'Shift-P' (press the 'Shift' key and the 'P' key) and 'PM' is changed to 'AM' by pressing 'Shift A' (press the 'Shift' key and the 'A' key).

- The 'End Time' is the time the incident was resolved. This is a required field.

- Enter the location where the incident occurred in the 'Location' field.

- Enter a brief description of the incident in the 'Description' field.

- Enter the SP's (or staff) ID in the ID field and press the Tab key. The remainder of the 'Personal Information' will be automatically entered.

Exhibit 7-3. Incident Form – vitals

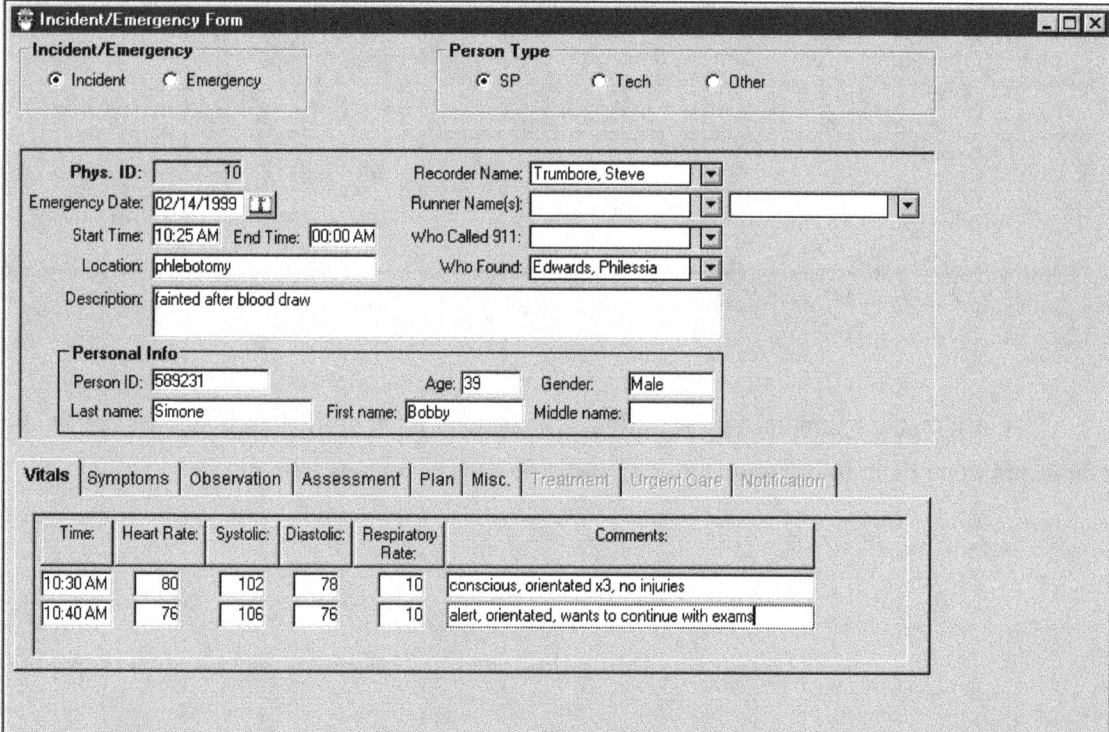

- To add a line to enter 'Vitals' information, right click (click the right button on the mouse) and select 'Add' or 'Insert.' This may also be used to delete a line.

- Enter the time the vital signs were taken and then enter the heart rate/minute, systolic and diastolic blood pressure, and respiratory rate/minute.

- Enter a comment to describe the SP's condition at the time the vital signs were taken. Add additional lines as necessary.

Exhibit 7-4. Incident Form – observations

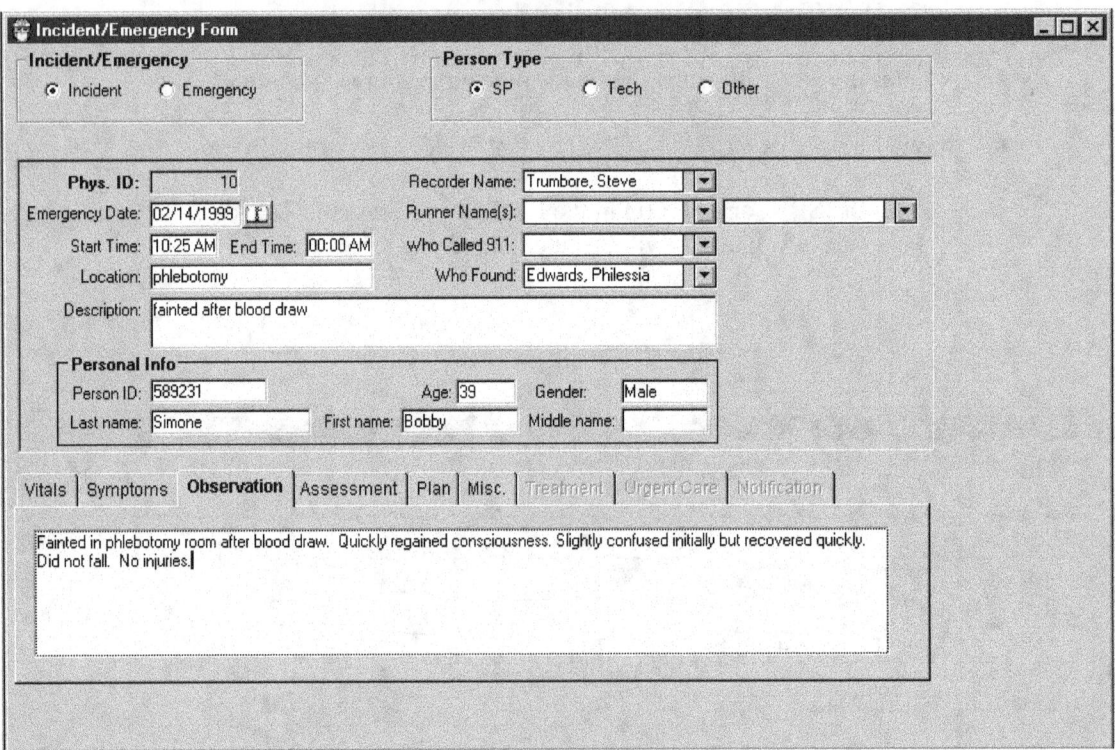

Click on the Symptoms, Observation, Assessment, Plan, or the miscellaneous (MISC.) tab to open the appropriate field. Information for each of the fields is entered as free text.

Exhibit 7-5. Incident Form – save

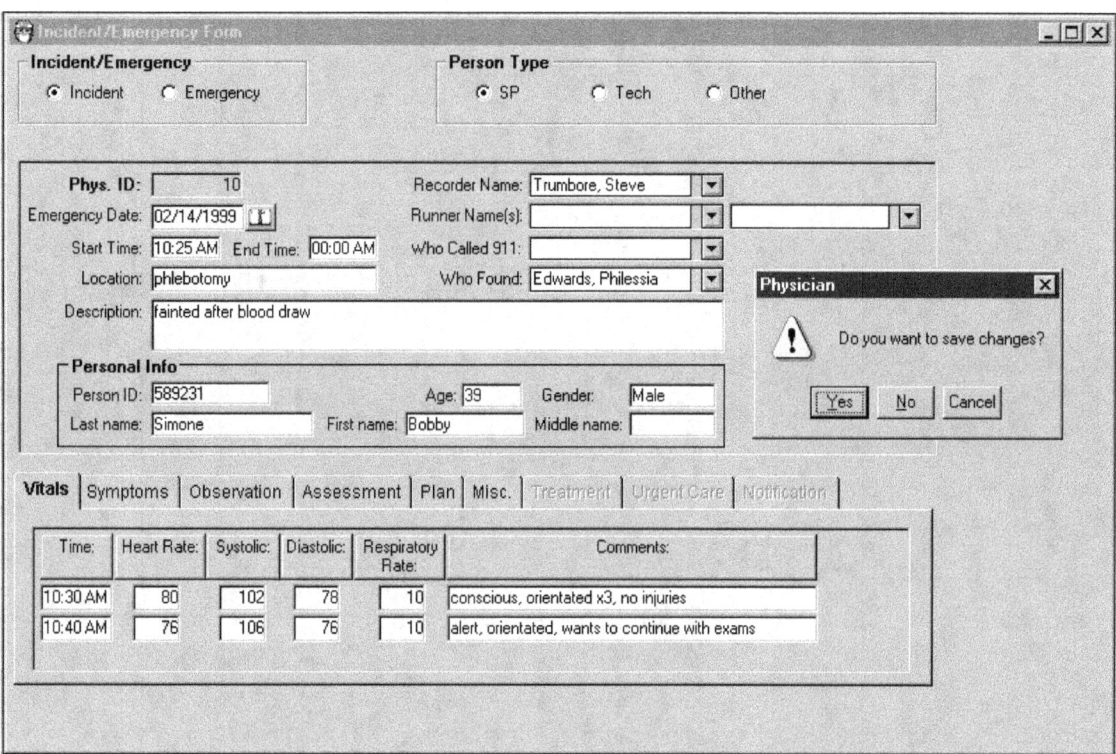

- Select 'File' and choose 'Save' to close and save the form.

- If you close without saving, a message will be displayed 'Do you want to save changes?'

- Click 'Yes' if you want to close and save the form or changes made to the form.

- Click 'No' if you want to close without saving the form or changes made to the form.

- Click 'Cancel' if you do not want to close the form at this time.

Exhibit 7-6. Incident Form – required fields

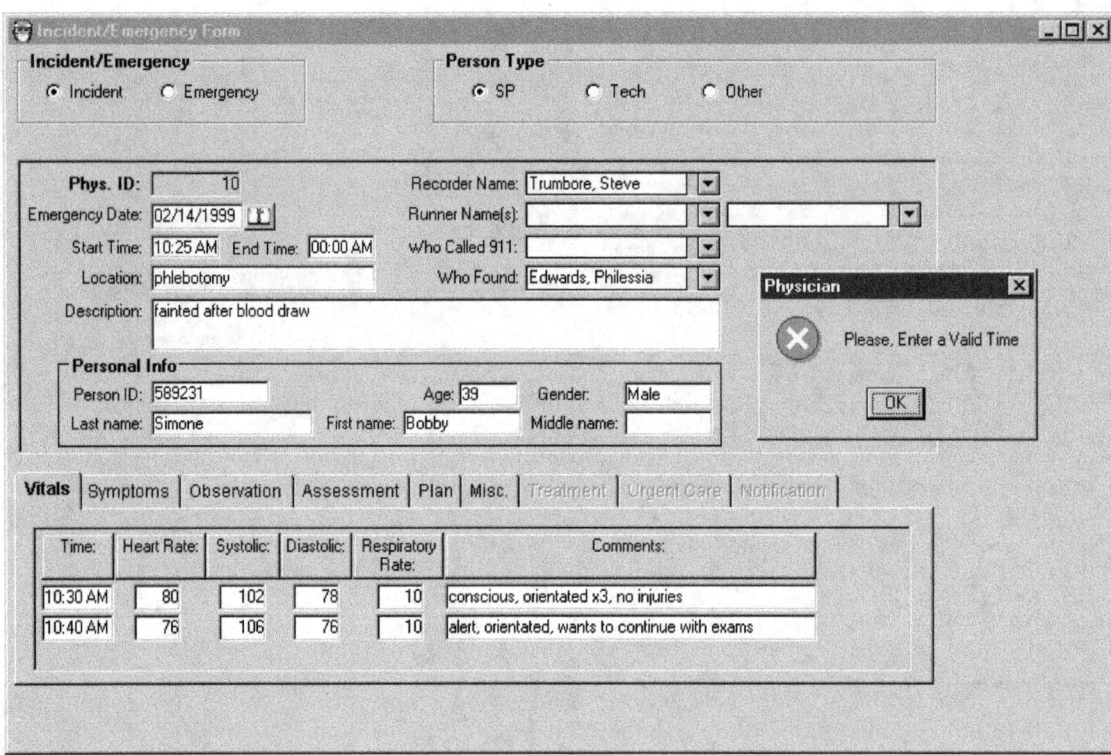

If you try to close the form without entering and 'End Time' a message will be displayed 'Please enter a valid time.' Click OK and enter the time the incident/emergency was completed.

If you try to close the form and the 'End Time' is not valid (end time must be later than start time), the above message will be displayed. Click OK and enter the correct time.

Exhibit 7-7. Incident Form tab marks – vitals

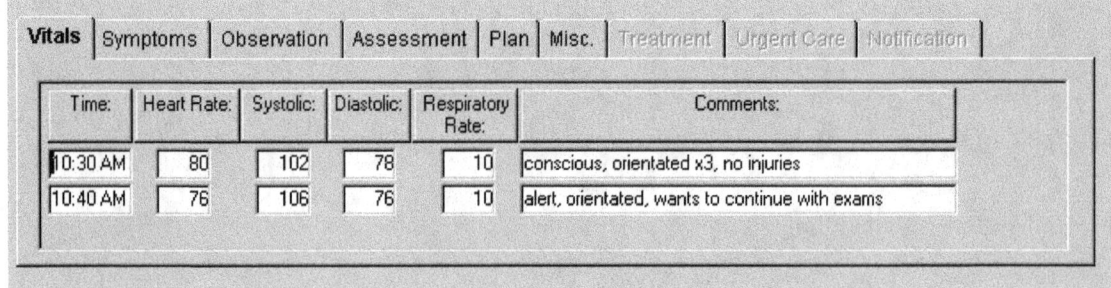

Tab for 'Vitals' for both the Incident and Emergency Forms.

Exhibit 7-8. Incident Form – symptoms

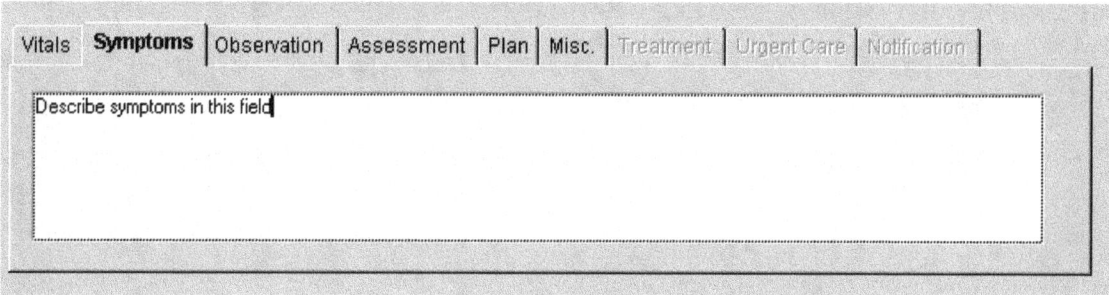

Tab for 'Symptoms' for both Incident and Emergency Forms.

Exhibit 7-9. Incident Form – observation

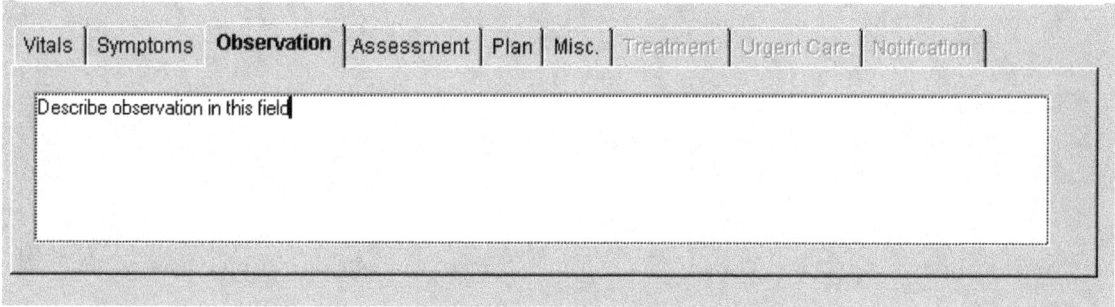

Tab for 'Observations' for both Incident and Emergency Forms.

Exhibit 7-10. Incident Form – assessment

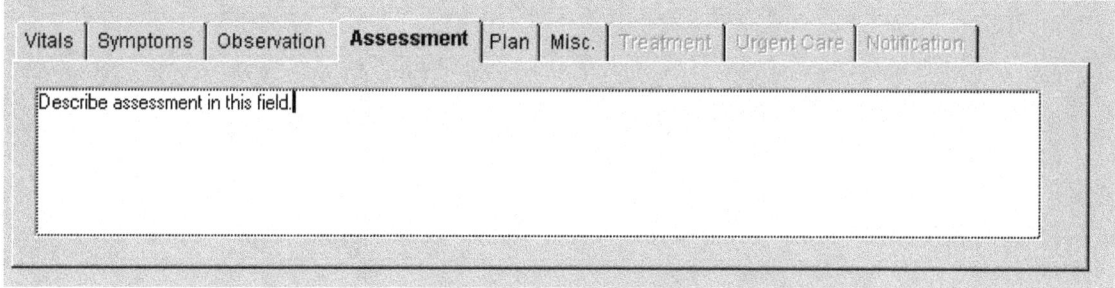

Tab for 'Assessment' for both Incident and Emergency Forms.

Exhibit 7-11. Incident Form – plan

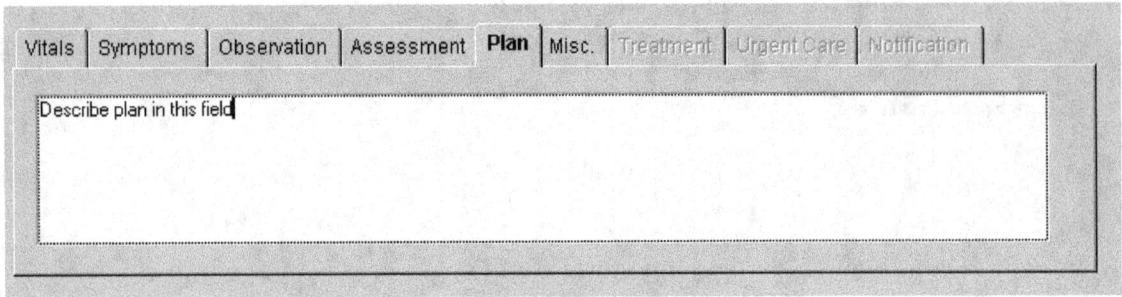

Tab for 'Plan' for both Incident and Emergency Forms.

Exhibit 7-12. Incident Form – miscellaneous

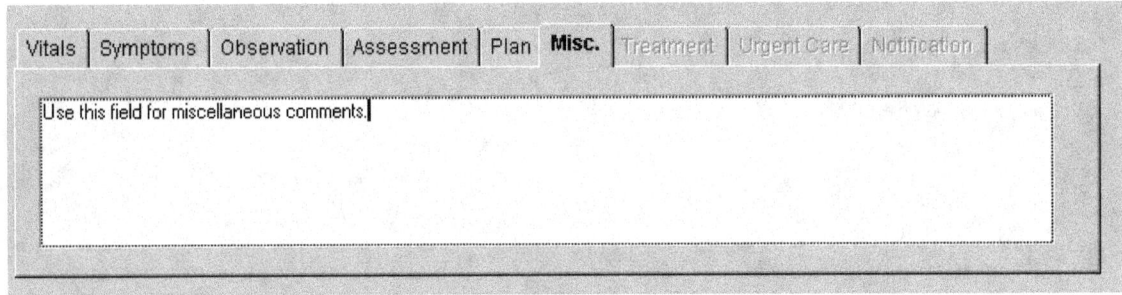

Tab for 'Miscellaneous' for both Incident and Emergency Forms.

7.1.1   Incident Report Hard-Copy Form

Exhibit 7-13. Incident Report hard-copy form

Incident Report for Bobby Simone   02/14/1999

General Information

Person Type: SP	Recorder Name: Trumbore, Steve
Emergency Date: 02/14/1999	Runner Name(s):
Start Time: 10:25 AM End Time: 10:50 AM	Who Called 911:
Location: phlebotomy	Who Found: Edwards, Philessia
Description: fainted after blood draw	

Personal Info

Person ID: 589231	Age: 39	Gender: Male
Last name: Simone	First name: Bobby	Middle name:

Symptoms

Describe symptoms in this field

Vitals

Time:	Heart Rate:	Systolic:	Diastolic:	Respiratory Rate:	Comments:
10:30 AM	80	102	78	10	conscious, orientated x3, no injuries
10:40 AM	76	106	76	10	alert, orientated, wants to continue with exams

Observations

Describe observation in this field

Assessment

Describe assessment in this field.

Plan

Describe plan in this field

Miscellaneose

Use this field for miscellaneous comments.

This is a hard-copy printout of an Incident Report form.

7.2   Emergency Forms

Exhibit 7-14. Emergency Form – blank

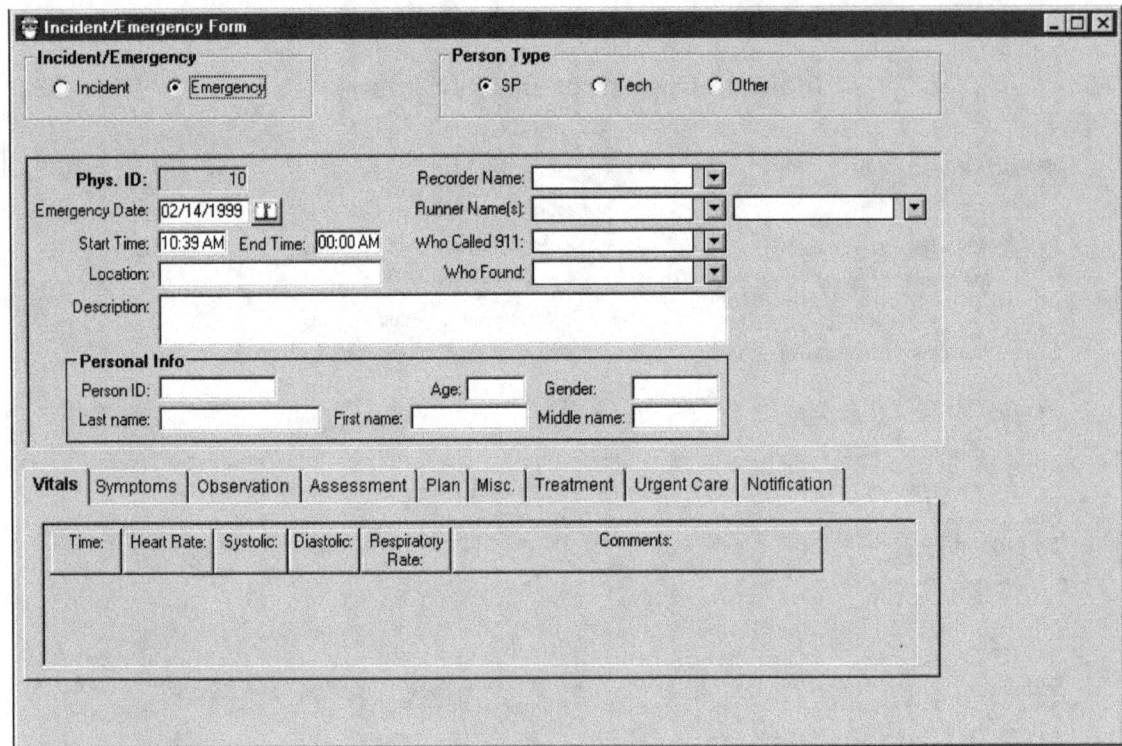

The data entry for this form is similar to data entry for the Incident Form.

- Select 'Incident' or 'Emergency' as appropriate.

- Select the 'Person Type.' The choices are 'SP,' 'Staff' or 'Other.' 'Other' may include visitors or guests.

The 'Date' is automatically entered as the current date. If the incident occurred on an earlier date, the date entered should be the date the incident occurred. The date is a required field.

The 'Start Time' is automatically entered as the time the form was opened. If the incident occurred at an earlier time, the time entered should be the time the incident started. The start time is a required field.

> NOTE: 'AM' is changed to 'PM' by pressing 'Shift-P' (press the 'Shift' key and the 'P' key) and 'PM' is changed to 'AM' by pressing 'Shift A' (press the 'Shift' key and the 'A' key.)

Exhibit 7-15. Emergency Form – data

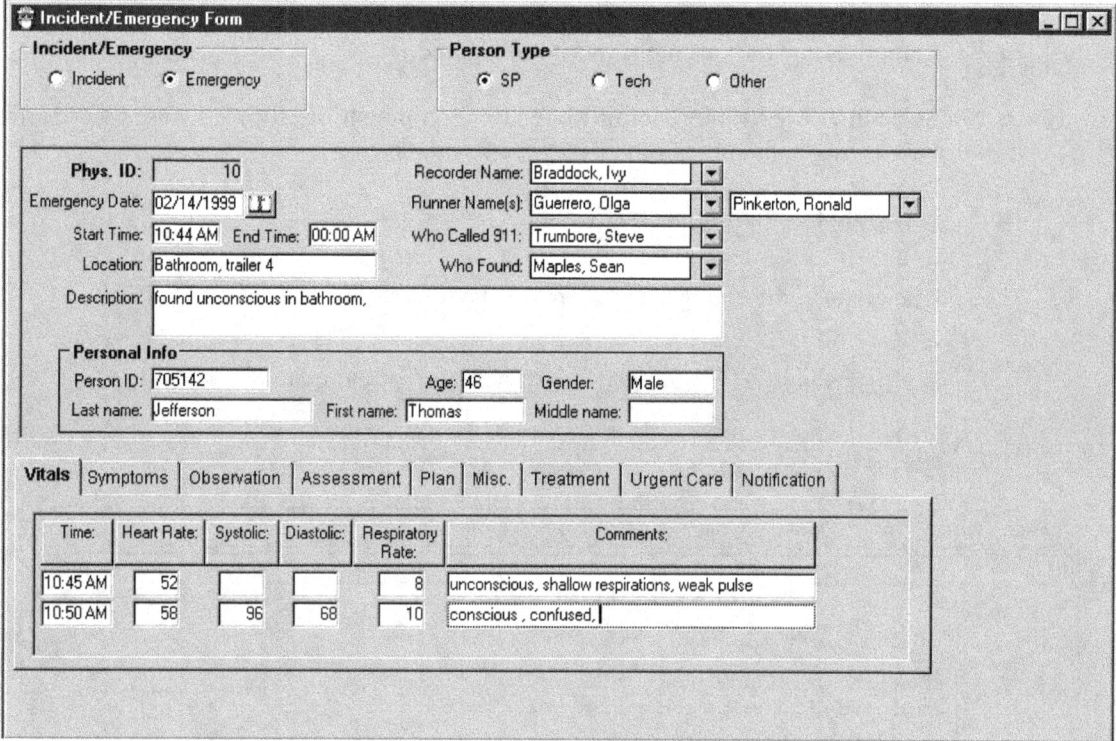

The 'End Time' is the time the incident was resolved. This is a required field.

- Enter the location where the incident occurred in the 'Location' field.

- Enter a brief description of the incident in the 'Description' field.

- Enter the SP's (or staff) ID in the ID field and press the Tab key. The remainder of the 'Personal Information' will be automatically entered.

- To add a line to enter 'Vitals' information, right click (click the right button on the mouse) and select 'Add' or 'Insert.' This may also be used to delete a line.

- Enter the time the vital signs were taken and then enter the heart rate/minute, systolic and diastolic blood pressure and respiratory rate/minute.

- Enter a comment to describe the SP's condition at the time the vital signs were taken.

- Add additional lines as necessary.

- Enter free text information in the Vitals, Symptoms, Observation, Assessment, Plan, and Miscellaneous fields.

- To add a line to enter 'Treatment' information, right click (click the right button on the mouse) and select 'Add' or 'Insert.' This may also be used to delete a line.

- Enter the time the treatment was administered.

- Select the 'Medication' administered or 'Equipment' used by clicking on the arrow to pull down the menu with the list of medications.

- Highlight the appropriate medication.

The medications in the emergency kit are displayed in Exhibits 7-16 and 7-17.

Exhibit 7-16. Emergency Report Form – treatment 1

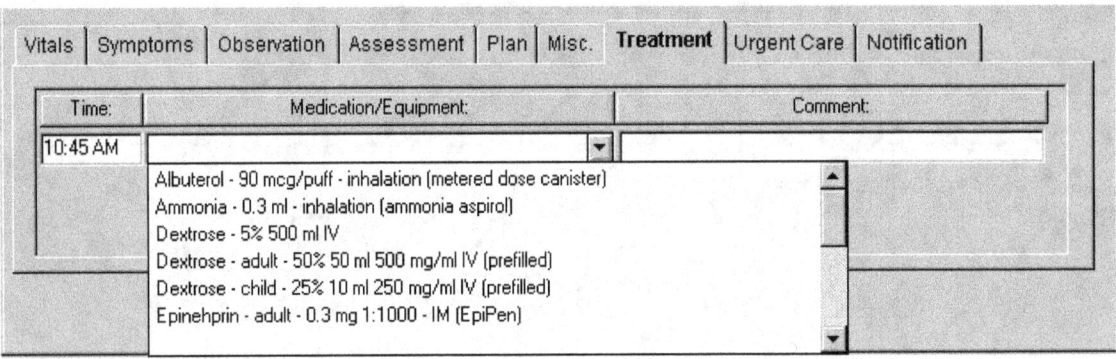

Exhibit 7-17. Emergency Report Form – treatment 2

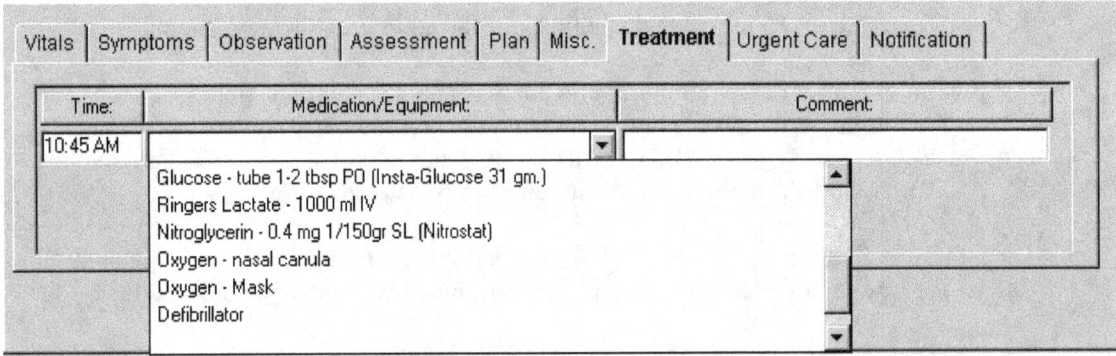

Additional medications or equipment in the pick list for Emergency Medications/Equipment.

Exhibit 7-18. Emergency Report Form – urgent care

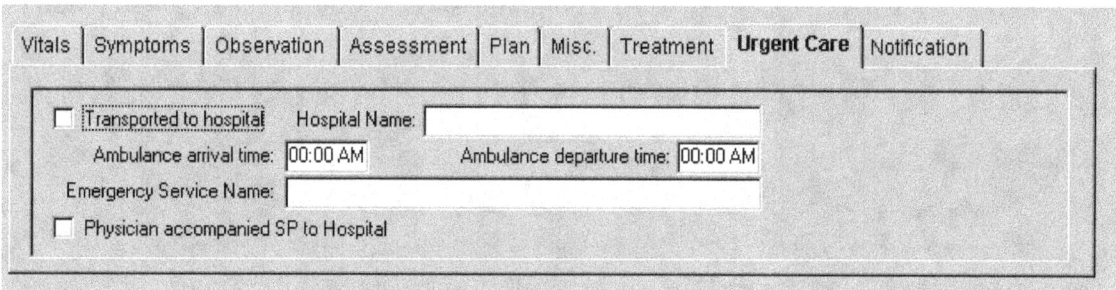

- If the SP needs to be transported to a hospital or clinic, click on the 'Urgent Care' tab.

- Check the box labeled 'Transported to hospital.'

- Enter the name of the hospital in the 'Hospital Name' field.

- Enter the arrival and departure time of the ambulance.

- Enter the name of the Emergency Service.

- Check the appropriate box if the physician accompanied the SP to the hospital.

Exhibit 7-19. Emergency Report Form – notification

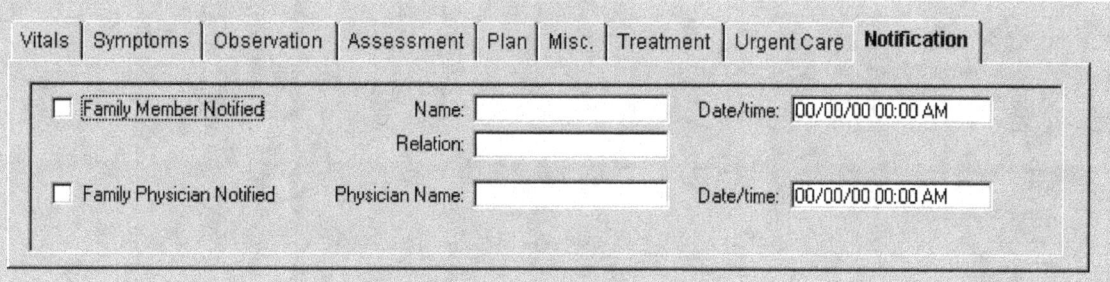

- Click on the 'Notification' tab and enter information about notification of family member and/or physician.

7.2.1 Emergency Report Hard-Copy Form

An example of the hard-copy printout of the Emergency Report form is displayed in Exhibits 7-20 and 7-21.

Exhibit 7-20. Emergency Report hard-copy form (page 1)

Emergency Report for Thomas Jefferson

02/14/1999

General Information

Person Type: SP	**Recorder Name:** Braddock, Ivy
Emergency Date: 02/14/1999	**Runner Name(s):** Guerrero, Olga Pinkerton, Ronald
Start Time: 10:44 AM **End Time:** 11:30 AM	**Who Called 911:** Trumbore, Steve
Location: Bathroom, trailer 4	**Who Found:** Maples, Sean
Description: found unconscious in bathroom,	

Personal Info

Person ID: 705142	**Age:** 46	**Gender:** Male
Last name: Jefferson	**First name:** Thomas	**Middle name:**

Symptoms

Vitals

Time:	Heart Rate:	Systolic:	Diastolic:	Respiratory Rate:	Comments:
10:45 AM	52			8	unconscious, shallow respirations, weak pulse
10:50 AM	58	96	68	10	conscious , confused,

Observations

Describe observations in this field.

Assessment

Describe assessment in this field.

Plan

Describe plan in this field.

Miscellaneose

Additional field for miscellaneous comments.

Treatment

Time:	Medication/Equipment:	Comment:
10:45 AM	Oxygen - nasal canula	

Exhibit 7-21. Emergency Report hard-copy form (page 2)

Emergency Report for Thomas Jefferson

02/14/1999

Urgent Care

☐ Transported to hospital   Hospital Name:

   Ambulance arrival time: 00:00 AM   Ambulance departure time: 00:00 AM

   Emergency service name:

☐ Physician accompanied SP to Hospital

Notification

☑ Family Member N   Name: Mary   Date/time: 02/14/99 11:00 AM

                           Relation: wife

☑ Family Physician Notified

              Family Physican Name: Comstock   Date/time: 02/14/99 11:30 AM

8. PHYSICIAN EQUIPMENT QUALITY CONTROL

8.1   Equipment and Room Set Up Checks

The equipment, room supplies, and room set up need to be checked on a regular basis. Some checks are completed daily and others need only be completed on a weekly basis or at the beginning of each stand. These checks include calibration checks, maintenance inspection of equipment and supplies, and preparation of the room and equipment for the session exams.

Each time you log onto the application, the system will remind you to do Quality Control (QC) checks if the checks have not been completed for that time period. The checks are to be completed daily, weekly, and/or every stand. If you do not have time to do the checks when you log on, you can bypass this message and complete the checks at a later time. However, this message will be displayed each time you log on until you have completed the checks for that time period. After you have completed the checks and entered this in the system, the message box with the reminder will not be displayed again until the appropriate time period has passed.

The daily, weekly, and once-a-stand checks are listed in the following sections.

8.1.1   Daily

Confirm the daily equipment checks for blood pressure measurement are complete.

- Check the shape of the meniscus (it should be rounded on the top).

- Check to see that the level of the mercury in the glass tube is zero.

- Check that the mercury rises easily in the tubing and does not bounce noticeably.

- Check for cracks in the glass manometer tube.

- Check that the cap at the top of the calibrated glass tube is secure.

- Check the pressure control valve for sticks or leaks. Use the following procedure to check for air leaks.

    - Connect the inflation system and wrap it around the calibration cylinder;

    - Inflate to 250 mm Hg;

- Open valve and deflate to 200 mmHg and close valve; and

- Wait for 10 seconds; if mercury column falls more than 10 mm Hg, there is an air leak in the system.

■ Check the stethoscope for cracks.

■ Wipe both sides of the blood pressure cuff with disinfectant wipes. Cuffs will be wiped after each use during the exam.

8.1.2 Weekly

■ Complete all daily checks.

■ Check the functioning of all emergency equipment.

8.1.3 Stand

■ Complete all daily checks.

■ Complete all weekly checks.

■ Remove bladders from BP cuff and wash the cuffs with soap and water. Allow the cuffs to dry completely.

8.2 Data Entry Screens for QC on Equipment

Exhibit 8-1. Quality Control reminder message box

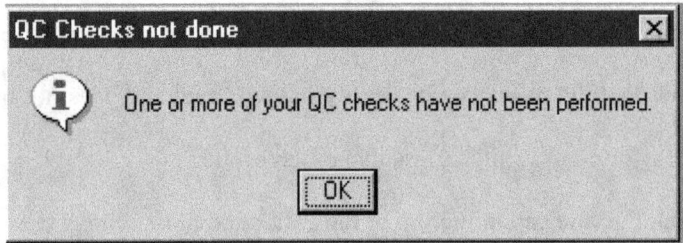

When you log onto the application before the Quality Control checks are performed, the system displays a message: 'One or more of your QC checks have not been performed.'

Click OK to this message.

Exhibit 8-2. Utilities menu to select Quality Control

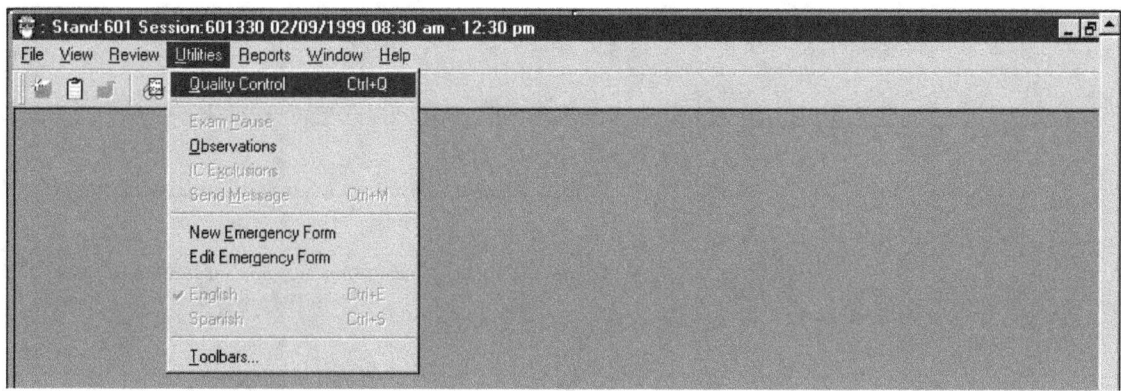

When you want to complete the QC checks, select 'Utilities'. Then select Quality Control from the menu.

Clicking on the QC icon from the Toolbar can also access the QC screens.

Exhibit 8-3. Quality Control log-on

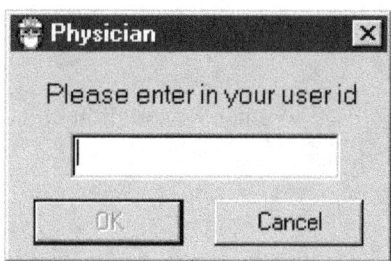

When QC is selected from the Utilities menu, the User ID entry box will be displayed.

Each physician will have a personal ID. This ID will be used to identify the person who completed the QC checks for this time period.

Enter your User ID and click OK.

If you do not want to do the QC checks at this time, click Cancel.

Exhibit 8-4. Quality Control daily checks (1)

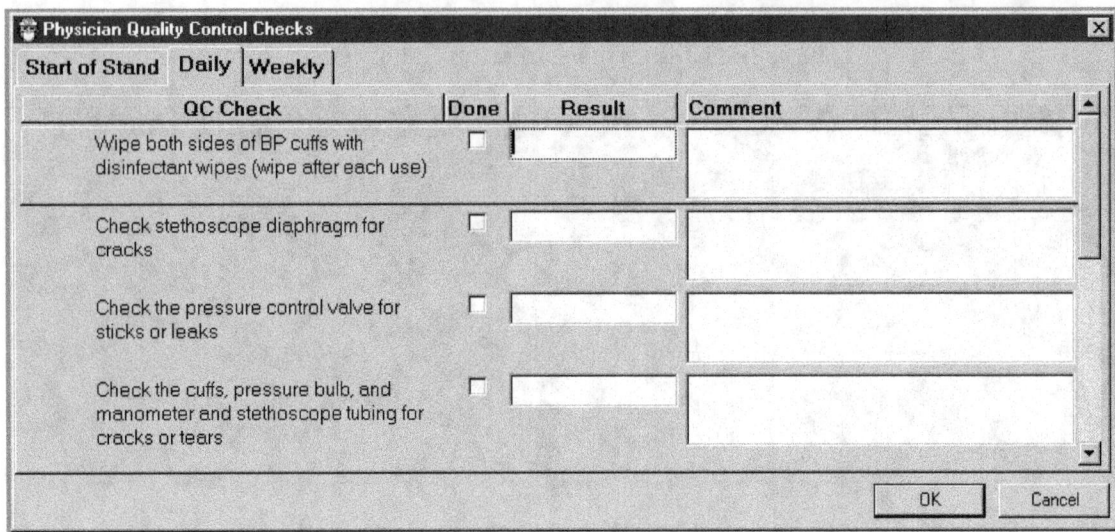

On the QC screens, check 'Done' for the listed items when that item has been completed.

You are not required to enter anything in the 'Result' or 'Comment' fields unless there is a problem.

The 'Result' field is used to enter values for selected QC items if required.

The 'Comments' field is used to enter information about problems encountered with the QC item check.

Exhibit 8-5. Quality Control daily checks (2)

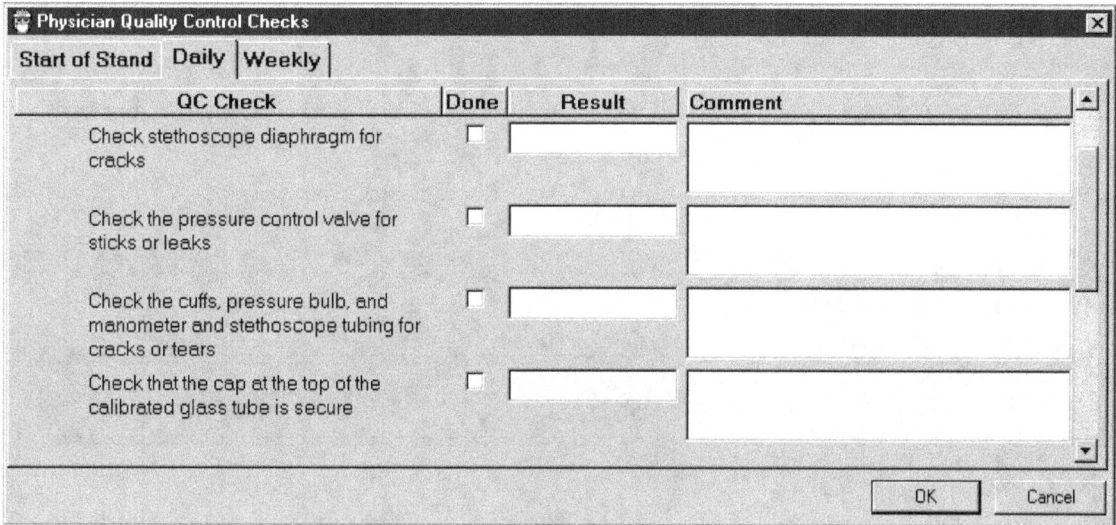

Use the scroll bar to move to the next items on the list.

Exhibit 8-6. Quality Control daily checks (3)

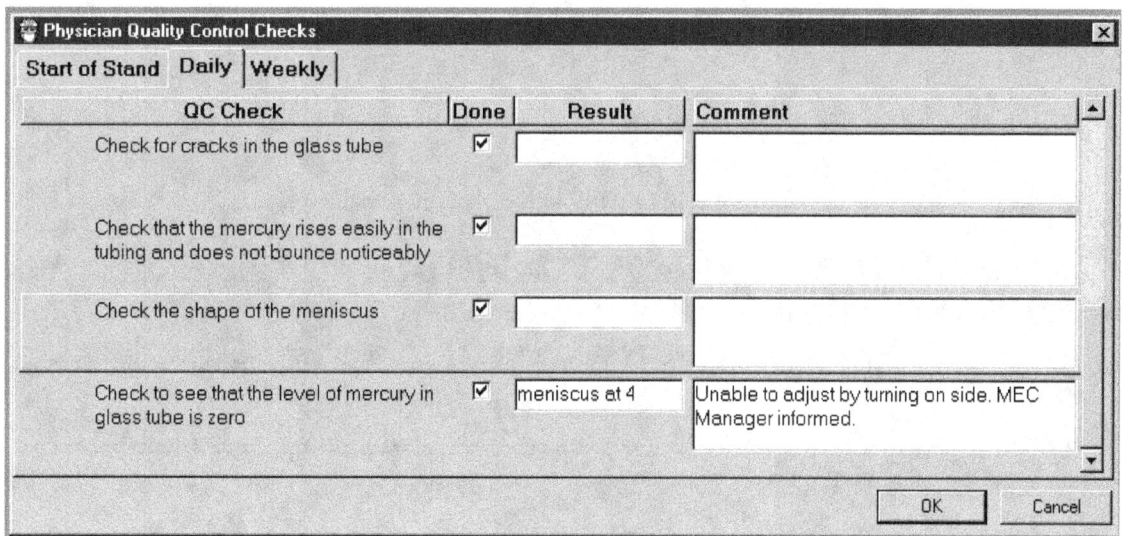

Use the scroll bar to move to the remaining items.

If there is a problem with one of the items, enter a value if appropriate and then enter a comment in the comment box briefly describing the nature of the problem.

Report the problem to the MEC manager. Note in the Comments field that the MEC manager has been informed.

When you are finished with the daily item checks, click OK to close the QC box.

Exhibit 8-7. Quality Control weekly checks

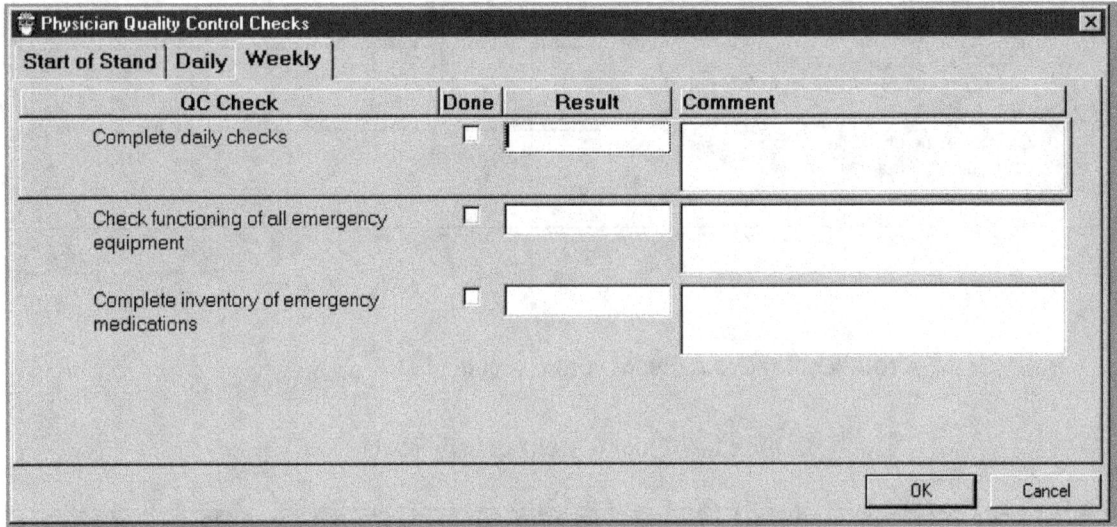

Check 'Done' for each item on the weekly checks when complete.

Exhibit 8-8. Quality Control stand checks

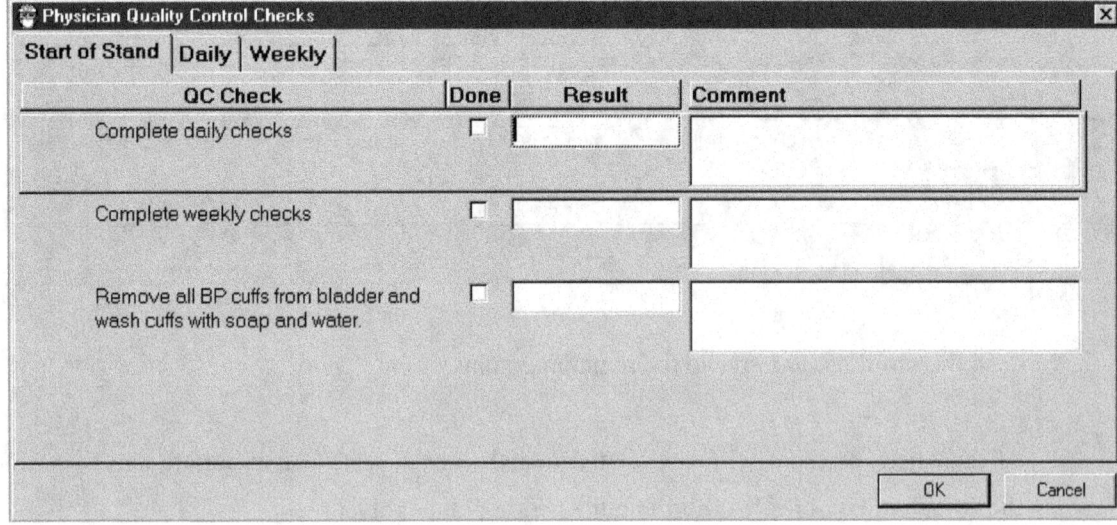

Complete all 'Start of Stand' checks.

'Start of Stand' checks include all daily and weekly checks.

Exhibit 8-9. Quality Control incomplete entry

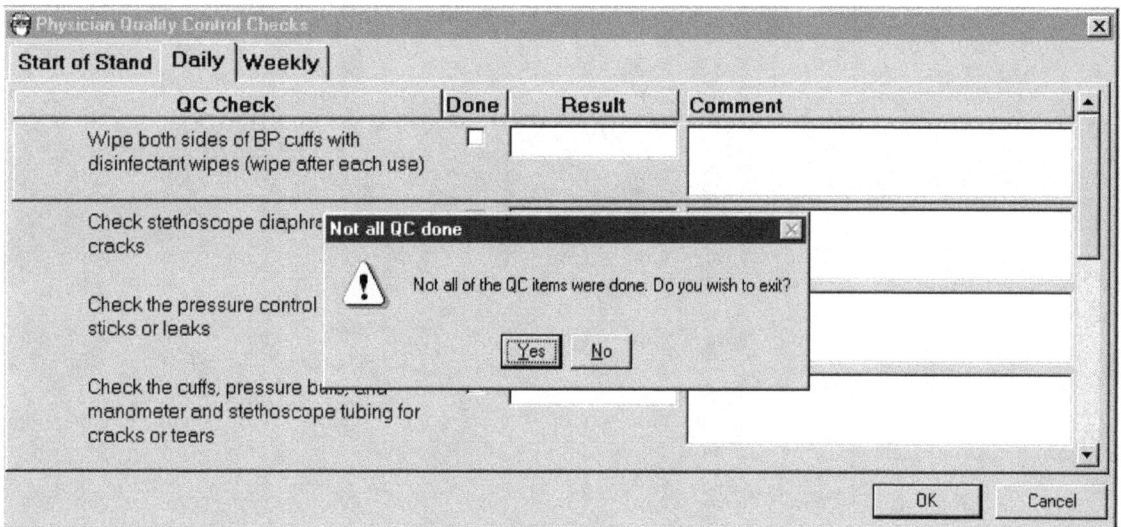

When you have completed all checks, click OK to close the QC box.

If you do not check that all items are complete, the system will display this message: 'Not all the QC items were done. Do you wish to exit?'

If you want to complete the items before exiting, click No' to this message and complete the items.

If you do not wish to exit without completing all the QC checks, click 'Yes' to this message.

If all QC items were not complete, the system will remind you each time you log on that the QC checks are not complete.

Appendix A
Child Blood Pressure Values

APPENDIX A. CHILD BLOOD PRESSURE VALUES
GIRLS - AGE 6

Percentile of height = 1 - 9%

Systolic (mm Hg)	Diastolic (mm Hg)			
	<67	67 - 70	71-85	≥ 86
< 104	1	2	3	4
104-107	2	2	3	4
108-129	3	3	3	4
≥ 130	4	4	4	4

Percentile of height = 10 - 24%

Systolic (mm Hg)	Diastolic (mm Hg)			
	<67	67 - 70	71 - 85	≥ 86
< 105	1	2	3	4
105-108	2	2	3	4
109-129	3	3	3	4
≥ 130	4	4	4	4

Percentile of height = 25 - 49%

Systolic (mm Hg)	Diastolic (mm Hg)			
	<68	68 - 71	72 - 85	≥ 86
< 106	1	2	3	4
106-109	2	2	3	4
110-129	3	3	3	4
≥ 130	4	4	4	4

Percentile of height = 50 - 74%

Systolic (mm Hg)	Diastolic (mm Hg)			
	<69	69 - 72	73 - 85	≥ 86
< 107	1	2	3	4
107-110	2	2	3	4
111-129	3	3	3	4
≥ 130	4	4	4	4

Child Blood Pressure Values
Girls - Age 6 (continued)

Percentile of height = 75 - 89%

Systolic (mm Hg)	Diastolic (mm Hg)			
	<69	69 - 72	73 - 85	≥ 86
< 109	1	2	3	4
109-111	2	2	3	4
112-129	3	3	3	4
← 130	4	4	4	4

Percentile of height = 90 - 94%

Systolic (mm Hg)	Diastolic (mm Hg)			
	<70	70 - 73	74 - 85	← 86
< 110	1	2	3	4
110-113	2	2	3	4
114-129	3	3	3	4
← 130	4	4	4	4

Percentile of height = 95 - 99%

Systolic (mm Hg)	Diastolic (mm Hg)			
	<71	71 - 74	75 - 85	← 86
< 111	1	2	3	4
111-113	2	2	3	4
114-129	3	3	3	4
← 130	4	4	4	4

Child Blood Pressure Values
Girls - Age 7

Percentile of height = 1 - 9%

Systolic (mm Hg)	Diastolic (mm Hg)			
	<69	69 - 72	73-85	← 86
< 106	1	2	3	4
106-109	2	2	3	4
110-129	3	3	3	4
← 130	4	4	4	4

Percentile of height = 10 - 24%

Systolic (mm Hg)	Diastolic (mm Hg)			
	<69	67 - 72	73 - 85	<86
< 107	1	2	3	4
107-109	2	2	3	4
110-129	3	3	3	4
← 130	4	4	4	4

Percentile of height = 25 - 49%

Systolic (mm Hg)	Diastolic (mm Hg)			
	<69	69 - 72	73-85	← 86
< 108	1	2	3	4
108-111	2	2	3	4
112-129	3	3	3	4
← 130	4	4	4	4

Percentile of height = 50 - 74%

Systolic (mm Hg)	Diastolic (mm Hg)			
	<70	70 - 73	74 - 85	← 86
< 109	1	2	3	4
109-112	2	2	3	4
113-129	3	3	3	4
← 130	4	4	4	4

Child Blood Pressure Values
Girls - Age 7 (continued)

Percentile of height = 75 - 89%

Systolic (mm Hg)	Diastolic (mm Hg)			
	<71	71 - 74	75 - 85	← 86
< 110	1	2	3	4
110-113	2	2	3	4
114-129	3	3	3	4
← 130	4	4	4	4

Percentile of height = 90 - 94%

Systolic (mm Hg)	Diastolic (mm Hg)			
	<72	72 - 75	76 - 85	← 86
< 112	1	2	3	4
112-114	2	2	3	4
115-129	3	3	3	4
← 130	4	4	4	4

Percentile of height = 95 - 99%

Systolic (mm Hg)	Diastolic (mm Hg)			
	<72	72 - 75	76 - 85	← 86
< 112	1	2	3	4
112-115	2	2	3	4
116-129	3	3	3	4
← 130	4	4	4	4

Child Blood Pressure Values
Girls - Age 8

Percentile of height = 1 - 9%

Systolic (mm Hg)	Diastolic (mm Hg)			
	<70	70 - 73	74-85	← 86
< 108	1	2	3	4
108-111	2	2	3	4
112-129	3	3	3	4
← 130	4	4	4	4

Percentile of height = 10 - 24%

Systolic (mm Hg)	Diastolic (mm Hg)			
	<70	70 - 73	74-85	← 86
< 109	1	2	3	4
109-111	2	2	3	4
112-129	3	3	3	4
← 130	4	4	4	4

Percentile of height = 25 - 49%

Systolic (mm Hg)	Diastolic (mm Hg)			
	<71	71 - 74	75 - 85	← 86
< 110	1	2	3	4
110-112	2	2	3	4
113-129	3	3	3	4
← 130	4	4	4	4

Percentile of height = 50 - 74%

Systolic (mm Hg)	Diastolic (mm Hg)			
	<71	71 - 74	75 - 85	← 86
< 111	1	2	3	4
111-114	2	2	3	4
115-129	3	3	3	4
← 130	4	4	4	4

Child Blood Pressure Values
Girls - Age 8 (continued)

Percentile of height = 75 - 89%

Systolic (mm Hg)	Diastolic (mm Hg)			
	<72	72 - 75	76 - 85	← 86
< 112	1	2	3	4
112-115	2	2	3	4
116-129	3	3	3	4
← 130	4	4	4	4

Percentile of height = 90 - 94%

Systolic (mm Hg)	Diastolic (mm Hg)			
	<73	73 - 75	76 - 85	← 86
< 113	1	2	3	4
113-116	2	2	3	4
117-129	3	3	3	4
← 130	4	4	4	4

Percentile of height = 95 - 99%

Systolic (mm Hg)	Diastolic (mm Hg)			
	<74	74 - 77	78 - 85	← 86
< 114	1	2	3	4
114-117	2	2	3	4
118-129	3	3	3	4
← 130	4	4	4	4

Child Blood Pressure Values
Girls - Age 9

Percentile of height = 1 - 9%

Systolic (mm Hg)	Diastolic (mm Hg)			
	<71	71 - 74	75-85	← 86
< 110	1	2	3	4
110-113	2	2	3	4
114-129	3	3	3	4
← 130	4	4	4	4

Percentile of height = 10 - 24%

Systolic (mm Hg)	Diastolic (mm Hg)			
	<72	72 - 75	76 - 85	<86
< 110	1	2	3	4
110-113	2	2	3	4
114-129	3	3	3	4
← 130	4	4	4	4

Percentile of height = 25 - 49%

Systolic (mm Hg)	Diastolic (mm Hg)			
	<73	73 - 76	77 - 85	← 86
< 112	1	2	3	4
112-114	2	2	3	4
115-129	3	3	3	4
← 130	4	4	4	4

Percentile of height = 50 - 74%

Systolic (mm Hg)	Diastolic (mm Hg)			
	<73	73 - 75	76 - 85	← 86
< 113	1	2	3	4
113-116	2	2	3	4
117-129	3	3	3	4
← 130	4	4	4	4

Child Blood Pressure Values
Girls - Age 9 (continued)

Percentile of height = 75 - 89%

Systolic (mm Hg)	Diastolic (mm Hg)			
	<74	74 - 77	78 - 85	← 86
< 114	1	2	3	4
114-117	2	2	3	4
118-129	3	3	3	4
← 130	4	4	4	4

Percentile of height = 90 - 94%

Systolic (mm Hg)	Diastolic (mm Hg)			
	<74	74 - 77	78 - 85	← 86
< 115	1	2	3	4
115-118	2	2	3	4
119-129	3	3	3	4
← 130	4	4	4	4

Percentile of height = 95 - 99%

Systolic (mm Hg)	Diastolic (mm Hg)			
	<75	75 - 78	79 - 85	← 86
< 116	1	2	3	4
116-118	2	2	3	4
119-129	3	3	3	4
← 130	4	4	4	4

Child Blood Pressure Values
Girls - Age 10

Percentile of height = 1 - 9%

Systolic (mm Hg)	Diastolic (mm Hg)			
	<73	73 - 76	77-89	←90
< 112	1	2	3	4
112-115	2	2	3	4
116-133	3	3	3	4
←134	4	4	4	4

Percentile of height = 10 - 24%

Systolic (mm Hg)	Diastolic (mm Hg)			
	<73	73 - 76	77-89	←90
< 112	1	2	3	4
112-115	2	2	3	4
116-133	3	3	3	4
←134	4	4	4	4

Percentile of height = 25 - 49%

Systolic (mm Hg)	Diastolic (mm Hg)			
	<73	73 - 76	77-89	←90
< 114	1	2	3	4
114-116	2	2	3	4
117-133	3	3	3	4
←134	4	4	4	4

Percentile of height = 50 - 74%

Systolic (mm Hg)	Diastolic (mm Hg)			
	<74	74 - 77	78 - 89	←90
< 115	1	2	3	4
115-118	2	2	3	4
119-133	3	3	3	4
←134	4	4	4	4

Percentile of height = 75 - 89%

Systolic (mm Hg)	Diastolic (mm Hg)			
	<75	75 - 78	79 - 89	← 90
< 116	1	2	3	4
116-119	2	2	3	4
120-133	3	3	3	4
← 134	4	4	4	4

Percentile of height = 90 - 94%

Systolic (mm Hg)	Diastolic (mm Hg)			
	<76	76 - 79	80 - 89	← 90
< 117	1	2	3	4
117-120	2	2	3	4
121-133	3	3	3	4
← 134	4	4	4	4

Percentile of height = 95 - 99%

Systolic (mm Hg)	Diastolic (mm Hg)			
	<76	76 - 79	80 - 89	← 90
< 118	1	2	3	4
118-121	2	2	3	4
122-133	3	3	3	4
← 134	4	4	4	4

Child Blood Pressure Values
Girls - Age 11

Percentile of height = 1 - 9%

Systolic (mm Hg)	Diastolic (mm Hg)			
	<74	74 - 77	78-89	←90
< 114	1	2	3	4
114-117	2	2	3	4
118-133	3	3	3	4
←134	4	4	4	4

Percentile of height = 10 - 24%

Systolic (mm Hg)	Diastolic (mm Hg)			
	<74	74 - 77	78 - 89	←90
< 114	1	2	3	4
114-117	2	2	3	4
118-133	3	3	3	4
←134	4	4	4	4

Percentile of height = 25 - 49%

Systolic (mm Hg)	Diastolic (mm Hg)			
	<75	75 - 78	79 - 89	←90
< 116	1	2	3	4
116-118	2	2	3	4
119-133	3	3	3	4
←134	4	4	4	4

Percentile of height = 50 - 74%

Systolic (mm Hg)	Diastolic (mm Hg)			
	<75	75 - 78	79 - 89	←90
< 117	1	2	3	4
117-120	2	2	3	4
121-133	3	3	3	4
←134	4	4	4	4

Percentile of height = 75 - 89%

Systolic (mm Hg)	Diastolic (mm Hg)			
	<76	76 - 79	80 - 89	← 90
< 118	1	2	3	4
118-121	2	2	3	4
122-133	3	3	3	4
← 134	4	4	4	4

Percentile of height = 90 - 94%

Systolic (mm Hg)	Diastolic (mm Hg)			
	<77	77 - 80	81 - 89	← 90
< 119	1	2	3	4
119-122	2	2	3	4
123-133	3	3	3	4
← 134	4	4	4	4

Percentile of height = 95 - 99%

Systolic (mm Hg)	Diastolic (mm Hg)			
	<77	77 - 80	81 - 89	← 90
< 120	1	2	3	4
120-123	2	2	3	4
124-133	3	3	3	4
← 134	4	4	4	4

Child Blood Pressure Values
Girls - Age 12

Percentile of height = 1 - 9%

Systolic (mm Hg)	Diastolic (mm Hg)			
	<75	75 - 77	79 - 89	←90
< 116	1	2	3	4
116-119	2	2	3	4
120-133	3	3	3	4
←134	4	4	4	4

Percentile of height = 10 - 24%

Systolic (mm Hg)	Diastolic (mm Hg)			
	<75	75 - 77	79 - 89	←90
< 116	1	2	3	4
116-119	2	2	3	4
120-133	3	3	3	4
←134	4	4	4	4

Percentile of height = 25 - 49%

Systolic (mm Hg)	Diastolic (mm Hg)			
	<76	76 - 79	80 - 89	←90
< 118	1	2	3	4
118-120	2	2	3	4
121-133	3	3	3	4
←134	4	4	4	4

Percentile of height = 50 - 74%

Systolic (mm Hg)	Diastolic (mm Hg)			
	<76	76 - 79	80 - 89	←90
< 119	1	2	3	4
119-122	2	2	3	4
123-133	3	3	3	4
←134	4	4	4	4

Child Blood Pressure Values
Girls - Age 12 (continued)

Percentile of height = 75 - 89%

Systolic (mm Hg)	Diastolic (mm Hg)			
	<77	77 - 80	81 - 89	← 90
< 120	1	2	3	4
120-123	2	2	3	4
124-133	3	3	3	4
← 134	4	4	4	4

Percentile of height = 90 - 94%

Systolic (mm Hg)	Diastolic (mm Hg)			
	<78	78 - 81	82 - 89	← 90
< 121	1	2	3	4
121-124	2	2	3	4
125-133	3	3	3	4
← 134	4	4	4	4

Percentile of height = 95 - 99%

Systolic (mm Hg)	Diastolic (mm Hg)			
	<78	78 - 81	82 - 89	← 90
< 122	1	2	3	4
122-124	2	2	3	4
125-133	3	3	3	4
← 134	4	4	4	4

Child Blood Pressure Values
Girls - Age 13

Percentile of height = 1 - 9%

Systolic (mm Hg)	Diastolic (mm Hg)			
	<76	76 - 79	80 - 91	← 92
< 118	1	2	3	4
118-120	2	2	3	4
121-143	3	3	3	4
← 144	4	4	4	4

Percentile of height = 10 - 24%

Systolic (mm Hg)	Diastolic (mm Hg)			
	<76	76 - 79	80 - 91	← 92
< 118	1	2	3	4
118-121	2	2	3	4
122-143	3	3	3	4
← 144	4	4	4	4

Percentile of height = 25 - 49%

Systolic (mm Hg)	Diastolic (mm Hg)			
	<77	77- 80	81 - 91	← 92
< 119	1	2	3	4
119-122	2	2	3	4
123-143	3	3	3	4
← 144	4	4	4	4

Percentile of height = 50 - 74%

Systolic (mm Hg)	Diastolic (mm Hg)			
	<78	78 - 81	82 - 91	← 92
< 121	1	2	3	4
121-124	2	2	3	4
125-143	3	3	3	4
← 144	4	4	4	4

Child Blood Pressure Values
Girls - Age 13 (continued)

Percentile of height = 75 - 89%

Systolic (mm Hg)	Diastolic (mm Hg)			
	<78	78 - 81	82 - 91	← 92
< 122	1	2	3	4
122-125	2	2	3	4
126-143	3	3	3	4
← 144	4	4	4	4

Percentile of height = 90 - 94%

Systolic (mm Hg)	Diastolic (mm Hg)			
	<79	79 - 82	83 - 91	← 92
< 123	1	2	3	4
123-126	2	2	3	4
127-143	3	3	3	4
← 144	4	4	4	4

Percentile of height = 95 - 99%

Systolic (mm Hg)	Diastolic (mm Hg)			
	<80	80 - 83	84 - 91	← 92
< 124	1	2	3	4
124-127	2	2	3	4
128-143	3	3	3	4
← 144	4	4	4	4

Child Blood Pressure Values
Girls - Age 14

Percentile of height = 1 - 9%

Systolic (mm Hg)	Diastolic (mm Hg)			
	<77	77 - 80	81 - 91	← 92
< 119	1	2	3	4
119-122	2	2	3	4
123-143	3	3	3	4
← 144	4	4	4	4

Percentile of height = 10 - 24%

Systolic (mm Hg)	Diastolic (mm Hg)			
	<77	77 - 80	81 - 91	← 92
< 120	1	2	3	4
120-123	2	2	3	4
124-143	3	3	3	4
← 144	4	4	4	4

Percentile of height = 25 - 49%

Systolic (mm Hg)	Diastolic (mm Hg)			
	<78	78 - 81	82 - 91	← 92
< 121	1	2	3	4
121-124	2	2	3	4
125-143	3	3	3	4
← 144	4	4	4	4

Percentile of height = 50 - 74%

Systolic (mm Hg)	Diastolic (mm Hg)			
	<79	79 - 82	83 - 91	← 92
< 122	1	2	3	4
122-126	2	2	3	4
127-143	3	3	3	4
← 144	4	4	4	4

Percentile of height = 75 - 89%

Systolic (mm Hg)	Diastolic (mm Hg)			
	<79	79 - 82	83 - 91	← 92
< 124	1	2	3	4
124-127	2	2	3	4
128-143	3	3	3	4
← 144	4	4	4	4

Percentile of height = 90 - 94%

Systolic (mm Hg)	Diastolic (mm Hg)			
	<80	80 - 83	84 - 91	← 92
< 125	1	2	3	4
125-128	2	2	3	4
129-143	3	3	3	4
← 144	4	4	4	4

Percentile of height = 95 - 99%

Systolic (mm Hg)	Diastolic (mm Hg)			
	<81	81 - 84	85 - 91	← 92
< 126	1	2	3	4
126-129	2	2	3	4
130-143	3	3	3	4
← 144	4	4	4	4

Child Blood Pressure Values
Girls - Age 15

Percentile of height = 1 - 9%

Systolic (mm Hg)	Diastolic (mm Hg)			
	<78	78 - 81	82 - 91	← 92
< 121	1	2	3	4
121-123	2	2	3	4
124-143	3	3	3	4
← 144	4	4	4	4

Percentile of height = 10 - 24%

Systolic (mm Hg)	Diastolic (mm Hg)			
	<78	78 - 81	82 - 91	← 92
< 121	1	2	3	4
121-124	2	2	3	4
125-143	3	3	3	4
← 144	4	4	4	4

Percentile of height = 25 - 49%

Systolic (mm Hg)	Diastolic (mm Hg)			
	<79	79- 82	83 - 91	← 92
< 122	1	2	3	4
122-125	2	2	3	4
126-143	3	3	3	4
← 144	4	4	4	4

Percentile of height = 50 - 74%

Systolic (mm Hg)	Diastolic (mm Hg)			
	<79	79 - 82	83 - 91	← 92
< 124	1	2	3	4
124-127	2	2	3	4
128-143	3	3	3	4
← 144	4	4	4	4

Child Blood Pressure Values
Girls - Age 15 (continued)

Percentile of height = 75 - 89%

Systolic (mm Hg)	Diastolic (mm Hg)			
	<80	80 - 83	84 - 91	← 92
< 125	1	2	3	4
125-128	2	2	3	4
129-143	3	3	3	4
← 144	4	4	4	4

Percentile of height = 90 - 94%

Systolic (mm Hg)	Diastolic (mm Hg)			
	<81	81 - 84	85 - 91	← 92
< 126	1	2	3	4
126-129	2	2	3	4
130-143	3	3	3	4
← 144	4	4	4	4

Percentile of height = 95 - 99%

Systolic (mm Hg)	Diastolic (mm Hg)			
	<82	82 - 85	86 - 91	← 92
< 127	1	2	3	4
127-130	2	2	3	4
131-143	3	3	3	4
← 144	4	4	4	4

Child Blood Pressure Values
Girls - Age 16

Percentile of height = 1 - 9%

Systolic (mm Hg)	Diastolic (mm Hg)			
	<79	79 - 82	83 - 97	← 98
< 122	1	2	3	4
122-124	2	2	3	4
125-149	3	3	3	4
← 150	4	4	4	4

Percentile of height = 10 - 24%

Systolic (mm Hg)	Diastolic (mm Hg)			
	<79	79 - 82	83 - 97	← 98
< 122	1	2	3	4
122-125	2	2	3	4
126-149	3	3	3	4
← 150	4	4	4	4

Percentile of height = 25 - 49%

Systolic (mm Hg)	Diastolic (mm Hg)			
	<79	79- 82	83 - 97	← 98
< 123	1	2	3	4
123-126	2	2	3	4
127-149	3	3	3	4
← 150	4	4	4	4

Percentile of height = 50 - 74%

Systolic (mm Hg)	Diastolic (mm Hg)			
	<80	80 - 83	84 - 97	← 98
< 125	1	2	3	4
125-127	2	2	3	4
128-149	3	3	3	4
← 150	4	4	4	4

Child Blood Pressure Values
Girls - Age 16 (continued)

Percentile of height = 75 - 89%

Systolic (mm Hg)	Diastolic (mm Hg)			
	<81	81 - 84	85 - 97	← 98
< 126	1	2	3	4
126-129	2	2	3	4
130-149	3	3	3	4
← 150	4	4	4	4

Percentile of height = 90 - 94%

Systolic (mm Hg)	Diastolic (mm Hg)			
	<82	82 - 85	86 - 97	← 98
< 127	1	2	3	4
127-130	2	2	3	4
131-149	3	3	3	4
← 150	4	4	4	4

Percentile of height = 95 - 99%

Systolic (mm Hg)	Diastolic (mm Hg)			
	<82	82 - 85	86 - 97	← 98
< 128	1	2	3	4
128-131	2	2	3	4
132-149	3	3	3	4
← 150	4	4	4	4

Child Blood Pressure Values
Girls - Age 17

Percentile of height = 1 - 9%

Systolic (mm Hg)	Diastolic (mm Hg)			
	<79	79- 82	83 - 97	←98
< 122	1	2	3	4
122-125	2	2	3	4
126-149	3	3	3	4
←150	4	4	4	4

Percentile of height = 10 - 24%

Systolic (mm Hg)	Diastolic (mm Hg)			
	<79	79 - 82	83 - 97	←98
< 123	1	2	3	4
123-125	2	2	3	4
126-149	3	3	3	4
←150	4	4	4	4

Percentile of height = 25 - 49%

Systolic (mm Hg)	Diastolic (mm Hg)			
	<79	79- 82	83 - 97	←98
< 124	1	2	3	4
124-126	2	2	3	4
127-149	3	3	3	4
←150	4	4	4	4

Percentile of height = 50 - 74%

Systolic (mm Hg)	Diastolic (mm Hg)			
	<80	80 - 83	84 - 97	←98
< 125	1	2	3	4
125-128	2	2	3	4
129-149	3	3	3	4
←150	4	4	4	4

Child Blood Pressure Values
Girls - Age 17 (continued)

Percentile of height = 75 - 89%

Systolic (mm Hg)	Diastolic (mm Hg)			
	<81	81 - 84	85 - 97	← 98
< 126	1	2	3	4
126-129	2	2	3	4
130-149	3	3	3	4
← 150	4	4	4	4

Percentile of height = 90 - 94%

Systolic (mm Hg)	Diastolic (mm Hg)			
	<82	82 - 85	86 - 97	← 98
< 128	1	2	3	4
128-130	2	2	3	4
131-149	3	3	3	4
← 150	4	4	4	4

Percentile of height = 95 - 99%

Systolic (mm Hg)	Diastolic (mm Hg)			
	<82	82 - 85	86 - 97	← 98
< 128	1	2	3	4
128-131	2	2	3	4
132-149	3	3	3	4
← 150	4	4	4	4

Child Blood Pressure Values
Boys - Age 6

Percentile of height = 1 - 9%

Systolic (mm Hg)	Diastolic (mm Hg)			
	<67	67 - 71	72-85	← 86
< 105	1	2	3	4
105-108	2	2	3	4
109-129	3	3	3	4
← 130	4	4	4	4

Percentile of height = 10 - 24%

Systolic (mm Hg)	Diastolic (mm Hg)			
	<68	68 - 71	72 - 85	← 86
< 106	1	2	3	4
106-109	2	2	3	4
110-129	3	3	3	4
← 130	4	4	4	4

Percentile of height = 25 - 49%

Systolic (mm Hg)	Diastolic (mm Hg)			
	<69	69 - 72	73 - 85	← 86
< 108	1	2	3	4
108-111	2	2	3	4
112-129	3	3	3	4
← 130	4	4	4	4

Percentile of height = 50 - 74%

Systolic (mm Hg)	Diastolic (mm Hg)			
	<70	71 - 73	74 - 85	← 86
< 110	1	2	3	4
110-113	2	2	3	4
114-129	3	3	3	4
← 130	4	4	4	4

Child Blood Pressure Values
Boys - Age 6 (continued)

Percentile of height = 75 - 89%

Systolic (mm Hg)	Diastolic (mm Hg)			
	<70	70 - 74	75 - 85	← 86
< 111	1	2	3	4
111-112	2	2	3	4
113-129	3	3	3	4
← 130	4	4	4	4

Percentile of height = 90 - 94%

Systolic (mm Hg)	Diastolic (mm Hg)			
	<71	71 - 75	76 - 85	← 86
< 113	1	2	3	4
113-116	2	2	3	4
117-129	3	3	3	4
← 130	4	4	4	4

Percentile of height = 95 - 99%

Systolic (mm Hg)	Diastolic (mm Hg)			
	<72	72 - 75	76 - 85	← 86
< 114	1	2	3	4
114-116	2	2	3	4
117-129	3	3	3	4
← 130	4	4	4	4

Child Blood Pressure Values
Boys - Age 7

Percentile of height = 1 - 9%

Systolic (mm Hg)	Diastolic (mm Hg)			
	<69	69 - 73	74-85	← 86
< 106	1	2	3	4
106-109	2	2	3	4
110-129	3	3	3	4
← 130	4	4	4	4

Percentile of height = 10 - 24%

Systolic (mm Hg)	Diastolic (mm Hg)			
	<70	70 - 73	74 - 85	<86
< 107	1	2	3	4
107-110	2	2	3	4
111-129	3	3	3	4
← 130	4	4	4	4

Percentile of height = 25 - 49%

Systolic (mm Hg)	Diastolic (mm Hg)			
	<71	71 - 74	75-85	← 86
< 109	1	2	3	4
109-112	2	2	3	4
113-129	3	3	3	4
← 130	4	4	4	4

Percentile of height = 50 - 74%

Systolic (mm Hg)	Diastolic (mm Hg)			
	<72	72 - 75	76 - 85	← 86
< 111	1	2	3	4
111-114	2	2	3	4
115-129	3	3	3	4
← 130	4	4	4	4

Percentile of height = 75 - 89%

Systolic (mm Hg)	Diastolic (mm Hg)			
	<72	72 - 76	77 - 85	← 86
< 113	1	2	3	4
113-115	2	2	3	4
116-129	3	3	3	4
← 130	4	4	4	4

Percentile of height = 90 - 94%

Systolic (mm Hg)	Diastolic (mm Hg)			
	<73	73 - 77	78 - 85	← 86
< 114	1	2	3	4
114-117	2	2	3	4
118-129	3	3	3	4
← 130	4	4	4	4

Percentile of height = 95 - 99%

Systolic (mm Hg)	Diastolic (mm Hg)			
	<74	74 - 77	78 - 85	← 86
< 115	1	2	3	4
115-118	2	2	3	4
119-129	3	3	3	4
← 130	4	4	4	4

Child Blood Pressure Values
Boys - Age 8

Percentile of height = 1 - 9%

Systolic (mm Hg)	Diastolic (mm Hg)			
	<71	71 - 74	75-85	← 86
< 107	1	2	3	4
107-110	2	2	3	4
111-129	3	3	3	4
← 130	4	4	4	4

Percentile of height = 10 - 24%

Systolic (mm Hg)	Diastolic (mm Hg)			
	<71	71 - 75	76-85	← 86
< 108	1	2	3	4
108-111	2	2	3	4
112-129	3	3	3	4
← 130	4	4	4	4

Percentile of height = 25 - 49%

Systolic (mm Hg)	Diastolic (mm Hg)			
	<72	72 - 75	76 - 85	← 86
< 110	1	2	3	4
110-113	2	2	3	4
114-129	3	3	3	4
← 130	4	4	4	4

Percentile of height = 50 - 74%

Systolic (mm Hg)	Diastolic (mm Hg)			
	<73	73 - 76	77 - 85	← 86
< 112	1	2	3	4
112-115	2	2	3	4
116-129	3	3	3	4
← 130	4	4	4	4

Percentile of height = 75 - 89%

Systolic (mm Hg)	Diastolic (mm Hg)			
	<74	74 - 77	78 - 85	← 86
< 114	1	2	3	4
114-117	2	2	3	4
118-129	3	3	3	4
← 130	4	4	4	4

Percentile of height = 90 - 94%

Systolic (mm Hg)	Diastolic (mm Hg)			
	<75	75 - 78	79 - 85	← 86
< 115	1	2	3	4
115-118	2	2	3	4
119-129	3	3	3	4
← 130	4	4	4	4

Percentile of height = 95 - 99%

Systolic (mm Hg)	Diastolic (mm Hg)			
	<75	75 - 78	79 - 85	← 86
< 116	1	2	3	4
116-119	2	2	3	4
120-129	3	3	3	4
← 130	4	4	4	4

Child Blood Pressure Values
Boys - Age 9

Percentile of height = 1 - 9%

Systolic (mm Hg)	Diastolic (mm Hg)			
	<72	72 - 75	76-85	← 86
< 109	1	2	3	4
109-112	2	2	3	4
113-129	3	3	3	4
← 130	4	4	4	4

Percentile of height = 10 - 24%

Systolic (mm Hg)	Diastolic (mm Hg)			
	<73	73 - 76	77 - 85	<86
< 110	1	2	3	4
110-113	2	2	3	4
114-129	3	3	3	4
← 130	4	4	4	4

Percentile of height = 25 - 49%

Systolic (mm Hg)	Diastolic (mm Hg)			
	<73	73 - 77	78 - 85	← 86
< 112	1	2	3	4
112-115	2	2	3	4
116-129	3	3	3	4
← 130	4	4	4	4

Percentile of height = 50 - 74%

Systolic (mm Hg)	Diastolic (mm Hg)			
	<74	74 - 78	79 - 85	← 86
< 113	1	2	3	4
113-116	2	2	3	4
117-129	3	3	3	4
← 130	4	4	4	4

Child Blood Pressure Values
Boys - Age 9 (continued)

Percentile of height = 75 - 89%

Systolic (mm Hg)	Diastolic (mm Hg)			
	<75	75 - 79	80 - 85	←86
< 115	1	2	3	4
115-118	2	2	3	4
119-129	3	3	3	4
←130	4	4	4	4

Percentile of height = 90 - 94%

Systolic (mm Hg)	Diastolic (mm Hg)			
	<76	76 - 79	80 - 85	←86
< 117	1	2	3	4
117-120	2	2	3	4
121-129	3	3	3	4
←130	4	4	4	4

Percentile of height = 95 - 99%

Systolic (mm Hg)	Diastolic (mm Hg)			
	<77	77 - 80	81 - 85	←86
< 117	1	2	3	4
117-120	2	2	3	4
121-129	3	3	3	4
←130	4	4	4	4

Child Blood Pressure Values
Boys - Age 10

Percentile of height = 1 - 9%

Systolic (mm Hg)	Diastolic (mm Hg)			
	<73	73 - 76	77-89	←90
< 110	1	2	3	4
110-113	2	2	3	4
114-133	3	3	3	4
←134	4	4	4	4

Percentile of height = 10 - 24%

Systolic (mm Hg)	Diastolic (mm Hg)			
	<73	73 - 76	77-89	←90
< 112	1	2	3	4
112-114	2	2	3	4
115-133	3	3	3	4
←134	4	4	4	4

Percentile of height = 25 - 49%

Systolic (mm Hg)	Diastolic (mm Hg)			
	<74	74 - 78	79-89	←90
< 113	1	2	3	4
113-116	2	2	3	4
117-133	3	3	3	4
←134	4	4	4	4

Percentile of height = 50 - 74%

Systolic (mm Hg)	Diastolic (mm Hg)			
	<75	75 - 79	80 - 89	←90
< 115	1	2	3	4
115-118	2	2	3	4
119-133	3	3	3	4
←134	4	4	4	4

Child Blood Pressure Values
Boys - Age 10 (continued)

Percentile of height = 75 - 89%

Systolic (mm Hg)	Diastolic (mm Hg)			
	<76	76 - 79	80 - 89	← 90
< 117	1	2	3	4
117-120	2	2	3	4
121-133	3	3	3	4
← 134	4	4	4	4

Percentile of height = 90 - 94%

Systolic (mm Hg)	Diastolic (mm Hg)			
	<77	77 - 80	81 - 89	← 90
< 118	1	2	3	4
118-121	2	2	3	4
122-133	3	3	3	4
← 134	4	4	4	4

Percentile of height = 95 - 99%

Systolic (mm Hg)	Diastolic (mm Hg)			
	<78	78 - 81	82 - 89	← 90
< 119	1	2	3	4
119-122	2	2	3	4
123-133	3	3	3	4
← 134	4	4	4	4

Child Blood Pressure Values
Boys - Age 11

Percentile of height = 1 - 9%

Systolic (mm Hg)	Diastolic (mm Hg)			
	<74	74 - 77	78-89	← 90
< 112	1	2	3	4
112-115	2	2	3	4
116-133	3	3	3	4
← 134	4	4	4	4

Percentile of height = 10 - 24%

Systolic (mm Hg)	Diastolic (mm Hg)			
	<74	74 - 78	79 - 89	← 90
< 113	1	2	3	4
113-116	2	2	3	4
117-133	3	3	3	4
← 134	4	4	4	4

Percentile of height = 25 - 49%

Systolic (mm Hg)	Diastolic (mm Hg)			
	<75	75 - 78	79 - 89	← 90
< 115	1	2	3	4
115-118	2	2	3	4
119-133	3	3	3	4
← 134	4	4	4	4

Percentile of height = 50 - 74%

Systolic (mm Hg)	Diastolic (mm Hg)			
	<76	76 - 79	80 - 89	← 90
< 117	1	2	3	4
117-120	2	2	3	4
121-133	3	3	3	4
← 134	4	4	4	4

Percentile of height = 75 - 89%

Systolic (mm Hg)	Diastolic (mm Hg)			
	<77	77 - 80	81 - 89	← 90
< 119	1	2	3	4
119-122	2	2	3	4
123-133	3	3	3	4
← 134	4	4	4	4

Percentile of height = 90 - 94%

Systolic (mm Hg)	Diastolic (mm Hg)			
	<78	78 - 81	82 - 89	← 90
< 120	1	2	3	4
120-123	2	2	3	4
124-133	3	3	3	4
← 134	4	4	4	4

Percentile of height = 95 - 99%

Systolic (mm Hg)	Diastolic (mm Hg)			
	<78	78 - 82	83 - 89	← 90
< 121	1	2	3	4
121-124	2	2	3	4
125-133	3	3	3	4
← 134	4	4	4	4

Child Blood Pressure Values
Boys - Age 12

Percentile of height = 1 - 9%

Systolic (mm Hg)	Diastolic (mm Hg)			
	<75	75 - 77	79 - 89	←90
< 115	1	2	3	4
115-118	2	2	3	4
119-133	3	3	3	4
←134	4	4	4	4

Percentile of height = 10 - 24%

Systolic (mm Hg)	Diastolic (mm Hg)			
	<75	75 - 77	79 - 89	←90
< 116	1	2	3	4
116-119	2	2	3	4
120-133	3	3	3	4
←134	4	4	4	4

Percentile of height = 25 - 49%

Systolic (mm Hg)	Diastolic (mm Hg)			
	<76	76 - 79	80 - 89	←90
< 117	1	2	3	4
117-120	2	2	3	4
121-133	3	3	3	4
←134	4	4	4	4

Percentile of height = 50 - 74%

Systolic (mm Hg)	Diastolic (mm Hg)			
	<76	77 - 80	81 - 89	←90
< 119	1	2	3	4
119-122	2	2	3	4
123-133	3	3	3	4
←134	4	4	4	4

Child Blood Pressure Values
Boys - Age 12 (continued)

Percentile of height = 75 - 89%

Systolic (mm Hg)	Diastolic (mm Hg)			
	<78	78 - 81	82 - 89	← 90
< 121	1	2	3	4
121-124	2	2	3	4
125-133	3	3	3	4
← 134	4	4	4	4

Percentile of height = 90 - 94%

Systolic (mm Hg)	Diastolic (mm Hg)			
	<78	78 - 82	83 - 89	← 90
< 123	1	2	3	4
123-125	2	2	3	4
126-133	3	3	3	4
← 134	4	4	4	4

Percentile of height = 95 - 99%

Systolic (mm Hg)	Diastolic (mm Hg)			
	<79	78 - 82	83 - 89	← 90
< 123	1	2	3	4
123-126	2	2	3	4
127-133	3	3	3	4
← 134	4	4	4	4

Child Blood Pressure Values
Boys - Age 13

Percentile of height = 1 - 9%

Systolic (mm Hg)	Diastolic (mm Hg)			
	<75	75 - 78	79 - 91	←92
< 117	1	2	3	4
117-120	2	2	3	4
121-143	3	3	3	4
←144	4	4	4	4

Percentile of height = 10 - 24%

Systolic (mm Hg)	Diastolic (mm Hg)			
	<76	76 - 79	80 - 91	←92
< 118	1	2	3	4
118-121	2	2	3	4
122-143	3	3	3	4
←144	4	4	4	4

Percentile of height = 25 - 49%

Systolic (mm Hg)	Diastolic (mm Hg)			
	<76	76- 80	81 - 91	←92
< 120	1	2	3	4
120-125	2	2	3	4
126-143	3	3	3	4
←144	4	4	4	4

Percentile of height = 50 - 74%

Systolic (mm Hg)	Diastolic (mm Hg)			
	<77	77 - 81	82 - 91	←92
< 122	1	2	3	4
122-125	2	2	3	4
126-143	3	3	3	4
←144	4	4	4	4

Child Blood Pressure Values
Boys - Age 13 (continued)

Percentile of height = 75 - 89%

Systolic (mm Hg)	Diastolic (mm Hg)			
	<78	78 - 82	83 - 91	← 92
< 124	1	2	3	4
124-127	2	2	3	4
128-143	3	3	3	4
← 144	4	4	4	4

Percentile of height = 90 - 94%

Systolic (mm Hg)	Diastolic (mm Hg)			
	<79	79 - 82	83 - 91	← 92
< 125	1	2	3	4
125-128	2	2	3	4
129-143	3	3	3	4
← 144	4	4	4	4

Percentile of height = 95 - 99%

Systolic (mm Hg)	Diastolic (mm Hg)			
	<80	80 - 83	84 - 91	← 92
< 126	1	2	3	4
126-129	2	2	3	4
130-143	3	3	3	4
← 144	4	4	4	4

Child Blood Pressure Values
Boys - Age 14

Percentile of height = 1 - 9%

Systolic (mm Hg)	Diastolic (mm Hg)			
	<76	76 - 79	80 - 91	←92
< 120	1	2	3	4
120-123	2	2	3	4
124-143	3	3	3	4
←144	4	4	4	4

Percentile of height = 10 - 24%

Systolic (mm Hg)	Diastolic (mm Hg)			
	<76	76 - 80	81 - 91	←92
< 121	1	2	3	4
121-124	2	2	3	4
125-143	3	3	3	4
←144	4	4	4	4

Percentile of height = 25 - 49%

Systolic (mm Hg)	Diastolic (mm Hg)			
	<77	77 - 80	81 - 91	←92
< 123	1	2	3	4
123-126	2	2	3	4
127-143	3	3	3	4
←144	4	4	4	4

Percentile of height = 50 - 74%

Systolic (mm Hg)	Diastolic (mm Hg)			
	<78	78 - 81	82 - 91	←92
< 125	1	2	3	4
125-127	2	2	3	4
128-143	3	3	3	4
←144	4	4	4	4

Child Blood Pressure Values
Boys - Age 14 (continued)

Percentile of height = 75 - 89%

Systolic (mm Hg)	Diastolic (mm Hg)			
	<79	79 - 82	83 - 91	←92
< 126	1	2	3	4
126-129	2	2	3	4
130-143	3	3	3	4
←144	4	4	4	4

Percentile of height = 90 - 94%

Systolic (mm Hg)	Diastolic (mm Hg)			
	<80	80 - 83	84 - 91	←92
< 128	1	2	3	4
128-131	2	2	3	4
132-143	3	3	3	4
←144	4	4	4	4

Percentile of height = 95 - 99%

Systolic (mm Hg)	Diastolic (mm Hg)			
	<80	80 - 84	85 - 91	←92
< 128	1	2	3	4
128-131	2	2	3	4
132-143	3	3	3	4
←144	4	4	4	4

Child Blood Pressure Values
Boys - Age 15

Percentile of height = 1 - 9%

Systolic (mm Hg)	Diastolic (mm Hg)			
	<77	77 - 80	81 - 91	←92
< 123	1	2	3	4
123-126	2	2	3	4
127-143	3	3	3	4
←144	4	4	4	4

Percentile of height = 10 - 24%

Systolic (mm Hg)	Diastolic (mm Hg)			
	<77	77 - 81	82 - 91	←92
< 124	1	2	3	4
124-127	2	2	3	4
128-143	3	3	3	4
←144	4	4	4	4

Percentile of height = 25 - 49%

Systolic (mm Hg)	Diastolic (mm Hg)			
	<78	78- 82	83 - 91	←92
< 125	1	2	3	4
125-128	2	2	3	4
129-143	3	3	3	4
←144	4	4	4	4

Percentile of height = 50 - 74%

Systolic (mm Hg)	Diastolic (mm Hg)			
	<79	79 - 82	83 - 91	←92
< 127	1	2	3	4
127-130	2	2	3	4
131-143	3	3	3	4
←144	4	4	4	4

Child Blood Pressure Values
Boys - Age 15 (continued)

Percentile of height = 75 - 89%

Systolic (mm Hg)	Diastolic (mm Hg)			
	<80	80 - 83	84 - 91	← 92
< 129	1	2	3	4
129-132	2	2	3	4
133-143	3	3	3	4
← 144	4	4	4	4

Percentile of height = 90 - 94%

Systolic (mm Hg)	Diastolic (mm Hg)			
	<81	81 - 84	85 - 91	← 92
< 131	1	2	3	4
131-134	2	2	3	4
135-143	3	3	3	4
← 144	4	4	4	4

Percentile of height = 95 - 99%

Systolic (mm Hg)	Diastolic (mm Hg)			
	<81	81 - 85	86 - 91	← 92
< 131	1	2	3	4
131-134	2	2	3	4
135-143	3	3	3	4
← 144	4	4	4	4

Child Blood Pressure Values
Boys - Age 16

Percentile of height = 1 - 9%

Systolic (mm Hg)	Diastolic (mm Hg)			
	<79	79 - 82	83 - 97	←98
< 125	1	2	3	4
125-128	2	2	3	4
129-149	3	3	3	4
←150	4	4	4	4

Percentile of height = 10 - 24%

Systolic (mm Hg)	Diastolic (mm Hg)			
	<79	79 - 82	83 - 97	←98
< 126	1	2	3	4
126-129	2	2	3	4
130-149	3	3	3	4
←150	4	4	4	4

Percentile of height = 25 - 49%

Systolic (mm Hg)	Diastolic (mm Hg)			
	<80	80- 83	84 - 97	←98
< 128	1	2	3	4
128-131	2	2	3	4
132-149	3	3	3	4
←150	4	4	4	4

Percentile of height = 50 - 74%

Systolic (mm Hg)	Diastolic (mm Hg)			
	<81	81 - 84	85 - 97	←98
< 130	1	2	3	4
130-133	2	2	3	4
134-149	3	3	3	4
←150	4	4	4	4

Percentile of height = 75 - 89%

Systolic (mm Hg)	Diastolic (mm Hg)			
	<82	82 - 85	86 - 97	←98
< 132	1	2	3	4
132-135	2	2	3	4
136-149	3	3	3	4
←150	4	4	4	4

Percentile of height = 90 - 94%

Systolic (mm Hg)	Diastolic (mm Hg)			
	<82	82 - 86	87 - 97	←98
< 133	1	2	3	4
133-135	2	2	3	4
136-149	3	3	3	4
←150	4	4	4	4

Percentile of height = 95 - 99%

Systolic (mm Hg)	Diastolic (mm Hg)			
	<83	83 - 86	87 - 97	←98
< 134	1	2	3	4
134-137	2	2	3	4
138-149	3	3	3	4
←150	4	4	4	4

Child Blood Pressure Values
Boys - Age 17

Percentile of height = 1 - 9%

Systolic (mm Hg)	Diastolic (mm Hg)			
	<81	81- 84	85 - 97	←98
< 128	1	2	3	4
128-131	2	2	3	4
132-149	3	3	3	4
←150	4	4	4	4

Percentile of height = 10 - 24%

Systolic (mm Hg)	Diastolic (mm Hg)			
	<81	81 - 84	85 - 97	←98
< 129	1	2	3	4
129-132	2	2	3	4
133-149	3	3	3	4
←150	4	4	4	4

Percentile of height = 25 - 49%

Systolic (mm Hg)	Diastolic (mm Hg)			
	<82	82- 85	86 - 97	←98
< 131	1	2	3	4
131-134	2	2	3	4
135-149	3	3	3	4
←150	4	4	4	4

Percentile of height = 50 - 74%

Systolic (mm Hg)	Diastolic (mm Hg)			
	<83	83 - 86	87 - 97	←98
< 133	1	2	3	4
133-135	2	2	3	4
136-149	3	3	3	4
←150	4	4	4	4

Child Blood Pressure Values
Boys - Age 17 (continued)

Percentile of height = 75 - 89%

Systolic (mm Hg)	Diastolic (mm Hg)			
	<84	84 - 87	88 - 97	← 98
< 134	1	2	3	4
134-139	2	2	3	4
140-149	3	3	3	4
← 150	4	4	4	4

Percentile of height = 90 - 94%

Systolic (mm Hg)	Diastolic (mm Hg)			
	<85	85 - 88	89 - 97	← 98
< 136	1	2	3	4
136-139	2	2	3	4
140-149	3	3	3	4
← 150	4	4	4	4

Percentile of height = 95 - 99%

Systolic (mm Hg)	Diastolic (mm Hg)			
	<85	85 - 88	89 - 97	← 98
< 136	1	2	3	4
136-139	2	2	3	4
140-149	3	3	3	4
← 150	4	4	4	4

Appendix B
Child Blood Pressure References

APPENDIX B. CHILD BLOOD PRESSURE REFERENCES

Blood Pressure - Children

Referral Levels:

Level 1	(category 4)	Indicates major medical findings that warrant immediate attention by a health care provider.
Level 2	(categories 3)	Indicates major medical findings that warrant attention by a health care provider within the next 2 weeks. These findings are expected to cause adverse effects within this time period and they have previously been undiagnosed, unattended, nonmanifested or not communicated to the examinee by his/her personal health care provider.
Level 3	(categories 1 & 2,)	Indicates no medical findings; minor medical findings that an examinee already knows about, and is under care for, or findings that do not require prompt attention by a medical provider.

Referral Comments for Blood Pressure (Children)

Referral Comments:

Statement for blood pressure in category 4	**Level 1 referral**	The participant's blood pressure is **very high** based on the 1996 update of the Task Force Report on High Blood Pressure in Children and Adolescents.*
Statement for blood pressure in category 3	**Level 2 referral**	The participant's blood pressure is **high** based on the 1996 update of the Task Force Report on High Blood Pressure in Children and Adolescents.*
Statement for blood pressure in category 2	**Level 3 no referral**	The participant's blood pressure is **normal but at the high end of normal** based on the 1996 update of the Task Force Report on High Blood Pressure in Children and Adolescents.*
Statement for blood pressure in category 1	**Level 3 - no referral**	The participant's blood pressure is **normal** based on the 1996 update of the Task Force Report on High Blood Pressure in Children and Adolescents.*

National High Blood Pressure Education Program Working Group on Hypertension Control in Children and Adolescents. Update on the 1987 Task Force Report on High Blood Pressure in Children and Adolescents: A Working Group Report from the National High Blood Pressure Education Program. *Pediatrics.* 1996;11:649-658.

Report of Findings Comments:

- Category 4   Your child's blood pressure today is **very high**.

- Category 3   Your child's blood pressure today is **high**.

- Category 2   Your child's blood pressure today is **normal but at high end of normal range**.

- Category 1   Your child's blood pressure today is **normal**.

Appendix C
Adult Blood Pressure Reference Table

APPENDIX C. ADULT BLOOD PRESSURE REFERENCE TABLE

Blood Pressure - Adults

Referral Levels and Referral Comments for Blood Pressure (Adults)

(Systolic mm Hg)	Diastolic (mm Hg)					
	≤ 84	85 - 89	90 - 99	100 - 109	110 - 119	≥ 120
≤ 129	1	2	3	4	5	6
130 – 139	2	2	3	4	5	6
140 – 159	3	3	3	4	5	6
160 – 179	4	4	4	4	5	6
180 – 209	5	5	5	5	5	6
≥ 210	6	6	6	6	6	6

From the Sixth Report of the Joint National Committee on Detection, Evaluation, and Treatment of High Blood Pressure

Level 1 (category 6) Indicates major medical findings that warrant immediate attention by a health care provider.

Level 2 (categories 4 & 5) Indicates major medical findings that warrant attention by a health care provider within the next 2 weeks. These findings are expected to cause adverse effects within this time period and they have previously been undiagnosed, unattended, nonmanifested or not communicated to the examinee by his/her personal health care provider.

Level 3 (categories 1, 2, & 3) Indicates no medical findings; minor medical findings that an examinee already knows about, and is under care for, or findings that do not require prompt attention by a medical provider.

Referral Comments:

Statement for blood pressure in category 6	**Level 1 referral**	The participant's blood pressure is **severely high** based on the Sixth Report of the Joint National Committee on Detection, Evaluation, and Treatment of High Blood Pressure.
Statement for blood pressure in category 5	**Level 2 referral**	The participant's blood pressure is **very high** based on the Sixth Report of the Joint National Committee on Detection, Evaluation, and Treatment of High Blood Pressure.
Statement for blood pressure in category 4	**Level 2 referral**	The participant's blood pressure is **moderately high** based on the Sixth Report of the Joint National Committee on Detection, Evaluation, and Treatment of High Blood Pressure.
Statement for blood pressure in category 3	**Level 3 - no referral**	The participant's blood pressure is **mildly high** based on the Sixth Report of the Joint National Committee on Detection, Evaluation, and Treatment of High Blood Pressure.
Statement for blood pressure in category 2	**Level 3 - no referral**	The participant's blood pressure is **normal but at the high end of the normal range** based on the Sixth Report of the Joint National Committee on Detection, Evaluation, and Treatment of High Blood Pressure.
Statement for blood pressure in category 1	**Level 3 - no referral**	The participant's blood pressure is **normal** based on the Sixth Report of the Joint National Committee on Detection, Evaluation, and Treatment of High Blood Pressure.

Report of Findings Comments:

- Category 6   Your blood pressure today is **severely high**.

- Category 5   Your blood pressure today is **very high**.

- Category 4   Your blood pressure today is **moderately high**.

- Category 3   Your blood pressure today is **mildly high**.

- Category 2   Your blood pressure today is **normal but at the high end of the normal range**.

- Category 1   Your blood pressure today is within the **normal range.**

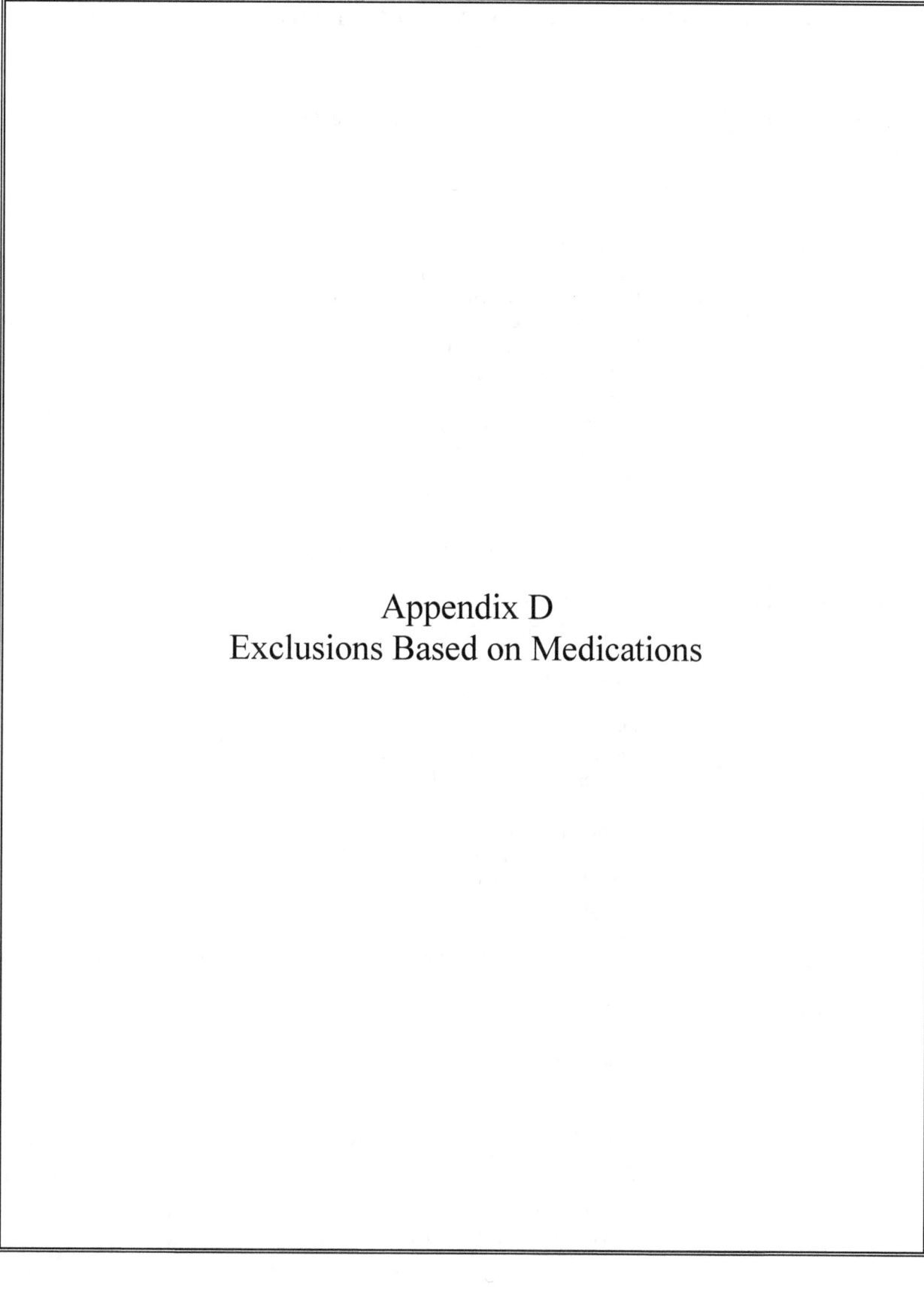

Appendix D
Exclusions Based on Medications

APPENDIX D. EXCLUSIONS BASED ON MEDICATIONS UPDATED 09/01/2000

SP medications are reviewed by the Physician and the SP is excluded from CV Fitness if he/she is taking any of the following medications.

Updated 09-01-2000

Calcium Channel-Blockers	Amlodipine (Norvasc)
	Bepridil (Vascor)
	Diltiazem (Cardizem, Dilacor, Tiazac)
	Felodipine (Plendil)
	Isradipine (Dyna Circ)
	Norvasc (Amlodipine)
	Nicardipine (Cardene)
	Nifedipine (Procardia, Adalat)
	Nimodipine (Nimotop)
	Nisoldipine (Sular)
	Posicor (Mibefradil)
	Tiazak (Diltiazem HCl)
	Verapamil (Covera, Verelan, Calan, Isoptin)
Anti Arrhythmics	Amiodarone (Cordarone)
	Bretylium (Bretylol)
	Disopyramide (Norpace)
	Encainide (Enkaid)
	Ethmozine (Moricizine)
	Flecanide (Tambocor)
	Lidocaine (Xylocaine, Xylocard)
	Metoprolol Succinate (Toprol-XL)
	Mexiletine (Mexitil)
	Moricizine (Ethmozine)
	Procainamide (Pronestyl, Procan SR)
	Propafenone (Rhythmol)
	Sotalol (Betapace)
	Tocainide (Tonocard)
	Quinidine (Quinora, Quinalan, Cardioquin, Quinidex, Quinaglute)
Beta Blockers	Acebutolol (Sectral)
	Atenolol (Tenormin)
	Betaxolol (Kerlone)
	Bisoprolol (Zebeta)
	Carteolol (Cartrol)
	Corzide *
	Esmolol (Brevibloc)
	Inderide *
	Labetalol (Normodyne)
	Lopressor Hydrochlorothiazide *

Beta Blockers (cont'd)	Metoprolol tartrate (Lopressor) Nadolol (Corgard) Penbutolol (Levatol) Pindolol (Visken) Propranolol (Inderal) Sotolol (Betapace) Tenorectic * Timolide * Timolol (Blocadren) Ziac * * Beta blocker/diuretic combinations
Eye Drops	Betoptic Eyedrops Timoptic Eyedrops
Nitrates and Nitroglycerin	Isosorbide dinitrate (Isordil, Diltrate) Isosorbide mononitrate (Ismo, Monoket) Nitroglycerin, translingual (Nitrostat, Nitrolingual spray) Nitroglycerin, transmucosal (Nitrogard) Nitroglycerin, topical (Nitrol, Nitro-Bid, Transderm Nitro, Nitro-Dur II, Nitrodisc, Minitran, Deponit, Nitroderm) Nitroglycerin, sustained release (Nitrong, Nitrocine, Nitroglyn) Pentaerythritol tetranitrate (Cardilate)
Digitalis	Digoxin (Lanoxin)
CNS Stimulant	Ma Huang (ephedrine)

Appendix E
Exclusions Based on Medical Conditions

APPENDIX E. EXCLUSIONS BASED ON MEDICAL CONDITIONS

From Responses to Household Questionnaire

Medical Conditions and Health Status (MCQ)

- MCQ.160b   (if 1, 7, or 9 exclude)   Congestive heart failure

- MCQ.160c   (if 1, 7, or 9 exclude)   Coronary heart disease

- MCQ.160d   (if 1, 7, or 9 exclude)   Angina pectoris

- MCQ.160e   (if 1, 7, or 9 exclude)   Myocardial infarction

- MCQ.160f   (if 1, 7, or 9 exclude)   Stroke

- MCQ.160g   (if 1, 7, or 9 exclude)   Emphysema

Physical Functioning - (PFQ) -

- PFQ.060b   (if 3, 4, 7, or 9, exclude)   Difficulty walking for a quarter mile (2-3 blocks)

- PFQ.060c   (if 3, 4, 7, or 9, exclude)   Difficulty walking up 10 steps without resting

- PFQ.060h   (if 3, 4, 7, or 9, exclude)   Walking from one room to another - same level

- PFQ060i   (if 3, 4, 7, or 9, exclude)   Standing up from an armless straight chair

- PFQ.067

    - =11   (if 2,3, or 4, exclude)   Back or Neck Problem

    - =15   (if 2,3, or 4, exclude)   Developmental Problems (Cerebral Palsy)

    - =17   (if 2,3, or 4, exclude)   Fractures, Bone/Joint Injury

    - =19   (if 2,3, or 4, exclude)   Heart Problem

    - =21   (if 2,3, or 4, exclude)   Lung/Breathing Problem

-	=25	(if 2,3, or 4, exclude)	Stroke Problem
-	=77	(if 2,3, or 4, exclude)	Refused
-	=99	(if 2,3, or 4, exclude)	Don't Know
■	PFQ.090	(if 1,7, or 9, exclude)	Use of a device such as a cane or wheelchair

Diabetes (DIQ)

■	DIQ.080	(if 1,7, or 9, exclude)	Retinopathy

Cardiovascular (CDQ)-

■	CDQ.030	(if 1, 7, or 9, exclude)	Stop when walking at own pace on level
■	CDQ.040	(if 1, 7, or 9, exclude)	SOB after walking 100 yards or few minutes on the level
■	CDQ.050	(if 1, 7, or 9, exclude)	PND
■	CDQ.060	(if 1, 7, or 9, exclude)	PND relieved by sitting on side of bed
■	CDQ.070	(if 1, 7, or 9, exclude)	Orthopnea

Respiratory Health (RDQ) -

■	RDQ.080	(if 12 or more attacks, 77, or 99 exclude)	Wheezing in past 12 months
■	RDQ.110	(if 1,7,or 9, exclude)	Wheezing that limits speech (last 12 months)

Vision (VIQ) -

■	VIQ.020	(if 1,7, or 9, exclude)	Blind
■	VIQ.030	(if 5,7, or 9, exclude)	Very poor eyesight

DSQ.240

- Medications will be available in SP History in Physician's Exam. Physician will check this list and exclude based on medication on the Exclusion list.

See Exclusionary Medication List:

Interviewer will have participant get medication bottles and will enter the complete product name of the medication in CAPI. This list of medications will be compared to the medications on the exclusion list - see Appendix E. Participants taking a medication that is on the exclusion medication list will be excluded from the CV Fitness component.

Appendix F
Hospitalization Exclusions from CV Fitness

APPENDIX F. HOSPITALIZATION EXCLUSIONS FROM CV FITNESS

- A recent significant change in the resting ECG suggesting infarction or other acute cardiac event.

- Recent complicated myocardial infarction

- Unstable angina

- Uncontrolled ventricular arrhythmia

- Uncontrolled atrial arrhythmia that comprimises cardiac function

- Third degree AV heart block

- Acute congestive heart failure

- Severe aortic stenosis

- Suspected or known dissecting aneurysm

- Active or suspected myocarditis or pericarditis

- Thrombophlebitis or intracardiac thrombi

- Recent systemic or pulmonary embolus

- Acute infections

- Significant emotional distress (psychosis)

- Moderate valvular heart disease

- Known electrolye abnormalities

- Fixed rate pacemaker

- Frequent or complex ventricular ectopy

- Ventricular aneurysm

- Uncontrolled metabolic disease (diabetes, thyrotoxicosis, myxedema, etc)

- Chronic infections disease (mononucleosis, hepatitis, AIDS)

- Neuromuscular, musculoskeletal, or rheumatoid disorders that are exacerbated by exercise

- Complicated or advanced pregnancy

See Safety/Exclusion Question 5: List of reasons for exclusion based on hospitalization from *ACSM Guidelines*, 5th edition, page 42.

Appendix G
Cardiovascular Safety and Exclusion Questions

APPENDIX G. CARDIOVASCULAR SAFETY AND EXCLUSION QUESTIONS

(Asked in Physician's Exam)

Shared questions asked in the Household Questionnaire (Relevant to CV Fitness):

- Do you have any amputations of your legs and feet other than toes?

- Yes   No   (If Yes, exclude from CV Fitness)

- How much do you weigh without shoes?

- _____ pounds   (If > 350, exclude from CV Fitness)

- Do you have a pacemaker or automatic defibrillator?

- Yes/No/Don't Know   (If Yes or Don't Know, exclude from CV Fitness)

Shared questions asked in MEC Exam:

- Are you currently pregnant? (Self-Report question for 16-49 years)

- Yes/ No (If Yes, exclude from Body Composition, ask follow-up question)

- How many weeks? _____ weeks   (If >12 weeks, exclude from CV Fitness)

CV Safety/Exclusion questions asked in the Physician's Exam:

- Have you been hospitalized in the past 3 months?

- Yes/No/Don't Know   (If Yes, and condition on exclusion list or Don't Know, exclude)

- **(12-19 years only)**   Has a doctor ever said you should not participate in sports or other activities because of a health condition?

- Yes/No/Don't Know   (If Yes or Don't Know, exclude)

- Has a doctor ever said you have a heart condition and that you should only do physical activity recommended by a doctor?

- Yes/No/Don't Know   (If Yes or Don't Know, exclude)

- **(20-49 years only)** Do you feel pain in your chest when you do physical activity?

- Yes/No/Don't Know (If Yes or Don't Know, exclude)

- **(20-49 years only)** In the past month, have you had chest pain when you were not doing physical activity? *(Probe: Have you seen a medical doctor about your chest pain? Did the doctor tell you that the chest pain was related to your heart?)*

- Yes/No/Don't Know (If Yes or Don't Know, exclude)

- Do you lose your balance because of dizziness? *(Probe: Is this an isolated incident or does it occur on a regular basis?)*

- Yes/No/Don't Know (If Yes or Don't Know, exclude)

- Do you ever lose consciousness? *(Probes: Did this occur as a result of illness or was it unexplained? Is this an isolated incident or does it occur on a regular basis?*

- Yes/No/Don't Know (If Yes or Don't Know, exclude)

- Do you have a bone or joint problem that could be made worse by walking? *(Probe: Do you think you can do the test without injuring yourself?*

- Yes/No/Don't Know (If Yes or Don't Know, exclude)

- Are you currently taking any prescription medications?

- Yes/No/Don't Know (If Yes, go to next question. If No, go to last question. If Don't Know, exclude.)

- Are you currently taking any prescription medications for your blood pressure?

- Yes/No/Don't Know (If Yes, go to next question. If No go to second last question. If Don't Know, exclude.)

- What is the name of this medication? _____.

- (If medication is on list, exclude. If not on list, go to next question.

- Are you taking any other medication for your blood pressure?

- Yes/No/Don't Know (Yes, go to next question/ No go to second last question./Don't Know, exclude.)

- What is the name of this medication? _____.

- (If medication is on list, exclude. If not on list, go to next question.

- Are you currently taking prescription medications for the following conditions:

    - Heart condition Yes/No/Don't Know (If Yes or Don't Know, exclude)

    - Prescription eye drops for glaucoma (If Yes or Don't Know, exclude)

- Do you know of any other reason why you should not do a treadmill test?

- Yes/No/Don't Know (If Yes or Don't Know, exclude)

Appendix H
Std Information Sheets and Role Plays

MEC INFORMATION SHEETS

INFECTIONS WITH HERPES SIMPLEX VIRUS TYPE 2

Mode of infection

- Almost always sexual

Laboratory assay used in NHANES

- Type specific immunodot assay using sera, which measures antibodies specific for HSV-2. This test result is an indicator of past infection.

Frequency

- Approximately 1 in 10 adolescents

- Increases with age among white adults to over 1 in 4 adults

- Increases with age among black adults to over 1 in 2 adults

Location of the initial infection and of symptoms

- Women

  - Skin around the vagina, urethra, and rectum

  - Skin of inner thighs and on the buttocks

  - In the vagina and on the cervix

- Men

  - Skin on and around the penis

  - Skin of inner thighs

  - Rectum and skin around the rectum and on the buttocks

Latent infection

- Most of the time, the virus remains dormant in nerve cells connected to the lower spinal cord.

- Symptoms occur when the virus begins to replicate in skin cells around the nerve endings.

Symptoms of uncomplicated infection

- Most infected individuals report no symptoms.

- Blisters that break to form multiple small tender sores that heal spontaneously within a week.

- Episodes recur with highly variable frequency, symptom-free intervals ranging from days to months.

Complications

- Occasionally, the sores are sufficiently painful to interfere with urination.

- Rarely, infection of the brain occurs.

- Rarely, babies born to infected women contract serious infections.

Diagnosis

- Blood tests to detect antibody

  - In NHANES, a special blood test is used that is not yet available to most physicians. Anticipated approval of this assay in the second quarter of 1999. The blood test detects antibody and is usually correct, but no test is 100% accurate.

  - Physicians can order blood tests, but they do not reliably distinguish between the type 2 herpes simplex virus infection and type 1 infection that is the infection that most commonly causes fever blisters of the mouth and is not usually sexually transmitted.

- Cultures and other tests detect the virus in blisters and sores, except during the later stage of healing.

- Frequently, the blisters, sores, and history of recurrences are characteristic, and the physician requires no laboratory test to make the diagnosis.

Note: except by using the NHANES type of blood test, the infection cannot be detected unless blisters or ulcers are present.

Treatment

- No treatment is curative.

- Anti-viral drugs suppress symptoms, which usually recur after the drug is stopped.

- Treatment of each recurrence, separately, is not usually worthwhile, because healing occurs before the drug can act.

Preventing infection of others

- Transmission-related factors

  - Intimate, usually sexual, contact is required.

  - Infected individuals are most infectious when they have sores, but they most often infect others when they are asymptomatic.

  - Infected individuals, who never have symptoms, often shed herpes virus, but how many are infectious is unknown.

- Prevention measures should be taken, but they are not entirely effective.

  - Visit a physician, who can help the infected person determine when a herpes outbreak is occurring.

  - Avoid intercourse during outbreaks.

  - Use condoms.

  - Make sex partners aware of need for preventive measures and residual risks.

INFECTIONS WITH HUMAN IMMUNODEFICIENCY VIRUS

Mode of infection

- Sexual transmission and percutaneous blood exposure (IV drug use, needle sticks in health care workers, etc.).

Laboratory assay used in NHANES

- Serum is screened for HIV-1 antibody using an FDA-licensed enzyme immuno assay kit. Repeatedly reactive specimens are then tested by an FDA-licensed Western blot assay.

Frequency

- Approximately 3 in 1,000 adults

- Approximately 2 in 1,000 white adults

- Approximately 11 in 1,000 black adults

- Approximately 4 in 1,000 Mexican American adults

Diagnosis

- Blood tests to detect antibody

Incubation (Infection to AIDS diagnosis)

- Median 8-10 years in untreated individual, but varies by age

- Treatment with HAART is altering the median incubation time.

Treatment

- HAART (highly active antiretroviral therapy), if given early, can slow or stop disease progression.

- Treatment of opportunistic infections as they occur.

Preventing infection of others

- Condom use has been demonstrated to be effective against transmission.

- Only abstinence or monogamous relationship (between two HIV negative partners) is totally effective in preventing exposure.

ROLE PLAY—SCENARIO 1:

Client

Sam is a 45 year old divorcé who left his former wife about a year ago. He was married for 20 years and has two children. He has never had an STD, just a urinary tract infection once. He has heard much about HIV/AIDS and is worried how to date safely in the '90s. He is a sample person for the NHANES survey and is willing to be tested for STDs. He is in general good health and looks forward to developing a new romantic relationship.

Counselor

You will be counseling Sam a 45 year old divorcé who has recently rejoined the dating scene. He is worried about HIV/AIDS and wants to become romantically involved again but safely. He is not very aware of the various types of STDs and the associated symptoms.

You will need to provide a smooth segue into this part of the physician's exam. Discuss the purpose of testing for STD/HIV and why these special tests have a different mechanism for reporting. Assure confidentiality of the survey and tests results. If asked, explain and educate Sam on the various STDs, risk behaviors associated with transmission, complications, testing methods, and possible treatments available if found to be infected. In closing, you will arrange for Sam to call to obtain his results if he wishes in a confidential manner.

Observer

As the observer, you are not to interrupt or engage in the counseling session. Take side notes of the counselor's ability to cover the major points listed:

- Smooth segue into STD/HIV component of physician's exam

- Assure confidential manner of testing and obtaining results